Cardiology of the horse

Commissioning Editor: *Robert Edwards, Joyce Rodenhuis*
Development Editor: *Louisa Welch*
Project Manager: *Janaki Srinivasan Kumar*
Designer: *Stewart Larking*
Illustration Manager: *Gillian Richards*

Cardiology of the horse

Second edition

Edited by

Celia M. Marr BVMS, MVM, PhD, DEIM, DipECEIM, MRCVS

Specialist in Equine Internal Medicine, Rossdale and Partners, Newmarket

I. Mark Bowen BVetMed, PhD, CertEM(IntMed), MRCVS

Associate Professor in Veterinary Internal Medicine, The University of Nottingham

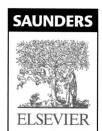

SAUNDERS

ELSEVIER

Edinburgh London New York Oxford Philadelphia St Louis Sydney Toronto 2010

SAUNDERS
ELSEVIER

First Edition © Harcourt Brace and Company 1999
Second edition © 2010, Elsevier Limited. All rights reserved.

ISBN 978-0-7020-2817-5

British Library Cataloguing in Publication Data
A catalogue record for this book is available from the British Library

Library of Congress Cataloging in Publication Data
A catalog record for this book is available from the Library of Congress

Notice
Knowledge and best practice in this field are constantly changing. As new research and experience broaden our knowledge, changes in practice, treatment and drug therapy may become necessary or appropriate. Readers are advised to check the most current information provided (i) on procedures featured or (ii) by the manufacturer of each product to be administered, to verify the recommended dose or formula, the method and duration of administration, and contraindications. It is the responsibility of the practitioner, relying on their own experience and knowledge of the patient, to make diagnoses, to determine dosages and the best treatment for each individual patient, and to take all appropriate safety precautions. To the fullest extent of the law, neither the Publisher nor the Editors assumes any liability for any injury and/or damage to persons or property arising out of or related to any use of the material contained in this book.

The Publisher

ELSEVIER your source for books, journals and multimedia in the health sciences
www.elsevierhealth.com

Working together to grow
libraries in developing countries
www.elsevier.com | www.bookaid.org | www.sabre.org
ELSEVIER   BOOK AID International   Sabre Foundation

The publisher's policy is to use **paper manufactured from sustainable forests**

Printed in China

Last digit is the print number: 9 8 7 6 5 4 3

Contents

v

Contents

Contents for the Website

Throughout the text, a DVD icon is used to direct the reader to digital case material on the accompanying website that is relevant to the topic under discussion. The website can be accessed at www.marrcardiology.com.

DIAGNOSTIC TECHNIQUES

Contents for the Website

Contents for the Website

Contents for the Website

Contributors

Fairfield T. Bain
Equine Sports Medicine & Surgery
Weatherford, Texas
USA

Karen Blissitt
Royal (Dick) School of Veterinary Studies
The University of Edinburgh
Large Animal Hospital
Easter Bush Veterinary Centre
Roslin, Midlothian
UK

Mark Bowen
The School of Veterinary Medicine and Science
The University of Nottingham Sutton Bonington Campus
Sutton Bonington
Leicestershire
UK

Janice McIntosh Bright
Colorado State University VTH
300 W. Drake
Fort Collins, CO
USA

Alistair Cox
Royal (Dick) School of Veterinary Studies
The University of Edinburgh
Large Animal Hospital
Easter Bush Veterinary Centre
Roslin, Midlothian
UK

Mary Durando
School of Veterinary Medicine
New Bolton Center
382 West Street Road
Kennett Square, PA
USA

Jonathan Elliott
Royal Veterinary College
Royal College Street
London
UK

David Evans
Faculty of Veterinary Science
The University of Sydney
Sydney NSW
Australia

Ursula Fogerty
Irish Equine Centre
Johnstown
Naas
County Kildare
Ireland

Alastair Foote
Rossdales Equine Hospital
Cotton End Road
Exning, Newmarket
Suffolk
UK

Gunther van Loon
Department of Internal Medicine and Clinical Biology of Large Animals
Salisburylaan 133
Ghent
Belgium

Gayle Hallowell
The School of Veterinary Medicine and Science
The University of Nottingham Sutton Bonington Campus
Sutton Bonington
Leicestershire
UK

Contributors

John Keen
Royal (Dick) School of Veterinary Studies
The University of Edinburgh
Large Animal Hospital
Easter Bush Veterinary Centre
Roslin, Midlothian
UK

Celia M. Marr
Rossdales Equine Hospital
Cotton End Road
Exning, Newmarket
Suffolk
UK

Elspeth Milne
Royal (Dick) School of Veterinary Studies
The University of Edinburgh
Large Animal Hospital
Easter Bush Veterinary Centre
Roslin, Midlothian
UK

Tony D. Mogg
The University of Sydney
University Veterinary Centre
410 Werombi Road
Camden
Australia

Cristobal Navas de Solis
School of Veterinary Medicine
New Bolton Center
382 West Street Road
Kennett Square, PA
USA

Mark Patteson
HeartVet Consultants
North Nibley, Dursley
Gloucestershire, UK

Richard Piercy
Department of Veterinary Clinical Sciences
Royal Veterinary College
Hawkshead Lane
North Mymms
Hertfordshire, UK

Virginia Reef
School of Veterinary Medicine
New Bolton Center
382 West Street Road
Kennett Square, PA
USA

Johanna Reimer
Rood and Riddle Equine Hospital
Lexington, KY
USA

Sheilah Robertson
Section of Anaesthesia and Pain Management
College of Veterinary Medicine
University of Florida
Gainesville FL
USA

Abby Sage
Blue Ridge Equine Clinic
4510 Mockernut Lane
Earlysville, VA 22936

Olga Seco
School of Veterinary Medicine
New Bolton Center
382 West Street Road
Kennett Square, PA
USA

William Thomas
Department of Medicine & Epidemiology
University of California
Davis, CA
USA

Claire Underwood
School of Veterinary Medicine
New Bolton Center
382 West Street Road
Kennett Square, PA
USA

Lesley Young
Specialist Equine Cardiology Services
Moat End
Dunstall Green Road
Ousden
Suffolk
UK

Glossary

Glossary of drug names (UK/US)

Adrenaline/epinephrine

Frusemide/furosemide

Guaiphenesin/guaifenesin

Lignocaine/lidocaine

Noradrenaline/norepinephrine

Thiopentone/thiopental

Dedication

In memory of Ian Marr and David and Jenny Bowen

"That best portion of a good man's life; his little, nameless, unremembered acts of kindness and love." William Wordsworth

Preface

Since the publication of the first edition of this book, significant advances continue to be made in equine cardiology. In that text, the focus was on the role of the clinician in the diagnosis of heart disease in horses. Recently epidemiological studies have provided a much fuller understanding on the prevalence and clinical impact of cardiac murmurs in equine athletes and in the older, general horse population while several new treatment options have been introduced. These are largely underpinned by work in the area of neuroendocrinology that not only informs our understanding of cardiac physiology and pathophysiology but also provides novel targets for therapeutic intervention. Electrocardioversion and electrical pacing are now feasible in equine patients and this introduces an exciting alternative to drug therapy in a variety of dysrhythmias.

New material has been included in this edition to reflect these developments, while maintaining the original format in which separate sections are devoted to (1) fundamental and applied physiology, (2) diagnostic methods and (3) clinical problems in equine cardiology. The hard copy has been supplemented with a series of clinical cases in digital format that have been selected to illustrate clinical problems with audio and video material. We hope this will greatly enhance the book's value to students and experienced clinicians alike. The clinical cases can be accessed through the website, www.marrcardiology.com.

Research in equine cardiology continues to be a vibrant area of endeavour for basic and clinical research workers across the world. In the UK, postgraduate clinical training programmes and fundamental and applied research have been generously supported by both the Horse Trust and the Horserace Betting Levy Board and we are delighted to have this opportunity to acknowledge the important contribution that these organizations have made towards a better understanding of cardiac disease and function in equine athletes and to the improvement in the welfare of horses with heart disease.

Finally, we would like to express our sincere thanks to the contributors, many of whom, once again, waited very patiently for this book to make its way through the editorial process and to the team at Elsevier who did what they could to speed this process up.

Celia M. Marr
I. Mark Bowen

Section | 1 |

Physiology, pathophysiology and pharmacology

Chapter | **1** |

Introduction to cardiac anatomy and physiology

Janice McIntosh Bright and Celia M Marr

> *I was almost tempted to think with Fracastorius that the motion of the heart was only to be comprehended by God.*
>
> William Harvey, 1628[1]

An appreciation of the anatomy of the heart and great vessels is central to the understanding of cardiac function and disease and for optimal interpretation of diagnostic techniques such as auscultation, echocardiography and radiography. This chapter also reviews cardiovascular physiology focusing on impulse conduction within the equine heart and on the heart as a muscular pump. Although clinically important parameters such as stroke volume, cardiac output and blood pressure are emphasized, these haemodynamic parameters are actually the ultimate functional expression of the biochemical and biophysical processes of myocyte excitation, contraction and relaxation.

ANATOMY OF THE HEART AND GREAT VESSELS (★ ET)

The heart can be regarded as a parallel pump system: deoxygenated blood returning from the body enters the right side from where it is directed via the pulmonary arterial system to the lungs for oxygenation. Oxygenated blood returns to the left side of the heart via the pulmonary veins and is then pumped to the body via the systemic arterial system. Deoxygenated blood returns via the systemic veins to the right side. The heart is located within the middle mediastinal space where its long axis is orientated at approximately 10° to vertical with its base lying dorsal and cranial to the apex. The apex is located above the last sternebra cranial to the sternal portion of the diaphragm. The heart consists of two atria and two ventricles, blood entering via the atria and leaving via the ventricles. The right atrium (RA) occupies the cranial part of the heart base and consists of two main parts, the larger part, the *sinus venarum cavarum*, into which the veins empty, and a conical out-pouching, the auricle. The auricle is triangular and broad-based and curves around the base of the heart towards the left ending cranial to the origin of the main pulmonary artery (Figs. 1.1 and 1.2). The cranial vena cava (draining structures of the head and neck) enters the most dorsal part of the RA, the caudal vena cava (draining abdominal structures) opens into the caudal part and the azygous vein (draining the caudal thorax) enters between the two cavae. The coronary sinus (draining the coronary circulation) opens into the RA ventral to the caudal vena cava. There are also several smaller veins that drain directly into the RA (see Figs. 1.1

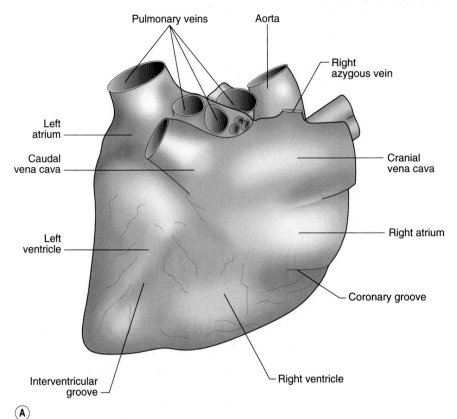

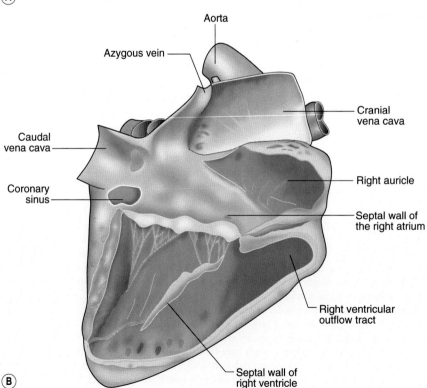

Figure 1.1 (A) The intact heart viewed from the right side: note the boundaries of the right atrium and ventricle and the left and right ventricle are delineated by the coronary and interventricular grooves, respectively. (B) The right aspect of the heart following removal of the right wall. Adapted with permission from Ghoshal NG. Equine heart and arteries. In: Getty R *Sisson and Grossman's The Anatomy of the Domestic Animals*, Vol 1, 5th ed. Philadelphia: WB Saunders, 1975:554–618.

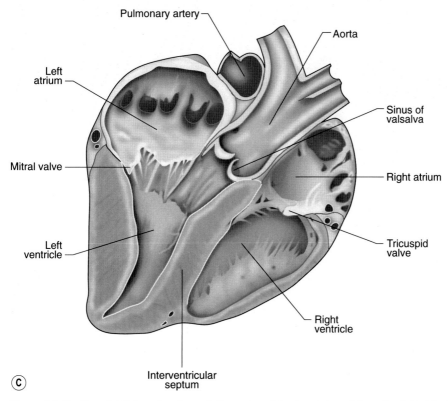

Figure 1.1 Continued (C) A section through the centre of the heart viewed from the right side. Adapted with permission from Ghoshal NG. Equine heart and arteries. In: Getty R (ed) *Sisson and Grossman's The Anatomy of the Domestic Animals*, Vol 1, 5th ed. Philadelphia: WB Saunders, 1975:554–618.

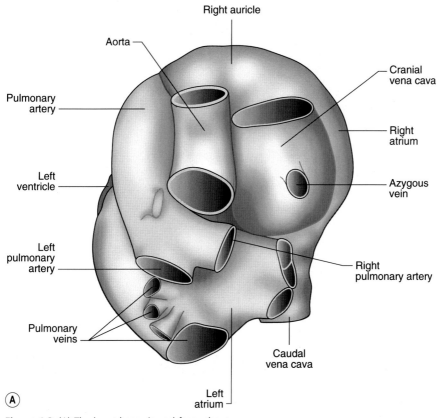

Figure 1.2 (A) The heart base viewed from above.

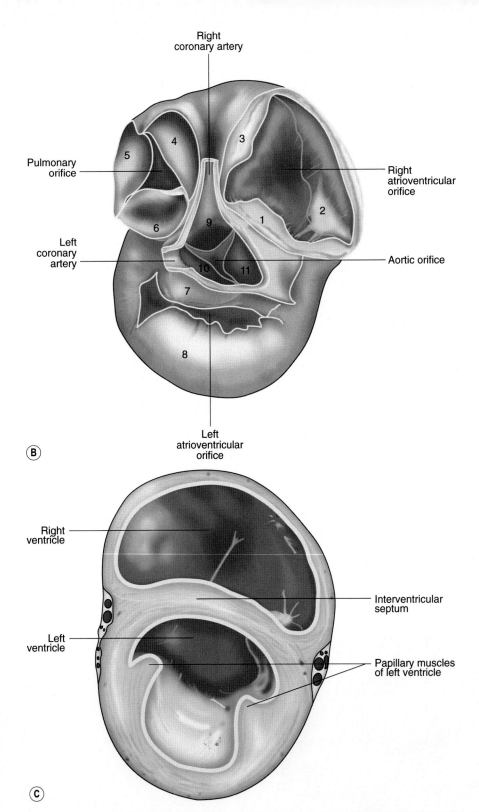

Figure 1.2 Continued (B) A cross-section through the heart base illustrating the valve leaflets: Tricuspid valve 1 = septal, 2 = right, 3 = left, Pulmonary valve 4 = right, 5 = left, 6 = intermediate, Mitral valve 7 = septal, 8 = nonseptal, Aortic Valve 9 = right coronary, 10 = left coronary, 11 = noncoronary. (C) A cross-section through the ventricles. Adapted with permission from Ghoshal NG. Equine heart and arteries. In: Getty R (ed) *Sisson and Grossman's The Anatomy of the Domestic Animals*, Vol 1, 5th ed. Philadelphia: WB Saunders, 1975:554–618.

and 1.2). On the internal surface of the RA there are pronounced ridges formed by extensive bands of pectinate muscles and dorsally these form the terminal crest at the base of the auricle (Fig. 1.3). The oval fossa is a diverticulum at the point of entrance of the caudal vena cava that is a remnant of the foramen ovale, the communication that exists between the two atria in the fetus.

The right atrioventricular (AV) or tricuspid valve forms the ventral floor of the RA and the entrance to the right ventricle (RV) (see Figs. 1.1 and 1.2). As its name suggests, the tricuspid valve is composed of three large leaflets: one is septal, one lies on the right margin (parietal) and the third lies between the AV opening and the right outflow tract (angular). The leaflets are anchored to the papillary muscles of the RV by a series of chordae tendineae. The RV is a crescent-shaped structure in cross-section and triangular when viewed from its inner aspect (see Fig. 1.2). It wraps around the cranial aspect of the heart and, in this respect, the convention derived from human anatomy ascribing the terms *right* and *left* to the heart, is rather misleading. In the horse, the heart would be better defined as having cranial and caudal components. The internal surface of the RV is trabeculated and moderator bands cross the lumen of the RV from the septum to the opposite wall carrying conduction tissue (see Fig. 1.3). These moderator bands vary in size greatly among individuals. Ventrally, the RV does not reach the heart's apex. It extends dorsally and to the left to form the right outflow tract leading to the main pulmonary artery (PA) via the pulmonary valve (right semilunar valve) valve (see Fig. 1.3). The pulmonary valve consists of three half-moon-shaped cusps, the right, left and intermediate, which occasionally have small fenestrations along their free edges and are attached to a fibrous ring at the base of the pulmonary artery. The PA arises from the left side of the RV and curves dorsally, caudally and medially to run under the descending aorta where it branches into left and right. The right PA passes over the cranial part of the left atrium and under the trachea while the left PA is in contact with the bulk of the dorsal surface of the left atrium (LA) (see Fig. 1.2).

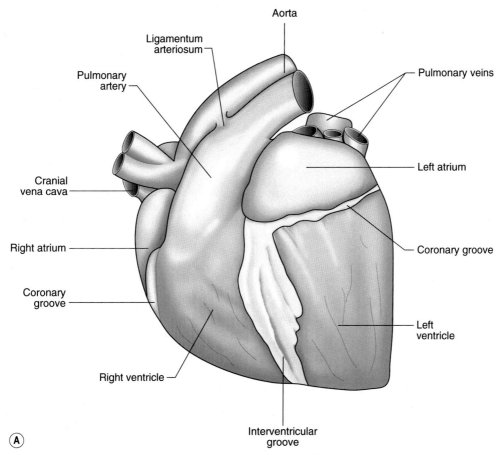

Aorta

Ligamentum arteriosum

Pulmonary artery

Pulmonary veins

Left atrium

Cranial vena cava

Right atrium

Coronary groove

Coronary groove

Left ventricle

Right ventricle

Interventricular groove

(A)

Figure 1.3 (A) The intact heart viewed from the left side. Note the boundaries of the left atrium and ventricle and the left and right ventricle are delineated by the coronary and interventricular groves respectively.

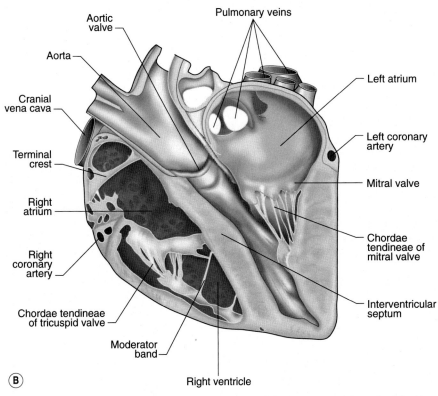

Figure 1.3 Continued (B) A section through the centre of the heart viewed from the left side. Adapted with permission from Ghoshal NG. Equine heart and arteries. In: Getty R (ed) *Sisson and Grossman's The Anatomy of the Domestic Animals*, Vol 1, 5th ed. Philadelphia: WB Saunders, 1975:554–618.

The LA forms the caudal part of the base of the heart and also has an auricle, extending laterally and cranially on the left side. The left auricle is more pointed than the right auricle and lacks a terminal crest (see Fig. 1.2). The LA lacks the extensive pectinate muscles that characterize the RA. Seven or eight pulmonary veins enter the LA around its caudal and right aspects. A depression may be appreciated on the septal surface, corresponding with the site of the fetal foramen ovale. The ventral floor of the LA consists of the left AV, mitral or bicuspid valve (see Figs. 1.1 to 1.3). This consists of two large leaflets, the septal and parietal leaflets which are larger and thicker than those of the tricuspid valve. The left ventricle (LV) is conical with walls approximately three times thicker than those of the RV, and it forms the bulk of the caudal aspect of the heart including the apex. The portion of the wall that forms the division between the LV and RV is called the interventricular septum while the remainder is termed the free wall. Arising from the free wall are two large papillary muscles that are symmetrically located to the left and right sides of the free wall and anchor the chordae tendineae of the mitral valve (see Fig. 1.2). The interventricular

septum (IVS) is mainly composed of muscular tissue, but at its most dorsal extent the membranous or nonmuscular septum is thinner and composed of more fibrous tissue. The left ventricular outflow tract lies in the centre of the heart and the aortic (left semilunar) valve consists of three half-moon-shaped cusps that are stronger and thicker than those of the pulmonary valve. The free edges often contain central nodules of fibrous tissue but may also have fenestrations. The cusps are attached to the fibrous and cartilaginous tissues that comprise the aortic annulus. The proximal segment of the aorta is the ascending aorta; it sweeps dorsally and cranially between the main PA on the left and the RA on the right. It then continues caudally and to the left as the descending aorta. The base of the aorta is bulbous in shape, and this bulbous portion is the sinus of Valsalva. The sino-tubular junction marks the point where the vessel becomes more tubular (see Figs. 1.1 and 1.3). To provide the blood to the myocardium, two coronary arteries arise from the right and left sinus of Valsalva. The most caudally located third part of the sinus lacks a coronary artery and is termed the septal (noncoronary) sinus. The same terminology is applied to the cusps of the aortic valve (see Fig. 1.2). The *ligamentum arteriosum* can be found in the site corresponding to the remnant of the *ductus arteriosus*, a vessel joining the PA to the descending aorta in the fetus (see Fig. 1.3).

The heart lies within the pericardial cavity that is comprised of the parietal pericardium and visceral pericardium (epicardium). The parietal pericardium attaches to the tunica externa of the proximal aorta, pulmonary artery, vena cavae and pulmonary veins. Between the parietal pericardium and visceral pericardium (epicardium) is a thin film of free serous fluid (pericardial fluid). The ventricular myocardium consists of muscle layers arranged both longitudinally and also spiralling circumferentially. The muscular tissue of the atria is separated from that of the ventricles by a fibrous skeleton that surrounds the atrioventricular orifices. The myocardium receives its blood supply from the coronary arteries and veins. There is an extensive autonomic nervous supply to the heart from the vagus nerve and sympathetic trunk (see Chapter 2).

ELECTRICAL PROPERTIES OF THE HEART

Contraction of cardiac myocytes occurs only in response to generation of action potentials in the cell membranes. Thus, normal mechanical function of the heart requires an orderly sequence of action potential generation and propagation through the atrial and ventricular myocardium. Spontaneous generation of an action potential without an external stimulus (automaticity) occurs normally as an inherent property of myocytes within the sinoatrial (SA) node, the atrioventricular (AV) node and the specialized conduction fibres of the His Purkinje system. However, cells of the SA node normally have the fastest rate of spontaneous action potential generation; consequently, the SA node is the site of impulse formation in the normal heart. The SA node is richly innervated by the parasympathetic and sympathetic nervous systems that provide stimuli to alter heart rate.

From the SA node, the impulse spreads over the atria to the AV node producing electrical potentials that inscribe a P wave on the surface electrocardiogram (ECG). Since spread of the cardiac impulse through the atria is in an overall direction that is dorsal to ventral, P waves are typically positive in a base apex ECG recording (see Chapter 6). The impulse is then conducted slowly through the AV node producing a delay recognized by an isoelectric segment (PR segment) on the ECG. The degree of AV conduction delay is influenced by autonomic tone with vagal tone reducing and sympathetic tone increasing rate of conduction. Autonomic tone, therefore, becomes an important determinant of heart rate in horses with dysrhythmias such as atrial fibrillation.

After relatively slow conduction through the AV node, the cardiac impulse is rapidly conducted over the bundle of His and Purkinje system to the terminal Purkinje fibres and the working ventricular myocytes. The equine Purkinje system is widely distributed throughout the right and left ventricular myocardium, penetrating the entire thickness of the ventricular walls. This vast distribution of the Purkinje system is physiologically important because the conduction velocity of working ventricular myocytes is approximately 6 times slower than conduction velocity of the Purkinje cells. Consequently, the time duration and sequence of ventricular activation and, ultimately, the surface ECG is affected. Specifically, the earliest phase of ventricular activation in horses consists of depolarization of a small apical region of the septum (Fig. 1.4). This early depolarization is often in an overall left to right and ventral direction. The electrical potentials generated from this early phase of ventricular activation may produce the

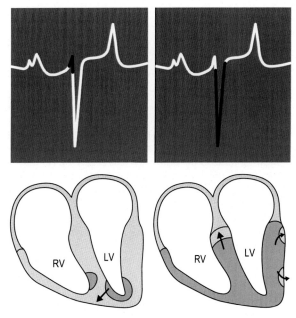

Figure 1.4 This figure illustrates the equine ventricular activation process. Areas of excited myocardium are shown in dark grey and the corresponding part of the ECG is shown in black. Arrows point in the overall direction of the wave of depolarization. During the earliest phase of activation (left panel) the septal myocardium begins to depolarize generating a variable vector often orientated ventrally and slightly rightward. During the next phase of ventricular activation the apical and middle thirds of the septum are excited simultaneously with the bulk of both ventricular walls; this phase generates no appreciable net electrical vector. The final phase of ventricular activation responsible for most of the QRS complex seen on the surface ECG is the result of spread of the impulse dorsally during excitation of the basilar third of the septum.

initial portion of the QRS complex on the surface ECG. However, there is significant variation in the direction of this early phase of ventricular activation, and in some horses the vectors of local electrical activity effectively cancel each other thereby eliminating any deflection on the surface ECG. Thus, the duration of QRS complexes in normal horses may vary from 0.08 to 1.4 seconds. Immediately after early ventricular activation of the apical portion of the septum, the major masses of both ventricles and the middle portion of the septum are depolarized with a single "burst" of activation that results from the vast distribution and penetration of the Purkinje fibres. Since this depolarization occurs without a spread of the impulse in any specific direction it contributes negligibly to genesis of the QRS complex on the ECG. The final phase of equine ventricular activation consists of depolarization of the basilar third of the septum, which occurs in an apical to basilar direction. This final phase of activation is responsible for generating most of the QRS complex and normally produces a negative deflection in a base apex recording (see Fig. 1.4).[2,3]

THE CARDIAC CYCLE

The cardiac cycle describes and relates temporally the mechanical, electrical and acoustical events that occur in the heart and great vessels. The cardiac cycle is usually described from onset of systole to end of diastole. It is helpful to describe the cardiac cycle with a diagram showing time on the horizontal axis (Fig. 1.5). An understanding of the cardiac cycle is essential for understanding function of the normal heart and for an appreciation of how various diseases disturb normal function.

The cardiac cycle is divided into ventricular systole and ventricular diastole. Systole is comprised of the isovolumic contraction phase and ventricular ejection. Diastole consists of the isovolumic relaxation phase, the rapid filling phase, diastasis and atrial contraction. It is helpful to recall that mechanical events are stimulated by electrical depolarization, and, thus, the mechanical events occur slightly after the electrical events on the cardiac cycle diagram.

Systole

Ventricular systole begins at the onset of the QRS complex, and mechanical systole begins slightly later with the onset of contraction and closure of the AV valves. During the isovolumic contraction phase of systole the intraventricular pressure rises rapidly, and when pressure in the left ventricle exceeds pressure in the aorta, the aortic valve opens and blood begins to flow into the aorta. Opening of the aortic valve marks the end of isovolumic contraction and the onset of ejection. The interval between the

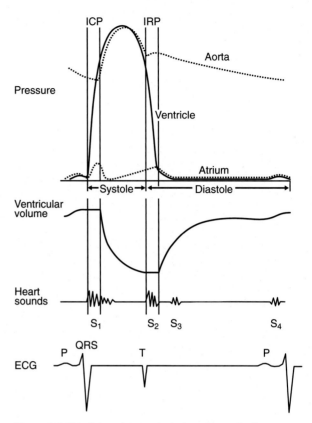

Figure 1.5 This figure shows a typical cardiac cycle diagram depicting important electrical, mechanical and acoustical events occurring on the left side of the heart using a common time axis. ICP = isovolumic contraction phase; IRP = isovolumic relaxation phase.

onset of the QRS complex and the onset of ejection is the pre-ejection period. The pre-ejection period includes both electromechanical delay and isovolumic contraction. During most of the ejection phase of systole left ventricular pressure exceeds aortic pressure. However, left ventricular pressure begins to decline during systole, and at the end of ejection aortic pressure exceeds ventricular pressure briefly. Aortic blood flow velocity reaches a peak during the first third of ejection and then decreases. Flow briefly reverses at the end of ejection abruptly closing the aortic valve. The interval between opening and closure of the aortic valve is the left ventricular ejection time. Closure of the aortic valve marks the end of systole.

Diastole

Ventricular diastole begins at aortic valve closure. The left ventricular pressure, which has been declining due to relaxation of the myocytes, continues to decline rapidly during early diastole, but ventricular volume remains constant because all of the cardiac valves are closed. This initial phase of diastole is, therefore, isovolumic relaxation, and the rate of intraventricular pressure decline during this phase of the cardiac cycle is determined by the rate of active relaxation of the myofibres. When left ventricular pressure drops below left atrial pressure, the mitral valve leaflets open and ventricular filling begins. Opening of the mitral valve marks the onset of the rapid filling phase of diastole during which filling occurs passively due to a difference in pressure between the ventricle and atrium that results largely from myocyte relaxation. The velocity of left ventricular inflow and the volume of blood transferred from the atrium to the ventricle during this early filling phase are largely determined by the increasing pressure gradient created by the continuing decline in tension in the ventricular myocytes at this time. As left ventricular pressure decline slows and ventricular filling progresses the atrioventricular pressure difference approaches zero and ventricular volume reaches a plateau. This phase of diastole is known as diastasis because minimal changes in intraventricular pressure and volume are occurring at this time. The duration of diastasis varies inversely with heart rate, and at resting heart rates in horses diastasis is the longest phase of diastole. Diastasis becomes progressively shorter as heart rate increases, but the shortening of diastasis from physiological increases in heart rate has a negligible effect on ventricular filling. Atrial systole is the final phase of ventricular diastole. This phase begins slightly after the P wave of the ECG. Atrial contraction recreates an atrioventricular pressure gradient that produces augmented LV filling. In healthy resting horses atrial systole has minimal effects on ventricular filling and cardiac performance. However, absence of atrial contraction or loss of atrioventricular synchrony in exercising horses has a considerable adverse effect on ventricular filling and cardiac output.

Although this discussion of the cardiac cycle has focused on events occurring on the left side of the circulation, events on the right side are nearly simultaneous and analogous. The main difference between the two sides of the heart is that the right ventricular and pulmonary artery peak systolic pressures are lower than the comparable left-sided pressures.

NORMAL HEART SOUNDS (EA)

During the cardiac cycle four heart sounds are generated as a result of rapid acceleration or deceleration of blood. Two, three or all four of these sounds may be heard in normal horses. Recognition and understanding of the normal heart sounds yields information regarding timing of murmurs and presence or absence of atrial contraction. Normally the first (S1) and second (S2) heart sounds are loudest and are audible in all normal animals. S1 is audible at the onset of mechanical systole and occurs in association with closure of the atrioventricular valves. S2 is heard at the end of systole with closure of the semilunar valves (see Fig. 1.5). In healthy horses S1 is the loudest of the normal heart sounds. It is also the longest in duration. S2 is a shorter, higher pitched sound. The third heart sound (S3), if audible, follows S2, and is associated with early ventricular filling (the rapid filling phase of diastole). The fourth heart sound (S4), if audible, is heard immediately prior to S1 and is associated with atrial contraction (late filling).

Typically, the normal heart sounds occur nearly simultaneously on the left and right sides of the heart. However, there are some conditions that may cause enough asynchrony that the first or second heart sounds are split into two components. An audible splitting of S1 is unusual in horses but generally not significant unless due to premature ventricular depolarizations or unless the split is mistaken for an audible S4 in horses with atrial fibrillation. S2 is frequently split in normal horses, and inspiration usually increases the degree of splitting in normal animals.

VENTRICULAR FUNCTION

Definitions

A discussion of ventricular performance requires at its onset clarification of terminology. Cardiac performance is a general term referring to the overall ability of the heart as an intact organ to pump blood for tissue needs. Cardiac performance is affected by a wide variety of both cardiac and extracardiac factors, including heart rate, contractility, valvular integrity, loading conditions and atrioventricular synchrony. The terms atrial function and ventricular function refer more specifically to the ability of each of these chambers to pump. Although various parameters, such as stroke volume and cardiac output, are used to describe and quantify ventricular function, these parameters actually reflect overall cardiac performance. Ventricular function is typically considered more important than atrial function in determining overall performance. However, atrial function can contribute significantly to cardiac output, particularly in exercising horses. Systolic performance and systolic function are terms referring to the ability of the ventricles to contract and eject blood, whereas diastolic performance and diastolic function refer to the ability of the ventricles to adequately relax and fill.

Ventricular systolic function

The major factors affecting ventricular systolic function are ventricular end-diastolic volume (preload), the inotropic or contractile state of the myocardium, impedance to ventricular outflow (afterload) and heart rate. Synchrony of interventricular and intraventricular contraction does not play a significant role in physiological alterations of ventricular function. However, synchrony may be abnormal in several cardiac diseases, and development of ventricular asynchrony has been shown to adversely affect systolic function, ventricular remodelling and mortality.[4]

Within a physiological range of end-diastolic volumes, as the ventricular volume (preload) increases, ensuing contractions become more forceful thereby increasing ejection pressure, stroke volume or both. In the words of Charles S. Roy, a 19th century physiologist, "the larger the quantity of blood which reaches the ventricles … the larger the quantity will be which it throws out."[5] This direct relationship between ventricular filling and cardiac performance enables the normal right and left ventricles to maintain equal minute outputs while their stroke outputs may vary considerably during normal respiration. In addition, cardiac output is augmented by an increase in preload in many conditions, including those associated with an increase in venous return and a decrease in peripheral vascular resistance, such as exercise, anaemia, fever and pregnancy. Thus, end-diastolic volume is an important determinant of ventricular systolic function and overall cardiac performance.

While there is strong evidence that the normal ventricle benefits from alterations in end-diastolic volume during normal resting circumstances or during exercise, the dilated failing ventricle has little, if any, preload reserve. Consequently, increases in filling do not produce increases in stroke volume in the failing heart. In pathologically dilated ventricles the direct correlation between end-diastolic volume and ventricular systolic function ceases to exist and both diastolic ventricular pressures and wall tension rise.

Afterload is the net force opposing myofibre shortening, and, although rather easily quantified in isolated cardiac muscle strips, measurement of afterload is significantly more challenging in the intact circulation. One approach for measurement of afterload in the clinical setting is to focus on vascular load by determining vascular resistance or arterial input impedance.[6] Impedance is a physiological parameter that incorporates pulsatile load as well as resistance. Under identical conditions of preload and inotropic state, increases in impedance reduce the degree of shortening of the myofibres and, hence, reduce stroke volume. An inverse relationship, therefore, exists between afterload and ventricular systolic function.

Inotropic state of the myocardium (myocardial contractility) also significantly affects ventricular function. It is important to note the distinction between the term myocardial function, which describes the inherent contractile state of the myocytes, and the term ventricular function, which describes overall pumping performance and is influenced by mechanical loading. Myocardial contractility may be altered by a variety of factors extrinsic to the myocardium, including autonomic output, circulating substances (hormones, pharmacological agents, endogenous and exogenous toxins, etc.), locally produced metabolites and pathological processes (ischaemia, acidosis, infarction, etc.). Myocardial contractility is difficult to quantify in the intact animal, and measurements of systolic ventricular function and contractility are often considered together. Fortunately, in most clinical situations quantification of myocardial contractility alone is unnecessary.

Ventricular diastolic function

Ventricular filling is a complex process affected primarily by venous return, atrioventricular valve function, atrial function, pericardial compliance, heart rate and myocardial relaxation and compliance. Although the importance of normal myocardial systolic function is easily and intuitively appreciated, the importance of normal diastolic function is often overlooked. Yet ventricular filling is extremely important physiologically because of the direct relationship between end-diastolic volume and systolic function. Inadequate end-diastolic volume will result in inadequate stroke volume and reduced coronary perfusion. Moreover, impaired left ventricular diastolic function, defined as inability of the ventricle to adequately fill without a compensatory increase in left atrial pressure, often results in pulmonary oedema and/or secondary right ventricular failure.

Two major factors affect ventricular diastolic performance: chamber compliance and myocardial relaxation. Reduced left ventricular (LV) chamber compliance (increased stiffness) produces an increase in the slope of the end-diastolic pressure–volume relationship. Thus, if ventricular compliance is reduced, a greater filling pressure is required to achieve a given end-diastolic volume. Most conditions that reduce ventricular compliance occur chronically and include reduction in LV lumen size, pathological hypertrophy, fibrosis, infiltrative diseases, pericardial tamponade or constriction, and disease or dilatation of the opposite ventricle.[7]

Diastolic function is also affected by the rate and the extent of myocardial relaxation. Myocardial relaxation is the energy-dependent process by which myocytes return to their original end-diastolic length and tension. With impaired relaxation the rate and extent of tension decline are diminished, resulting in a reduced rate of LV pressure decline and, hence, decreased early ventricular filling. In the intact heart relaxation is affected by loading conditions, synchrony of contraction and relaxation, and by the intracellular processes controlling calcium ion reuptake and cross-bridge inactivation.[8] Myocardial relaxation may change acutely in response to hypoxia, ischaemia, altered afterload, tachycardia, catecholamines and various pharmacological agents. Furthermore, myocardial relaxation may vary independently and in the opposite direction from changes in the inotropic state. For example, calcium channel blocking agents enhance relaxation but reduce contractility. In contrast, catecholamines have both positive lusitropic and positive inotropic effects.

Disease processes that produce diastolic dysfunction include pressure overload states with myocardial hypertrophy or fibrosis (aortic and pulmonic stenosis, systemic or pulmonary hypertension), ischaemic heart disease, constrictive pericarditis and primary or secondary hypertrophic cardiomyopathy. Most of these disorders are uncommon in horses. Nonetheless, recent data suggest that altered diastolic function may occur in horses following prolonged high-intensity exercise, particularly when superimposed with thermal stress.[9] Furthermore, some data suggest that dynamic exercise training may enhance LV diastolic function in human and equine athletes[10] (J. M. Bright & C. M. Marr, unpublished data).

ATRIAL FUNCTION

Because ventricular end-diastolic volume affects the contractile force of the ventricles and maximal stroke volume, atrial systolic function may significantly influence cardiac performance. Normally, atrial systole increases ventricular filling immediately prior to ventricular systole, thereby augmenting end-diastolic volume without the deleterious energetic sequelae of maintaining high filling pressures throughout diastole. In normal resting horses the overall effect of atrial systole on circulatory function is negligible, but normal atrial systolic function is essential for maximal performance in exercising horses.[11,12]

Two adverse haemodynamic consequences will arise from loss of the atrial "kick"; there will be an increase in mean atrial pressure as well as a decrease in ventricular end-diastolic volume and pressure. Various dysrhythmias, including atrial fibrillation, ventricular tachycardia or high-degree AV conduction block, can produce loss of effective atrial systole resulting in poor exercise tolerance, weakness or syncope. Both atrial fibrillation and paroxysmal ventricular tachycardia have been noted to cause impaired exercise performance in otherwise normal horses.[13]

Atrial function is not static; both systolic and diastolic function of the atria may be altered by many of the same factors that affect ventricular function, including atrial preload, impedance to atrial emptying, the inotropic state of the atrial myocytes and atrial compliance.[14–17] Furthermore, enhanced atrial function has been described as an important compensatory mechanism in patients with chronic heart failure.[18]

ASSESSMENT OF VENTRICULAR FUNCTION AND CARDIAC PERFORMANCE

Evaluation of myocardial systolic and diastolic function in an intact research animal or patient is problematic because the various determinants of ventricular function cannot be easily controlled or held constant. Quantifying cardiac performance of client-owned horses is also hampered by the frequently limited ability to use invasive or costly procedures. This discussion will briefly address those indexes most often used for assessment of ventricular function in clinical and clinical research settings.

In hospital or clinical research settings the method(s) used to identify ventricular dysfunction or to quantify cardiac performance should be selected with careful consideration of the question(s) being addressed as well as the overall usefulness, safety, limitations and cost of each procedure. If, for example, the quantitative information needed to answer a clinical or research question can be obtained by an extremely safe procedure such as Doppler echocardiography or exercise treadmill testing, there is little justification for cardiac catheterization or nuclear angiocardiography.

Pressure and flow data

Catheterization of the pulmonary artery by the Swan-Ganz technique[19] may be done relatively easily in standing horses using percutaneous catheter introduction into a jugular vein. The catheter can be used to measure pressures in the right atrium, right ventricle and pulmonary artery, and to obtain cardiac output measurements by the thermodilution, dye dilution or Fick methods. It is usually not possible to obtain measurements of pulmonary capillary wedge pressures in adult horses using standard-length commercially available catheters. However, when the pulmonary vascular bed, mitral valve and left ventricle function normally, the pulmonary artery diastolic pressure approximates the pulmonary capillary wedge pressure, and, therefore, the mean left atrial pressure.[20] A more accurate measurement of LV filling pressure is obtained by retrograde placement of a catheter into the left ventricle via the carotid artery for measurement of end-diastolic pressure. Normally the right atrial mean pressure approximates the right ventricular filling pressure. Pressure data from normal, resting horses is shown in Table 1.1.

Cardiac output, though one of the simplest and most traditional measurements of cardiac performance, provides little specific information regarding myocardial contractility because cardiac output, in addition to being affected by systolic and diastolic myocardial function, is also affected by loading conditions, atrioventricular

Table 1.1 Haemodynamic data obtained from healthy adult resting horses*

VARIABLE	VALUES	REFERENCE
Heart rate (beats/min)	32 ± 2	43
Mean right atrial pressure (mmHg)	8 ± 2, 10 ± 4	43, 44
RV end-diastolic pressure (mmHg)	11 ± 6, 22 ± 5	44, 32
RV peak systolic pressure (mmHg)	51 ± 9	44
RV dP/dt$_{max}$ (mmHg/s)	477 ± 84	32
Pulmonary artery systolic pressure (mmHg)	42 ± 3, 45 ± 9	43, 44
Pulmonary artery diastolic pressure (mmHg)	24 ± 2, 22 ± 8	43, 44
Mean pulmonary artery pressure (mmHg)	31 ± 2, 30 ± 8	43, 44
Pulmonary capillary wedge pressure (mmHg)	16 ± 4	32
Carotid artery systolic pressure (mmHg)	144 ± 17	44
Carotid artery diastolic pressure (mmHg)	98 ± 14	44
Carotid artery mean pressure (mmHg)	124 ± 13	44
Thermodilution cardiac output (L/min)	19.9 ± 7.4	26
Dye-dilution cardiac output (L/min)	40 ± 11	44

*Values from references 43 and 44 are mean ± SEM; those from references 26 and 32 are mean ± SD.

RV = right ventricular; dP/dt$_{max}$ = maximum rate of pressure increase during isovolumic contraction.

synchrony, valvular integrity and heart rate. Nonetheless, cardiac output is an important circulatory parameter that is relatively easy to obtain either serially at rest, during or after surgery or drug administration, or in combination with an exercise procedure.

Three methods commonly used to determine cardiac output are the Fick method, the thermodilution method and the lithium dilution method. The Fick method requires analysis of respiratory gases as well as analysis of arterial and mixed venous (pulmonary arterial) oxygen content.[21] Furthermore, the Fick method of cardiac output determination requires steady-state circulatory conditions. The thermodilution method of cardiac output measurement also requires placement of a pulmonary artery catheter but does not require analysis of respiratory gases or an arterial blood sample. Moreover, thermodilution cardiac output determinations do not require steady-state conditions. The thermodilution method has been shown to slightly overestimate (4.58%) true cardiac output.[22] Traditionally the lithium dilution method requires a central catheter, for the injection of lithium, and an arterial catheter for its sampling. It has been demonstrated that injection of lithium into a peripheral vein, such as the jugular vein, is a reliable alternative to both the Fick method and thermodilution method in both exercising and anaesthetized horses and may be a more appropriate method for assessment of cardiac output in client-owned horses.[23,24] A

further method of cardiac output determination based on arterial pulse contour has been described in anaesthetized horses and provides good agreement with the lithium dilution method but has not been evaluated in conscious horses.[25]

Radionuclide ventriculographic assessment of cardiac output in horses may be made using either gated or first-pass nuclear angiocardiographic techniques. However, gated studies are rarely done because anaesthesia is required to adequately immobilize the patient for the gated image acquisitions. First-pass studies may be done without anaesthesia and provide both left and right ventricular activity curves from which several indexes of systolic and diastolic ventricular function are derived. Radionuclide ventriculography, although noninvasive, requires costly equipment and considerable expertise. It also involves the use of ionizing radiation. Furthermore, first-pass radionuclide ventriculography in horses is generally limited to no more than two studies in a 24-hour period.[26] Figure 1.6 illustrates sequential images obtained from the first-pass nuclear angiocardiographic study of a normal, adult horse. The LV and right ventricular (RV) activity–time curves generated from the study are also shown.

Cardiac output can also be determined noninvasively by several echocardiographic techniques[27,28] (see Chapter 9) Doppler echocardiographic determination of cardiac

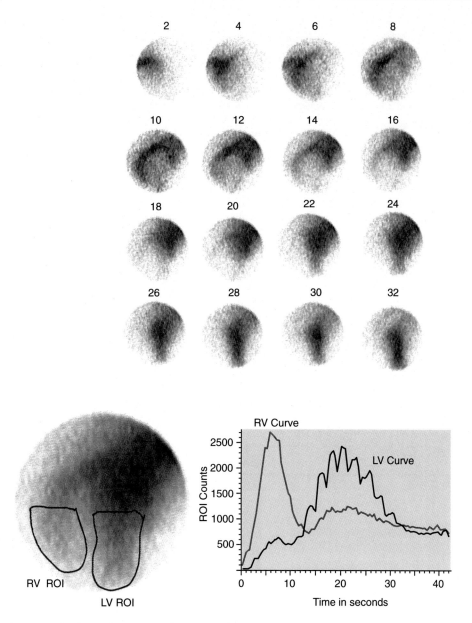

Figure 1.6 This figure demonstrates first pass nuclear ventriculography obtained from a normal horse. The top portion of the figure shows sequential images at 2 second intervals as the radioactive bolus passes through the right atrium, right ventricle, lungs, left atrium and left ventricle. A region of interest (ROI) is drawn over the area of the right ventricle (RV) and the left ventricle (LV) so that computer-generated activity-time curves may be derived.

output requires multiplication of the Doppler-derived aortic or pulmonary artery flow velocity time integral by the cross-sectional area of the vessel, and there are several potential sources of error inherent in this technique. These sources of potential error include inaccurate measurement of vessel diameter from the M-mode or two-dimensional echocardiographic images and failure to obtain parallel alignment of the Doppler beam with blood flow. However, one comparison of the pulsed Doppler and thermodilution measurements of cardiac output in horses has shown no significant differences between these two techniques.[29]

Contractility indexes

Measurement of the inherent inotropic state of the myocardium is often desirable, particularly in research settings. However, in clinical situations it is usually not necessary to obtain measurements of contractility that are load independent: if preload reserve has been fully utilized, reduced myocardial contractility will produce an "afterload mismatch" in the resting state such that ejection parameters will be depressed.

Therefore, in resting horses, the most feasible and practical method of evaluating LV systolic function is by determination of ejection phase indexes based on echocardiographic measurement of LV chamber size. Such indexes include the percent decrease of the LV minor axis (fractional shortening), the percent decrease in the LV end-diastolic volume (ejection fraction) and the mean velocity of circumferential fibre shortening (mean VCF). Fractional shortening is most commonly used. Table 1.2 contains a summary of normal echocardiographic indexes of systolic function obtained from resting horses. It is important to recognize that all ejection phase indexes will be reduced by an increase in afterload as well as by a decrease in inotropic state. Thus, in situations of acute aortic or mitral regurgitation, the ejection phase indexes of systolic function are unreliable due to afterload

mismatch. In contrast, the systolic unloading of the left ventricle that occurs with chronic mitral regurgitation may produce a normal or near normal shortening fraction, even when myocardial contractility is depressed. (ET, VMD)

Pulsed Doppler measurements of the velocity of blood flow in the aortic root or pulmonary artery may also be used to obtain several indexes of LV systolic function (see Table 1.2). These Doppler-derived indexes include peak and mean velocity, acceleration and ejection time.[30] With reduced inotropic state, velocities are reduced, ejection time is shortened and the rate of acceleration of the blood cells decreases. However, these same changes also occur with increased afterload. Furthermore, velocities can be accurately recorded only when the Doppler beam is oriented nearly parallel (±20 degrees) to the direction of blood flow. In horses the available acoustic windows are more limited than in people and dogs, and optimal alignment is less easily achieved.[31] (ET)

Tissue velocity imaging (TVI) is a Doppler echocardiographic modality that measures the velocity of selected areas of the myocardium, and TDI provides a sensitive and noninvasive method of assessing systolic function in people and dogs.[32,33] Preliminary data obtained from horses suggest that spectral TVI can also be used to quantify systolic function in horses and may possibly be useful

Table 1.2 Doppler echocardiographic indexes of ventricular systolic function in healthy adult horses

VARIABLE	VALUES	REFERENCE
LV fractional shortening (%)	32–45 (min–max)	27
	37.0 ± 3.9 (mean ± SD)	45
	46.0 ± 1.6 (mean ± SD)	46
Velocity of circumferential fibre shortening (mm/s)	1.16 ± 0.7 (mean ± SD)	46
LV ejection time (s) (M-mode)	0.49 ± 0.02 (mean ± SD)	46
Peak velocity RV outflow (m/s)	0.78–1.04 (min–max)	47
Peak velocity LV outflow (m/s)	1.29–4.17 (min–max)	47
Acceleration of RV outflow (m/s^2)	2.99–6.71 (min–max)	47
Acceleration of LV outflow (m/s^2)	5.19–10.8 (min–max)	47
RV pre-ejection period (s)	0.02–0.10 (min–max)	47
LV pre-ejection period (s)	0.04–0.11 (min–max)	47
RV ejection time (s)	0.45–0.58 (min–max)	47
LV ejection time (s) (pulsed Doppler)	0.41–0.55 (min–max)	47
Maximal systolic myocardial velocity caudal LVW (pulsed TDI) (m/s)	0.099 ± 0.028 (mean ± SD)	31

LV = left ventricular; RV = right ventricular; LVW = left ventricular wall; TDI = tissue Doppler imaging.

as an alternative or adjunct to postexercise echocardiographic testing.[34] (ET)

As in other species, quantitative assessment of right ventricular (RV) function is problematic in horses because of the complex shape and asynchronous contraction pattern of this ventricle. High-fidelity recording of the RV pressure with a micromanometer can be used to obtain the maximal rate of pressure rise (dP/dt_{max}) as an index of RV contractility.[35] Alternatively, radionuclide ventriculography provides a noninvasive means of computing the RV ejection fraction.

Indexes of diastolic function

Diastolic myocardial function, like systolic myocardial function, may be expected to deteriorate in diseased hearts and perhaps, to, improve with exercise training. Classically, clinical evaluation of diastolic function has relied on invasive measurement of ventricular pressure or nuclear angiographic demonstration of volume changes with time.[36,37] M-mode echocardiography has been used to measure various diastolic time intervals such as the relaxation time index.[38] More recently, pulsed Doppler evaluation of RV and LV filling patterns and diastolic time intervals has become a clinically useful means of noninvasively assessing diastolic function.[39-44] The most frequently used Doppler echocardiographic indexes of diastolic function include peak and mean velocities of early (passive) ventricular filling (peak and mean E-wave velocities), peak and mean velocities of late (atrial systolic) ventricular filling (peak and mean A-wave velocities), the deceleration time of early inflow, the rate of deceleration of early inflow, and the ratio of the peak early to peak late inflow velocities (E/A). Isovolumic relaxation time (IVRT) is obtained from a pulsed Doppler recording showing simultaneously LV inflow and outflow.

Two distinct Doppler patterns of abnormal LV filling have been noted in people[44] and in cats.[45] One pattern of abnormal transmitral flow is attributed to impaired LV relaxation and is characterized by prolongation of the isovolumic relaxation time and deceleration time, with a reduction of early (E) and increase in late (A) filling velocities. The second pattern is believed to reflect markedly increased LV or pericardial stiffness and is characterized by a shortened or normal IVRT, a decrease in the time (increase in rate) of deceleration and increased early (E) with reduced late (A) velocities. Table 1.3 contains a summary of available data pertaining to Doppler indexes of diastolic function in normal horses.

Table 1.3 Doppler echocardiographic indexes of ventricular diastolic function in healthy adult horses

VARIABLE	VALUES	REFERENCE
Peak velocity early (E wave)		
RV filling (m/s)	0.77–1.05 (min–max)	47
LV filling (m/s)	0.41–1.12 (min–max)	47
Peak velocity late (A wave)		
RV filling (m/s)	0.48–1.07 (min–max)	47
LV filling (m/s)	0.24–0.63 (min–max)	47
E/A ratio transtricuspid flow	0.87–1.97 (min–max)	47
E/A ratio transmitral flow	0.95–3.56 (min–max)	47
E wave deceleration time		
Transtricuspid flow (s)	0.16–0.34 (min–max)	47
Transmitral flow (s)	0.14–0.27 (min–max)	47
Transmitral E wave deceleration (m/s^2)	−1.72 ± 0.78 (mean ± SD)	9
LV isovolumic relaxation time (ms)	140 ± 24 (mean ± SD)	9
Maximal myocardial velocity caudal LVW (pulsed TDI) (m/s)		
Early diastole (E' wave)	−0.160 ± 0.090 (mean ± SD)	31
Late diastole (A' wave)	0.051 ± 0.043 (mean ± SD)	31
RV = right ventricular; LV = left ventricular; LVW = left ventricular wall; TDI = tissue Doppler imaging.		

REFERENCES

1. Harvey W. Exercitatio de Motu Cordis et Sanguinis in Animalibus, 1628 CD Leake (trans.). Springfield, IL: Charles C, Thomas, 1928.

2. Hamlin RL, Scher AM. Ventricular activation process and genesis of QRS complex in the goat. Am J Physiol 1961;200:223–228.

3. Fregin GF. Electrocardiography. Vet Clin North Am Eq Prac 1985;1:419–432.

4. Bax JJ, Abraham T, Barold SS, Breithardt OA, Fung JW, Garrigue S, et al. Cardiac resynchronization therapy part 1 – issues before device implantation. J Am Coll Cardiol 2005;46:2153–2167.

5. Roy CS. On the influences which modify the work of the heart. J Physiol (London) 1878;1:452–496.

6. Nichols WW, Pepine CJ. Left ventricular afterload and aortic input impedance: implications of pulsatile blood flow. Prog Cardiovasc Dis 1982;24:293–306.

7. Schlant RC, Sonnenblick EH. Normal physiology of the cardiovascular system. In: Schlant RC, Alexander RW, editors. The Heart: Arteries and Veins. 8th ed. New York: McGraw-Hill; 1994. p. 113–151.

8. Lorrell BH. Significance of diastolic dysfunction of the heart. Annu Rev Med 1991;42:411–436.

9. Marr CM, Bright JM, Martin DJ, Harris PA, Roberts CA. Pre- and post exercise echocardiography in horses performing treadmill exercise in cool and hot/humid conditions. Proceedings 5th International Conference on Equine Exercise Physiology, Japan, 1998.

10. Brandao MU, Wajngarten M, Rondon E, Giorgi MC, Hironaka F, Negrao CE. Left ventricular function during dynamic exercise in untrained and moderately trained subjects. J Appl Physiol 1993;75:1989–1995.

11. Deem DA, Fregin GF. Atrial fibrillation in horses: a review of 106 clinical cases with consideration of prevalence, clinical signs, and prognosis. J Am Vet Med Assoc 1982;180:261–265.

12. Marr CM, Reef VB, Reimer JM, Sweeney RW, Reid SW. An echocardiographic study of atrial fibrillation in horses: before and after conversion to sinus rhythm. J Vet Intern Med 1995;9:336–340.

13. McGuirk SM, Muir WW. Diagnosis and treatment of cardiac arrhythmias. Vet Clin North Am Eq Prac 1985;1:353–370.

14. Hoit BD, Shao Y, Gabel M, Walsh RA. Influence of acutely altered loading conditions on left atrial appendage flow velocities. J Am Coll Cardiol 1994;24:1117–1123.

15. Hoit BD, Shao Y, Gabel M, Walsh RA. In vivo assessment of left atrial contractile performance in normal and pathological conditions using a time-varying elastance model. Circulation 1994;89:1829–1838.

16. Nishikawa Y, Roberts JP, Tan P, Klopfenstein CE, Klopfenstein HS. Effect of dynamic exercise on left atrial function in conscious dogs. J Physiol Lond 1994;481:457–468.

17. Thomas JD, Weyman AE. Echocardiographic Doppler evaluation of left ventricular diastolic function: physics and physiology. Circulation 1991;84:977–990.

18. Dernellis J, Stenfanadis C, Toutouzas P. From science to bedside: the clinical role of atrial function. Eur Hear J 2000;2(Suppl. K):K48–K57.

19. Swan HJC, Ganz W, Forrester J, Marcus H, Diamond G, Chonette D. Catheterization of the heart in human beings with the use of a flow-directed balloon tipped catheter. N Engl J Med 1970;283:447–451.

20. Goldenheim PD, Homayoun K. Cardiopulmonary monitoring of critically ill patients. New Engl J Med 1984;311:776–780.

21. Rushmer RF. Hemodynamic Measurements: Cardiovascular Dynamics. Philadelphia: WB Saunders; 1976. p. 36–75.

22. Dunlop CI, Hodgson DS, Chapman PL, Grandy JL, Waldron RD. Thermodilution estimation of cardiac output at high flows in anesthetized horses. Am J Vet Res 1991;52:1893–1898.

23. Durando MM, Corley KTT, Boston RC, Berks EK. Cardiac output determination by use of lithium dilution during exercise in horses. Am J Vet Res 2008;69(8):1054–1060.

24. Linton RA, Young LE, Marlin DJ, Blissitt KJ, Brearley JC, Jonas MM, et al. Cardiac output measured by lithium dilution, thermodilution, and transesophageal Doppler echocardiography in anesthetized horses. Am J Vet Res 2000;61(7):731–737.

25. Hallowell GD, Corley KT. Use of lithium dilution and pulse contour analysis cardiac output determination in anaesthetized horses: a clinical evaluation. Vet Anaesth Analg 2005;32(4):201–211.

26. Koblick PD, Hornof WJ. Diagnostic radiology and nuclear cardiology: their use in assessment of equine cardiovascular disease. Vet Clin North Am Eq Prac 1985;1:289–310.

27. Blissett KJ, Yound LE, Jones RS, Darke PG, Utting J. Measurement of cardiac output in standing horses by Doppler echocardiography and thermodilution. Equine Vet J 1997;29:18–25.

28. Giguère S, Bucki E, Adin DB, et al. Cardiac output measurement by partial carbon dioxide rebreathing, 2-dimensional echocardiography, and lithium-dilution method in anesthetized neonatal foals. J Vet Intern Med 2005;19:737–743.

29. Stadler P, Kindel N, Deegen E. A comparison of cardiac stroke volume determination using the thermodilution method and PW-Doppler echocardiography for the evaluation of systolic heart function in the horse. DTW 1994;101:312–315.

30. Young LE, Long KJ, Darke PGG, Jones RS, Utting J. Effects of detomidine, dopamine and dobutamine on selected Doppler echocardiographic variables in the horse. Br J Anaesthesia 1992;69:16 (abstr).

31. Marr CM. Equine echocardiography – sound advice at the heart of the matter. Br Vet J 1994;150:527–545.

32. Waggoner AD, Bierig SM. Tissue Doppler imaging: a useful echocardiographic method for the cardiac sonographer to assess systolic and diastolic ventricular function. J Am Soc Echocardiogr 2001;14:1143–1152.

33. Chetboul V, Sampedrano CC, Testault I, Pouchelon JL. Use of tissue Doppler imaging to confirm the diagnosis of dilated cardiomyopathy in a dog with equivocal echocardiographic findings. J Am Vet Med Assoc 2004;225:1877–1880.

34. Sepulveda MF, Perkins JD, Bowen IM, Marr CM. Demonstration of regional differences in equine ventricular myocardial velocity in normal 2-year-old thoroughbreds with Doppler tissue imaging. Equine Vet J 2005;37:222–226.

35. Nollet H, Van Loon G, Deprez P, Sustronk B, Muylle E. Use of right ventricular pressure increase rate to evaluate cardiac contractility in horses. Am J Vet Res 1999;60:1508–1512.

36. Mirsky I. Assessment of diastolic function: suggested methods and future considerations. Circulation 1984;69:836–840.

37. Bonow RO. Radionuclide angiographic evaluation of left ventricular diastolic function. Circulation 1991;84(Suppl.):1-208–1-215.

38. Hanrath P, Mathey DG, Siegert R, Bleifeld W. Left ventricular relaxation and filling pattern in different forms of left ventricular hypertrophy: an echocardiographic study. Am J Cardiol 1980;45:15–23.

39. Lewis JF, Spirito P, Pelliccia A, Maron BJ. Usefulness of Doppler echocardiographic assessment of diastolic filling in distinguishing "athlete's heart" from hypertrophic cardiomyopathy. Br Heart J 1992;68:296–300.

40. Myreng Y, Smiseth OA. Assessment of left ventricular relaxation by Doppler echocardiography: comparison of isovolumic relaxation time and transmitral flow velocities with time constant of isovolumic relaxation. Circulation 1990;81:260–266.

41. DeMaria AN, Wisenbaugh T. Identification and treatment of diastolic dysfunction: role of transmitral Doppler recordings. J Am Coll Cardiol 1987;9:1106–1107.

42. DeMaria AN, Wisenbaugh TW, Smith MD, Harrisson MR, Berk MR. Doppler echocardiographic evaluation of diastolic dysfunction. Circulation 1991;84(Suppl.):1-288–1-295.

43. Ren J-F, Pancholy SB, Iskandrian AS, Lighty GW Jr., Mallavarapu C, Segal BL. Doppler echocardiographic evaluation of the spectrum of left ventricular diastolic dysfunction in essential hypertension. Am Heart J 1994;127:906–913.

44. Oh JK, Seward JB, Tajik AJ. Assessment of Ventricular Function. The Echo Manual. Boston: Little, Brown; 1994. p. 39–50.

45. Bright JM, Herrtage ME. Doppler echocardiographic assessment of diastolic function in normal cats and cats with hypertrophic cardiomyopathy. J Am Soc Echo 1995;8:383 (abstract).

Chapter | 2 |

Neuroendocrine control of cardiovascular function: physiology and pharmacology

Jonathan Elliott and Mark Bowen

CHAPTER CONTENTS

INTRODUCTION

The function of the cardiovascular system is to ensure that the tissues of the body are supplied with adequate blood flow in order to satisfy their requirements for oxygen and energy substrates and to ensure that metabolic waste products do not accumulate. Arterial blood pressure is the driving force for blood flow around the circulatory system and is closely regulated at a stable level despite large changes in the demand of the body organs for blood flow, depending on the metabolic state of the tissues (e.g. resting versus exercising muscle).

Certain intrinsic properties of the cardiovascular system ensure that demand for blood flow is met by its supply. For example, the heart functions as a demand pump – the more blood which returns to it (venous return) and stretches the heart in diastole, the larger the stroke volume which is ejected per beat (Starling's law of the heart). Tissue blood flow can also be regulated by local metabolites, which relax precapillary sphincters and reduce resistance to blood flow in actively metabolizing tissues. It is important to recognize that the cardiovascular system is

integrated closely with the respiratory and renal systems; the former ensures efficient oxygenation of the blood and excretion of carbon dioxide, the latter is involved in the long-term regulation of body fluid volume and hence vascular filling pressure in general and arterial blood pressure in particular.

Neurohormonal and paracrine mechanisms heighten the response of the cardiovascular system to changes in tissue demand for blood flow, ensure the system functions in the most efficient way possible from minute to minute and from hour to hour and allow the body to compensate in extreme conditions. In addition, the metabolic pathways involved in the generation and breakdown of these chemical mediators and the receptors that they utilize to produce their responses are all targets that can be exploited pharmacologically to treat cardiovascular diseases.

Much knowledge of cardiovascular physiology and pharmacology comes from the study of experimental animals and man. The importance of some of the more recently discovered mechanisms (which are the main focus of this chapter) in the horse, remains to be established. Where studies have been undertaken in the horse, these will be reviewed.

NEURONAL REGULATION OF THE CARDIOVASCULAR SYSTEM

Neuronal innervation of the cardiovascular system means that blood pressure can be tightly regulated on a beat-to-beat basis by the parasympathetic nervous system, which brings about changes in heart rate (chronotropic effects), and by the sympathetic nervous system, which brings about changes in both heart rate and contractility (inotropic effects) through innervation of the heart and changes in blood pressure through innervation of the vasculature. These control mechanisms are integrated by the brain stem.

Central nervous control

A full discussion of the central nervous system (CNS) control of the cardiovascular system is beyond the scope of this chapter,[1] and the following is a simplified account. Baroreceptors (stretch receptors) which detect high pressure within the vascular system are present in the walls of conductance vessels (aortic arch and carotid sinus) and those which determine low pressure (central volume receptors) are in atrial tissue (primarily at its junction with the great veins), pulmonary arteries and ventricles. Afferent inputs to the CNS are transmitted via the glossopharyngeal and vagal nerves which terminate in the *nucleus tractus solitarius* (NTS). The NTS also receives much information from other areas of the CNS (hypothalamus, cerebellum and cortex) involved to some extent in cardiorespiratory control. Integration of this information occurs in the NTS before it is relayed to the efferent cardiovascular control areas in the medulla of the brain stem (such as the nucleus ambiguus, rostral ventrolateral medulla) which initiate adjustments in vascular tone, heart rate and force of cardiac muscle contraction, mediated via the sympathetic and parasympathetic nervous systems, in order to normalize arterial blood and vascular filling pressures and make them appropriate for the physiological state of the animal.

Drugs which influence CNS control of the cardiovascular system

A number of drugs which are used clinically will affect the activity of centres within the brain controlling the cardiovascular system. Alpha$_2$-adrenoceptor agonists, for example, increase vagal tone to the heart and reduce sympathetic tone to the blood vessels, in part by their effects within the regulatory areas of the brain.[2] These actions give rise to the undesirable side effects of bradycardia and hypotension (following transient hypertension) when these drugs are used as analgesic sedatives.

Cardiac glycosides (e.g. digoxin) also have effects on the afferent nerves and the higher centres controlling the cardiovascular system, in addition to their direct effects on the heart and vasculature. Their effects can be very complex, depending on the physiological state of the animal treated, but generally include an increase in parasympathetic tone to the heart and increased baroreceptor stimulation, which produces reflex reduction in sympathetic vasoconstrictor nerve activity.[3] Individual variability in the response to cardiac glycosides could well reflect the degree of activation of the putative natural hormone "endogenous digitalis-like substance" which binds to the same receptors.[4]

Control of vascular tone

Vasomotor nerves

The categories of vasomotor nerves currently recognized are presented in Table 2.1. Efferent nervous control of the vascular system is primarily by the sympathetic vasoconstrictor nerves which tonically increase vascular smooth muscle tone throughout the circulatory system. The postganglionic noradrenergic neurones are distributed to all tissues innervating both arterioles and venules and increasing vascular tone by the action of noradrenaline on α_1-adrenoceptors. The density of sympathetic innervation and of α_1-adrenoceptors varies with different vascular beds. There is also clear evidence that sympathetic nerves supplying different vascular beds can be preferentially or even exclusively controlled by neurones in the medulla, according to the integrated afferent input.[5] Other vasomotor nerves are not tonically active or distributed in such a widespread fashion, but are stimulated under appropriate circumstances (see Table 2.1).[6]

Co-transmission in perivascular nerves

Sympathetic vasoconstrictor nerves also release adenosine 5' triphosphate (ATP), which is packaged in both large and small dense core vesicles with noradrenaline, and neuropeptide Y (NPY). NPY is preferentially localized in large vesicles.[7]

In some blood vessels, part or all of the vasoconstrictor response to perivascular nerve stimulation can be shown to be due to ATP, which acts on vascular smooth muscle receptors, distinct from α_1-adrenoceptors, namely P2x-purinoceptors. A prazosin-resistant component of the response of equine digital artery to perivascular nerve stimulation has been reported,[8] which shows characteristics of a purinergic response. The physiological importance of the purinergic component of sympathetic vasoconstrictor nerves is difficult to establish in vivo. Species differences and differences between vascular beds within a given species complicate the situation, making generalizations difficult to apply. There may be a greater purinergic component in small as opposed to large vessels.[9,10]

Neuropeptide Y (NPY) is a 36 amino acid peptide which, in addition to its presence in sympathetic vasoconstrictor nerves, is also found in areas of the brain involved in cardiovascular control and may play an important role in modulating the sympathetic nervous control of blood pressure.[11] NPY is preferentially released by high-frequency stimulation of perivascular nerves and has both direct vasoconstrictor effects (mediated via smooth muscle Y1 receptors) and potentiates the action of noradrenaline and ATP. These vasoconstrictor actions of NPY are most evident in vessels with wide neuromuscular junctions (i.e. larger vessels).

The concept of cotransmission in sympathetic vasoconstrictor nerves and other vasomotor nerves (see Table 2.1)

Table 2.1 Categories and properties of vasomotor nerves

CATEGORY OF NERVE	DISTRIBUTION	LEVEL OF ACTIVITY	NEUROTRANSMITTER
Vasoconstrictor sympathetic	Widespread throughout the vascular system (arterioles and venules) although density varies with the vascular bed	Tonically active, a major determinant of peripheral resistance, controlled by the brain stem	Noradrenaline Cotransmitters ATP and NPY are also important
Vasodilator sympathetic	Supply vascular beds of skeletal muscles in some species (carnivores) and sweat glands	Not tonically active, cause vasodilatation in readiness for exercise, influenced by the cerebral cortex	Acetylcholine (cholinergic fibres) Cotransmitter vasoactive intestinal polypeptide (VIP) is also important
Vasodilator parasympathetic	Glandular tissues Colonic and gastric mucosa Genital erectile tissue	Not tonically active – fire when organ function demands an increase in blood flow	Acetylcholine Cotransmitter VIP may play the more prominent role
"Sensory-motor" nerves (vasodilatory)	Nociceptive C fibres, responsible for part of the vasodilatory response in inflamed tissues (particularly skin)	Axon reflex occurs as a result of stimulation of sensory nerve (antidromic activation)	Sensory neurotransmitters Substance P and calcitonin gene-related peptide

provides the potential for greater complexity and fine tuning of control via multiple interactions between neurotransmitters. Actions at the presynaptic nerve membrane should also be mentioned here, as neuromodulatory actions occur often via receptors which differ from those on the postsynaptic membrane.[12] The complexity of this system is illustrated in Table 2.2, which lists some of the receptors found on the presynaptic membrane of sympathetic vasoconstrictor nerves.

Drugs which influence vasomotor nerve function

Most drugs have been developed to target the sympathetic vasoconstrictor nerves, as the therapeutic aim has been to reduce vascular resistance and increase venous capacitance, either in the management of hypertension or congestive heart failure. Antagonists with selectivity for α_1-adrenoceptors have proved to be the class which produce the least side effects. Nonselective α-adrenoceptor antagonists were less effective and caused more reflex tachycardia because blockade of presynaptic α_2-adrenoceptors increased the release of noradrenaline at all sympathetic postganglionic nerve synapses. Alpha$_1$-adrenoceptor antagonists are effective at reducing vasomotor tone initially. Indeed, a first-dose severe hypotensive effect can be a problem. With repeated dosing, however, the effect is reduced. This may well be due to physiological tolerance, via activation of other endogenous vasocon-

strictor systems, which might include increased importance of the cotransmitters (ATP and NPY) utilized by these nerves.[13] Drugs which inhibit the effects of ATP and NPY at their respective vascular receptors are under development but are not yet sufficiently well understood or developed for clinical use to be contemplated.[14–16]

Nervous control of cardiac function

Heart rate and inotropic state of the cardiac muscle are also influenced by the autonomic nervous system. Vagal tone predominates at rest in the horse to give a slow resting heart rate. Acetylcholine is the neurotransmitter involved and acts at M2-muscarinic receptors on cells of the sinoatrial and atrioventricular nodes. M2-receptors are not found on target cells of other organs, but do occur on the nerve terminals of parasympathetic postganglionic nerves where they inhibit acetylcholine release and at some autonomic ganglia, on the cell body of the postganglionic neurone, where their activation hyperpolarizes and reduces transmission. Direct innervation of ventricular muscle by the parasympathetic nervous system is sparse in most species.

By contrast, the distribution of cardiac sympathetic nerves is much more widespread, allowing this system to influence not only heart rate but also the inotropic state of cardiac muscle. Resting cardiac sympathetic tone in equine hearts is thought to be extremely low. The original concept that noradrenaline acts exclusively on β_1-

Table 2.2 Presynaptic receptors which modulate sympathetic vasoconstrictor nerves

RECEPTOR	ENDOGENOUS LIGAND	NEUROMODULATORY EFFECT
α_2-Adrenoceptors	Noradrenaline, adrenaline	Inhibits transmitter release
P_1-Purinoceptors	Adenosine (formed from ATP)	Inhibits transmitter release
Y_2-Receptors	NPY	Inhibits transmitter release (small vessels particularly)
DA_2-receptors	Dopamine	Inhibits transmitter release
β_2-Adrenoceptors	Adrenaline (circulating hormone)	Facilitates transmitter release
AT_1-receptors	Angiotensin II (circulating hormone)	Facilitates transmitter release
$5-HT_3$-receptors	5-HT released from platelets or from perivascular nerves	Facilitates transmitter release

adrenoceptors to mediate the effects of sympathetic stimulation, namely increased heart rate and force of contraction, is too simplistic. Although β_1-adrenoceptors predominate in all species including the horse,[17] β_2-adrenoceptors are found in the myocardium, particularly in atria and nodal tissue in man, rabbit and cat[18] and horse,[19] and probably explains why drugs with mixed β_1- and β_2-adrenoceptor agonist actions (e.g. isoprenaline) increase heart rate more effectively than those selective for β_1-adrenoceptors (e.g. dobutamine). In some species, there is good evidence that with chronic high levels of stimulation, the proportion of β_2-adrenoceptors in relation to β_1-adrenoceptors increases, while the overall number of β-adrenoceptors and their efficiency of coupling to cyclic AMP production decreases.[20] This phenomenon is less clear in the horse, and in 10 horses with congestive heart failure the density of β-adrenoceptors was unchanged and the density of β_2-adrenoceptors was increased only in five horses.[17] Beta-adrenoceptors have been implicated in cardiac remodelling leading to left ventricular enlargement and the β-adrenoceptor antagonists have been shown to reverse these effects in both pressure and volume loading.[21-25] As such, this class of agent may have potential therapeutic value in the horse with cardiac hypertrophy. In addition, α_1-adrenoceptors can be demonstrated in cardiac muscle. Stimulation of these receptors is thought to contribute, in a small way, to the positive inotropic effect of sympathetic nerve stimulation (with no effect on heart rate), but this contribution may increase in importance in disease states, when downregulation of the β_1-adrenoceptors occurs, and may also increase the tendency for dysrhythmias to develop in hearts driven by high sympathetic tone.[18] Alpha$_1$-adrenoceptors have also been implicated in the development of myocardial fibrosis during cardiac remodelling and offer potential targets for therapeutic intervention[23] although there is no clinical evidence to support their use in this way in any species.

HORMONAL CONTROL OF THE CARDIOVASCULAR SYSTEM

The key hormones currently thought to be involved in regulation of the cardiovascular system are summarized in Table 2.3. It is not possible to review these systems in any detail here, and areas with potential therapeutic importance will be focused on.

The renin–angiotensin–aldosterone system

The kidney responds to reduced perfusion, reduced solute filtration and increased sympathetic nerve stimulation by producing an enzyme, renin, which is secreted by modified smooth muscle cells of the afferent arterioles in the juxtaglomerular apparatus.[26] Renin then acts on its circulating substrate to produce angiotensin I, which is converted to the active hormone angiotensin II by the enzyme angiotensin-converting enzyme (ACE) present on endothelial cells, particularly in the lung (Fig. 2.1).

This is the conventional view of the way angiotensin II is produced, where it is thought to function in an endocrine fashion as a defence against hypovolaemia, hypotension and circulatory shock. There is good evidence for the local presence of renin (or renin-like enzyme activity), angiotensinogen and ACE, leading to local production of angiotensin II, in a number of tissues, including the myocardium, kidney and brain.[27] In the myocardium, upregulation of the system is thought to occur in response to increased ventricular wall stress[28] and may be important in the development of cardiac enlargement and fibrosis.[29-33] The effects of angiotensin II are summarized in Table 2.3. Aldosterone is synthesized in response to angiotensin II and acts via mineralocorticoid receptors to pre-

Table 2.3 Hormones of key importance in the control of the cardiovascular system

HORMONE	CARDIOVASCULAR AND RENAL EFFECTS
Adrenaline (and noradrenaline)	Increase heart rate and force of contraction (β_1) Increase vascular resistance, decrease venous capacitance (α_1 on vascular smooth muscle, β_2 on sympathetic nerve terminals) Increase blood flow to skeletal and cardiac muscle (β_2)
Angiotensin II	Increase vascular resistance, decrease venous capacitance (receptors on vascular smooth muscle and on sympathetic nerve terminals which increase noradrenaline release) Increase heart rate and force of contraction and stimulate cardiac muscle cell hypertrophy Enhance sodium retention by the kidney (direct effect in proximal tubule and mediated via aldosterone in distal tubule) Increase thirst and possibly salt appetite, enhance ADH secretion (effects on the brain produced by circulating angiotensin II or by angiotensin II produced in the brain)
Antidiuretic hormone (vasopressin)	Increase water retention by the kidney (V_2-receptors) Vasoconstriction (V_1-receptors on vascular smooth muscle) seen at higher ADH concentrations
Aldosterone Natriuretic peptides (ANP and BNP)	Increase sodium retention and potassium excretion by the kidney Increase salt and water excretion by the kidney (direct effects and inhibition of aldosterone secretion) Inhibit renin and ADH secretion Inhibit the peripheral and central actions of angiotensin II Vasodilatation (modest) of resistance blood vessels Increase in capillary permeability – reduction in circulating volume
Endogenous digitalis-like substances	Uncertain physiologic importance, may inhibit salt re-absorption by the kidney (natriuretic effect)

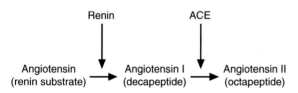

Figure 2.1

serve sodium by inducing reabsorption from the distal nephron. This results in an increase in circulating volume, and an increase in preload in the compensated diseased heart. However, volume overload ultimately leads to volume-induced hypertrophy, myocardial remodelling and fibrosis[34] and therefore inhibition of the actions of aldosterone, either by blocking production or its receptors, could reduce progression of cardiac disease.

Aldosterone has been proposed as a biomarker of severity of cardiac failure since its concentrations correlate with severity of disease in human patients,[35] although not in dogs with mitral valve regurgitation.[36,37] In the horse, increased serum concentrations of aldosterone have been reported in association with valvular regurgitation of the mitral, aortic and tricuspid valve.[38] Although this study

failed to differentiate the underlying disease it did show higher aldosterone concentrations in animals with significant left ventricular enlargement. Some horses with both atrial and ventricular enlargement had aldosterone concentrations similar to normal horses and in our laboratory horses with aortic valve regurgitation had no increase in serum activities of plasma renin, concentrations of angiotensin II or aldosterone (unpublished observations). It is not clear where these differences in study results arise although this may suggest that in certain forms of cardiac disease in the horse activation of the renin–angiotensin system is not important. Indeed, horses with compensated aortic valve regurgitation have increased systolic pressure due to increased end-diastolic volume (preload), such that there is no stimulation of renin release from the kidneys since systolic pressures are normal.

Drugs which affect the renin–angiotensin–aldosterone system

The clinical indications for interfering with this system pharmacologically are in hypertension and congestive heart failure; they potentially have a role in blocking or offsetting the remodelling effects of cardiac disease. In

Table 2.4 Therapeutic strategies for inhibition of the renin–angiotensin system

DRUG TARGET	EXAMPLES
Inhibition of renin secretion	β-Adrenoceptor antagonists (e.g. propranolol)
Inhibition of renin activity	Competitive renin inhibitors (e.g. enalkiren and remikiren)
Inhibition of angiotensin II formation	ACE inhibitors (captopril, enalapril, benazepril)
Inhibition of angiotensin II's effects	Competitive angiotensin II receptor antagonists (e.g. losartan)
Inhibition of aldosterone effects	Mineralocorticoid receptor antagonists, e.g. spironolactone

these diseases, inhibition of the system may produce beneficial effects. A number of therapeutic strategies might be employed, which are summarized in Table 2.4.

Much attention has been given to the development of inhibitors of ACE and these drugs have proven very successful in the management of congestive heart failure and have also been increasingly used as antihypertensive drugs in human medicine. They have been evaluated in the horse, where they resulted in modest benefits in cardiac function in asymptomatic horses with mitral valve regurgitation.[39] The oral bioavailability of enalapril is poor and has not demonstrated anti-ACE activity following oral dosing in the horse.[40,41] ACE is a nonspecific peptidyl-dipeptide hydrolase which also participates in the inactivation of bradykinin and encephalins. Some of the effects of ACE inhibitors may result from an increase of these mediators and the adverse effects of ACE inhibitors, such as dry cough and proinflammatory properties, have been attributed to the nonspecific action of ACE.[42] Renin inhibitors have been developed, but their usefulness may be limited by the body's ability to produce more renin when the system is perturbed and so overcome the effects of these inhibitors. Nonpeptide angiotensin II receptor antagonists have been evaluated in human clinical trials with losartan. This drug is selective for the AT1-angiotensin receptors and seems to inhibit most if not all of the effects of angiotensin II.[42] Although this drug causes regression of left ventricular hypertrophy in treated patients, which is superior to treatment with β-adrenoceptor blockers,[43] and a reduction in the occurrence of atrial fibrillation,[44,45] there is no improvement in survival over the use of ACE inhibitors (captopril) in patients with congestive heart failure.[46] One limitation of ACE inhibitors is the phenomenon of "aldosterone escape," whereby aldosterone concentrations increase despite ACE inhibition. This is reported in up to 40% of human patients treated.[34] The use of mineralocorticoid receptor antagonists therefore have potential synergistic effects with ACE inhibitors as well as diuretic effects, which, classically, was the reason for using them in patients with heart failure. The use of sprinolactone in combination with standard therapy has

been shown to result in an improvement in survival in human patients with severe heart failure.[47] Mineralocorticoid receptor antagonists also have potential antifibrotic effects in the remodelled heart as demonstrated by animal models of cardiac remodelling, in elderly human patients by improvement in diastolic function but not in Mainecoon cats with hypertrophic cardiomyopathy.[48-50] It has not been evaluated in the horse, but may prove to be a cost effective alternative to ACE inhibition in horses with heart failure.

Natriuretic peptides

The natriuretic peptides are released from the myocardium and have a range of effects both locally and within distant tissues. Predominantly the natriuretic hormones have cardioprotective effects, both in terms of changes in preload and in cardiac remodelling. Three natriuretic peptides (products of different genes) have thus far been discovered, all sharing a common 17 amino acid ring structure closed by a disulphide bond between two cysteine residues.[51] The sites of production, structures and factors controlling secretion of these peptides are summarized in Table 2.5.

Both ANP and BNP are released in response to cardiac chamber enlargement (atrial and ventricular, respectively), are released into the circulation and act on distant target sites; this is summarized in Table 2.3. The increase in ANP and BNP in cardiac enlargement has led to investigation of these as biomarkers of the severity of disease and are correlated with severity in human patients and dogs with cardiac enlargement[52-56] but not in horses.[57] Both peptides activate the natriuretic peptide receptors A and B (NPR-A and NPR-B), which mediate their effects on renal, endocrine and vascular systems. Both receptors possess guanylate cyclase activity, which raises intracellular cyclic GMP concentrations upon receptor activation. CNP has a low affinity for NPR-A receptors and is thought to produce its effects by binding to the NPR-B receptor, although the functional significance of CNP is far from clear. Unlike ANP and BNP, CNP probably acts in a paracrine fashion

Table 2.5 Properties of natriuretic peptides

PROPERTY	ATRIAL NATRIURETIC PEPTIDE (ANP)	BRAIN NATRIURETIC PEPTIDE (BNP)	C-NATRIURETIC PEPTIDE (CNP)
Site of production	Stored in granules of atrial tissue as pro-ANP Ventricular muscle can produce ANP when heart diseased Also present in the brain – particularly areas involved in blood pressure regulation May also be produced locally in the kidney	Produced primarily by ventricular muscle (despite name). Not stored in granules but secreted constitutively Atria can produce BNP but in smaller quantities than ventricles	Most abundant source is the brain Also produced by endothelium of blood vessels
Structure	Pro-ANP – 126 amino acids α-ANP (ANP_{99-126}) and (ANP_{1-98}) secreted by atria $ANP_{102-126}$ and $ANP_{103-126}$ produced in the brain Urodilantin (ANP_{95-126}) produced in the kidney Structure conserved across species	Pro-BNP – 108 amino acids BNP-32 (BNP_{77-108}) is secreted by ventricular and atrial cells Structure not conserved among species	Pro-CNP – 103 amino acids CNP-53 (CNP_{51-103}) and CNP-22 (CNP_{82-103}) both occur Structure is conserved across species
Stimuli for secretion	Increased atrial transmural pressure. Increased heart rate Ventricular production increases in heart failure	Increased stretch of the ventricles. Secretion is increased particularly in states of ventricular overload and hypertrophic cardiomyopathy	Unknown but may include cytokines CNP is not thought to circulate but may have effects local to its site of production

rather than entering the circulation and producing its effects at a distant site.

Natriuretic peptides are removed from the circulation by binding to a cell surface receptor which is termed NPR-C (clearance receptor). The peptides are then internalized and degraded by cellular lysosomal enzymes. ANP has the highest affinity for the NPR-C receptor, followed by CNP with BNP having the lowest affinity. An alternative means of removal of the peptides is through metabolic degradation via enzymes on the surface of cells. Neutral endopeptidase-24.11 (NEP; a Zn^{2+}-metallopeptidase) cleaves a peptide bond within the ring structure, destroying biological activity. NEP is present in many tissues but is particularly abundant in the kidney at the glomerulus, in renal vascular smooth muscle cells and on the brush borders of tubular cells. NEP has the highest affinity for CNP followed by ANP and then BNP. The same enzyme is capable of metabolizing a number of endogenous peptide mediators including encephalins.[58] The half-life of ANP in plasma is about 3 minutes, whereas that of BNP is approximately 20 minutes, a difference which presumably reflects the affinity of each peptide for the clearance receptor and the NEP enzyme.

Drugs acting on the natriuretic peptide system

As the natriuretic peptides have opposite actions to the renin–angiotensin system, therapeutically it would be desirable to enhance their effects in patients with hypertension or congestive heart failure. Currently, investigations have concentrated on inhibiting the breakdown of the peptides through the use of neutral endopeptidase (NEP) inhibitors. One such drug, candoxatril, has been shown to have similar effects to ACE inhibitors in improving clinical signs of congestive heart failure in human patients in a small-scale clinical trial,[59] but in another increased blood pressure in patients treated with this drug.[60] The combined effect of vasopeptidase inhibitors, drugs that show both NEP and ACE inhibition, shows clinical benefits compared to ACE inhibition alone[61-64] but they have not been evaluated in clinical use in veterinary medicine.

LOCAL REGULATION OF THE CARDIOVASCULAR SYSTEM BY THE ENDOTHELIUM

The endothelium plays an important role in the control of vascular function through the release of a range of local mediators in response to vasoactive mediators, changes in blood flow or oxygenation. The endothelial cell senses and integrates these local inputs by varying the mediators it produces, and contributes to the local regulation of blood flow in a major way.[7] The endothelium generates both vasodilator and vasoconstrictor mediators (Table 2.6).

Nitric oxide

Endothelial cells lining the cardiovascular system are thought to continuously produce the free radical gas nitric oxide (NO) as a result of the action of a constitutive enzyme present in the endothelial cells called endothelial nitric oxide synthase (eNOS). This enzyme, when activated by a rise in intracellular calcium ion concentration, catalyses the conversion of the amino acid L-arginine to NO and l-citrulline. L-arginine is actively taken up into endothelial cells to provide substrate for this reaction, and the product, L-citrulline, can be recycled, being converted back into L-arginine. Under normal circumstances, production of NO by endothelial cells is not limited by supply of substrate.

Endothelium-derived NO (EDNO) permeates biological membranes without hindrance and enters adjacent vascular smooth muscle cells, binding to the haem iron of the soluble enzyme, guanylate cyclase (GC). Activation of this enzyme maintains elevated concentrations of cyclic GMP within the vascular smooth muscle cell which results in tonic relaxation of the cell.[65]

Table 2.6 Important vasoactive mediators released by the endothelium[65]

VASODILATORS	VASOCONSTRICTORS
Nitric oxide	Endothelin (peptide)
Prostacyclin	Arachidonic acid metabolites
Endothelium-dependent hyperpolarizing factor (chemical nature unknown)	A diffusible factor released from hypoxic endothelial cells (unidentified)

Structural analogues of L-arginine, such as NG monomethyl-L-arginine, which inhibit production of EDNO by competing with L-arginine for the eNOS enzyme, cause a rise in total peripheral resistance and arterial blood pressure in vivo in most species examined. Transgenic mice have been produced which lack the eNOS enzyme and have a mean arterial blood pressure of 35% higher than their wild-type counterparts.[66] Thus, the concept of "tonic vasodilatation" of the circulation has emerged, much in the same way as we think of tonic vasoconstriction provided by sympathetic vasoconstrictor nerves (see above).

Continuous production of EDNO probably results from tonic activation of endothelial cells caused by blood flowing across their surfaces, activation of eNOS occurring as a result of the shear forces sensed by endothelial cells.[67] The exact mechanism by which this occurs is unknown but will involve an increase in cytosolic calcium concentration as eNOS is a calcium-calmodulin-activated enzyme. It is clear that this mechanism allows EDNO to modulate pressure–flow relationships within resistance arterioles, ensuring they relax in response to increased intraluminal pressure.

NO production is also stimulated by chemical agents which act via endothelial cell surface receptors. Many also interact with receptors on vascular smooth muscle to cause vasoconstriction, an effect which is functionally antagonized by EDNO (Table 2.7). Excellent examples include 5-hydroxytryptamine and ADP, which are released when platelets aggregate. Not only does EDNO production limit the vasoconstriction these mediators cause, it also inhibits platelet adhesion and is synergistic with prostacyclin in preventing platelet aggregation. The importance of receptor-mediated EDNO release by some mediators, such as acetylcholine and substance P, has been questioned, as these mediators are released from nerves on the adventitial side of blood vessels. Nevertheless, it has been clearly demonstrated that some endothelial cells can synthesize and release acetylcholine, substance P and 5-hydroxytryptamine. Thus, locally produced mediators, which are released under certain conditions (e.g. hypoxia), may play an important role in stimulating EDNO production.[7] Equine digital blood vessels have been shown to produce EDNO in response to acetylcholine and bradykinin.[68]

The discussion so far has centred on NO produced by endothelial cells under normal conditions. Other constitutive NOS isoforms exist, the best characterized being neuronal NOS, which is regulated in an identical manner and subserves functions in the central and peripheral nervous systems. Another major group of NOS enzymes are the inducible isoforms (iNOS). Expression of these enzymes is induced by cytokines (interleukin 1β, interferon gamma and tumour necrosis factor) and by endotoxin. The activity of iNOS is not regulated by cytosolic free calcium ion concentration. These enzymes generate

Table 2.7 Some important examples of chemical mediators which activate endothelial cells and stimulate the release of nitric oxide

ENDOGENOUS VASODILATORS (EFFECT MEDIATED IN PART BY EDNO)	ENDOGENOUS VASOCONSTRICTORS (EFFECT MODULATED BY EDNO)
Acetylcholine (M_3-receptors)	Adrenaline (α_2-adrenoceptors)
Bradykinin (B_2-receptors)	5-Hydroxytryptamine (5-HT_1-like receptors)
Histamine (H_1- or H_2-receptors)	ADP and ATP (P_{2Y}-purinoceptors)
Substance P	Vasopressin (V_1-receptors – present in coronary and cerebral vessels)
Vasoactive intestinal polypeptide	Endothelin (ET_B-receptors)
	Angiotensin II (AT_1-receptors)

Note: The receptor presence and type involved may vary with species and with the vascular bed involved – these examples are merely illustrative.

NO at a much greater, uncontrolled rate when compared with constitutive NOS. iNOS enzymes are important for the immune response – generation of large amounts of NO can kill invading organisms and unwanted cells, but can also be induced in the vasculature under certain circumstances (see below).

Pathophysiology of nitric oxide

Lack of production of EDNO might contribute to a number of diseases involving the vascular system, including atherosclerosis, hypertension, congestive heart failure and diabetes mellitus (vascular complications).[69] Endothelial dysfunction is also thought to be of importance in reperfusion injury which is evident in cases of myocardial infarction. An inflammatory response occurs during reperfusion with the adhesion of leucocytes to endothelial cells. Leucocytes are known to produce factors which neutralize NO, including superoxide anions and an unidentified peptide mediator.[70]

Excess production of NO occurs in gram-negative septic shock when iNOS is produced in endothelial cells and vascular smooth muscle cells, resulting in a vasodilated circulation which is hyporesponsive to pressor agents. iNOS production in myocardial cells may result from cytokine generation during inflammation and lead to poor systolic function.

Pharmacology of nitric oxide

Nitrovasodilators (e.g. glyceryl trinitrate; GTN) are currently used to deliver NO to vascular smooth muscle in conditions where the endogenous mediator may be lacking (coronary artery disease, congestive failure), and have been used in the management of equine laminitis,[71] although the ability of GTN to induce peripheral digital vascular dilation has been questioned by a failure to improve perfusion to the digit in horses with cold-induced digital vasoconstriction.[72] Organic nitrates are metabolized by vascular smooth muscle cells, releasing nitric oxide local to its site of action. Newer generation NO donors are under development, and these may lack some of the problems of tolerance that have hampered the older nitrovasodilators.

The supply of L-arginine to endothelial cells of vessels in the early stages of atheroma development appears to be rate limiting, such that supplementation of L-arginine can boost production of NO by the endothelium.[73] Supply of L-arginine is not normally rate limiting for the production of EDNO by eNOS for the reasons discussed above. The reason why L-arginine boosts NO production by vessels undergoing atheromatous change is poorly understood and is the subject of intense investigation.

Other therapeutic advances in the field of NO biology are aimed at inhibiting excessive NO production. The induction of iNOS can be inhibited by glucocorticoids, perhaps explaining the efficacy of these drugs if given in anticipation of septic shock. Selective iNOS inhibitors may be ideal in the treatment of septic shock, restoring vascular tone and arterial blood pressure. So far, they lack selectivity and thus are disadvantaged by the side effects which result from inhibition of constitutive forms of NOS, such as tissue ischaemia.[65]

Endothelins

Endothelins 1 and 3 (ET-1 and ET-3) are peptides (21 amino acids), discovered by Yanagisawa et al,[74] as products of cultured endothelial cells with extremely potent and long-lasting vasoconstrictor properties. The peptides are produced from larger peptide precursors (prepro-endothelin and pro-endothelin) by a neutral metallo-protease called endothelin-converting enzyme

(ECE[75]). The peptides are not stored in granules but synthesized and secreted by cells constitutively. Messenger RNA for the precursor of ET-1 is inherently unstable, allowing regulation of gene expression to closely control ET-1 secretion. ET gene expression can be upregulated by a number of factors, including hypoxia, shear stress and vasopressin. Atrial natriuretic peptide (ANP) can inhibit ET secretion by endothelial cells. More than 80% of the ET-1 secreted is released from the endothelial cell surface facing the vascular smooth muscle, thus ET-1 functions locally with little entering the circulation.

Although the endothelium is a major site of ET-1 secretion, it is clear that ETs are secreted by a variety of cells, including those in the central and peripheral nervous system (where ET-3 appears to predominate), kidney, heart, gut and adrenals.[76] The precise physiological roles of ETs in these tissues remain to be fully elucidated.

ETs have profound cardiovascular, renal and endocrine effects, the physiological significance of which remains to be established. Potent and long-lasting vasoconstriction of arterial and venous tissue, positive inotropic and chronotropic actions (in isolated cardiac tissue) and mitogenic effects on vascular smooth muscle and myocardial cells are the main cardiovascular effects. The effects of ET on renal function are extremely complex and depend on whether the peptide is generated local to its site of action or is delivered to the kidney from the general circulation. Reduced salt and water excretion can result in the latter case. Endocrine effects include stimulation of release of aldosterone, adrenaline, ADH (ET3 is located in the posterior pituitary gland) and ANP (which may represent an important negative feedback system because ANP inhibits ET secretion by endothelial cells).

Two different types of ET receptor have been cloned from the cardiovascular system.[77] ETA receptors are found in vascular smooth muscle and mediate contraction. Endothelial cells possess ETB receptors, which stimulate the production of NO. Arterial vascular smooth muscle thus far seems to possess predominantly ETA receptors, whereas venous vascular smooth muscle may, in addition, have a novel ETB receptor subtype linked to venoconstriction. The receptor types in cardiac muscle have not been well studied.

Excessive production of ET has been detected in a number of disease states in human patients and in horses. In particular ET-1 has been shown to induce vasoconstriction in both digital and pulmonary vasculature[78–80] and its concentrations increased in endotoxaemia and carbohydrate loading[81,82] and may be important in the pathogenesis of both laminitis and exercise-induced pulmonary haemorrhage. The vasoconstrictor and mitogenic effects of ET may contribute to the generation of hypertension and atherosclerosis. ET secretion increases in pacing-induced congestive heart failure in dogs and may contribute to increased cardiac workload due to vasoconstriction and salt retention. In addition, ET may stimulate myocardial hypertrophy. ET has also been implicated in vasospastic diseases (acute myocardial infarction, cerebral vasospasm and Reynaud's disease). Concentrations of ET are also increased in diabetes mellitus and endotoxaemia.

Pharmacology of endothelin

The greatest therapeutic indication will be for drugs which inhibit ET. Thus, potential drugs include endothelin-converting enzyme (ECE) inhibitors and ET receptor antagonists. Most progress has been made with receptor antagonists where the development of non-peptide analogues of ET will allow these agents to be given orally. Selective inhibitors of ETA and ETB receptors are available. Bosentan, a non-peptide ETA/ETB receptor antagonist has shown great promise in experimental models of heart failure but offered no haemodynamic benefits in human patients with heart failure; it was associated with an increased risk of adverse effects.[83–85] The use of selective ETA receptor antagonists may overcome some of these limitations of non-selective effects of these agents and have been shown to promote vasodilation in carbohydrate-induced models of laminitis in the horse when administered with GTN.[86]

CONCLUSIONS

The complexity of regulatory factors within the cardiovascular system is enormous, allowing tremendous flexibility in the control of this system. The more we discover, the more questions there seem to be to answer. The large number of mediators and variety of receptors involved allow endless possibilities for drug development.

REFERENCES

1. Dampney RAL. Functional organisation of central pathways regulating the cardiovascular system. Physiol Rev 1994;74: 323–364.

2. Rosendorff C. α-adrenoceptors in hypertension. J Cardiovasc Pharmacol 1986;8(suppl 2):S3–S7.

3. Lewis RP. Digitalis: a drug that refuses to die. Crit Care Med 1990;18:S5–S13.

4. Doris PA. Regulation of Na,K-ATPase by endogenous ouabain-like materials. Proc Soc Exp Biol Med 1994;205:202–212.

5. Dampney RAL. Functional organisation of central pathways

regulating the cardiovascular system. Physiol Rev 1994;74: 323–363.

6. Levick JR. Control of blood vessel. In: An Introduction to Cardiovascular Physiology. Oxford: Butterworth-Heinemann; 1991. p. 178–202.

7. Burnstock G, Ralevic V. New insights into the local regulation of blood flow by perivascular nerves and endothelium. Br J Plast Surg 1994;47:527–543.

8. Bryant CE, Elliott J, Clarke KC, Soydan J. Characterisation of alpha-adrenoceptors in the hind limb venous system of the horse. Br J Pharmacol 1992;107:376P.

9. Gitterman DP, Evans RJ. Nerve evoked P2X receptor contractions of rat mesenteric arteries; dependence on vessel size and lack of role of L-type calcium channels and calcium induced calcium release. Br J Pharmacol 2001; 132(6):1201.

10. Lamont C, Vial C, Evans RJ, Wier WG. P2X1 receptors mediate sympathetic postjunctional Ca²⁺ transients in mesenteric small arteries. Am J Physiol Heart Circ Physiol 2006;291(6):H3106– H3113.

11. Walker P, Grouzmann E, Burnier M, Waeber B. The role of neuropeptide Y in cardiovascular regulation. Trends Pharmacol Sci 1991;12:111–115.

12. Starke K, Gothert M, Kilbinger H. Modulation of neurotransmitter release by presynaptic autoreceptors. Physiol Rev 1989; 69:864–989.

13. von Kügelgen I, Starke K. Noradrenaline-ATP co-transmission in the sympathetic nervous system. Trends Physiol Sci 1991;12: 319–324.

14. Grundemar L, Håkanson R. Neuropeptide Y effector systems: perspectives for drug development. Trends Pharmacol Sci 1994;15: 153–159.

15. Kennedy C, IJzerman A. Adenosine and ATP: from receptor structure to clinical applications. Trends Pharmacol Sci 1994;15:311– 312.

16. Huang EY, Li JY, Tan PP, et al. The cardiovascular effects of PFRFamide and PFR(Tic)amide, a possible agonist and antagonist of neuropeptide FF (NPFF). Peptides 2000;21(2):205–210.

17. Horn J, Bailey S, Berhane Y. Density and binding characteristics of beta-adrenoceptors in the normal and failing equine myocardium. Equine Vet J 2002; 34(4):411–416.

18. Vaughan Williams EM. Adrenergic arrhythmogenicity. In: Vaughan Williams EM, editor. Antiarrhythmic Drugs. Handbook of Experimental Pharmacology. vol 89. Berlin: Springer Verlag; 1990. p. 303–308.

19. Toneke K. Beta-adrenoceptors in equine trachea and heart. Vet Res Commun 1999;23(1):41–51.

20. Brodde OE. β₁ and β₂-adrenoceptors in the human heart: properties, function and alterations in chronic heart failure. Pharmacol Rev 1991;43:203–242.

21. Kiriazis H, Wang K, Xu Q, et al. Knockout of beta(1)- and beta(2)-adrenoceptors attenuates pressure overload-induced cardiac hypertrophy and fibrosis. Br J Pharmacol 2008;153(4): 684–692.

22. Pacca SR, de Azevedo AP, De Oliveira CF, et al. Attenuation of hypertension, cardiomyocyte hypertrophy, and myocardial fibrosis by beta-adrenoceptor blockers in rats under long-term blockade of nitric oxide synthesis. J Cardiovasc Pharmacol 2002; 39(2):201–207.

23. Perlini S, Ferrero I, Palladini G, et al. Survival benefits of different antiadrenergic interventions in pressure overload left ventricular hypertrophy/failure. Hypertension 2006;48(1):93–97.

24. Zhang S, Rodriguez R, Scholz PM, Weiss HR. Functional interaction of a beta-adrenergic agonist and cyclic GMP phosphodiesterase inhibitor in control and hypertrophic cardiomyocytes. Pharmacology 2006;76(2):53–60.

25. Plante E, Lachance D, Champetier S, et al. Benefits of long-term beta-blockade in experimental chronic aortic regurgitation. Am J Physiol Heart Circ Physiol 2008;294(4):H1888–H1895.

26. Vallotton MB. The renin-angiotensin system. Trends Pharmacol Sci 1987;8:69–74.

27. Ganong WF. Origin of the angiotensin II secreted by cells. Proc Soc Exp Biol Med 1994;205: 213–219.

28. Dzau VJ. Autocrine and paracrine mechanisms in the pathophysiology of heart failure. Am J Cardiol 1992;70:4C–11C.

29. Ainscough JF, Drinkhill MJ, Sedo A, et al. Angiotensin II type-1 receptor activation in the adult heart causes blood pressure-independent hypertrophy and cardiac dysfunction. Cardiovasc Res 2009;81(3):592–600.

30. Guy JL, Lambert DW, Turner AJ, Porter KE. Functional angiotensin-converting enzyme 2 is expressed in human cardiac myofibroblasts. Exp Physiol 2008;93(5):579–588.

31. Kassab S, Garadah T, Abu-Hijleh M, et al. The angiotensin type 1 receptor antagonist valsartan attenuates pathological ventricular hypertrophy induced by hyperhomocysteinemia in rats. J Renin Angiotensin Aldosterone Syst 2006;7(4):206–211.

32. De Mello WC, Specht P. Chronic blockade of angiotensin II AT1-receptors increased cell-to-cell communication, reduced fibrosis and improved impulse propagation in the failing heart. J Renin Angiotensin Aldosterone Syst 2006;7(4):201–205.

33. Nemer M, Dali-Youcef N, Wang H, et al. Mechanisms of angiotensin II-dependent progression to heart failure. Novartis Found Symp 2006;274:58–68; discussion 68–72, 152–155, 272–276.

34. Struthers AD. The clinical implications of aldosterone escape in congestive heart failure. Eur J Heart Fail 2004;6(5):539–545.

35. Zannad F. Aldosterone and heart failure. Eur Heart J 1995;16(suppl N):98–102.

36. Haggstrom J, Hansson K, Kvart C, et al. Effects of naturally acquired decompensated mitral valve regurgitation on the renin-angiotensin-aldosterone system and atrial natriuretic peptide concentration in dogs. Am J Vet Res 1997;58(1):77–82.

37. Pedersen HD, Olsen LH, Mow T, Christensen NJ. Neuroendocrine changes in Dachshunds with mitral valve prolapse examined under different study conditions. Res Vet Sci 1999;66(1):11–17.

38. Gehlen H, Sundermann T, Rohn K, Stadler P. Aldosterone plasma concentration in horses with heart valve insufficiencies. Res Vet Sci 2008;85(2):340–344.

39. Gehlen H, Vieht JC, Stadler P. Effects of the ACE inhibitor quinapril on echocardiographic variables in horses with mitral valve insufficiency. J Vet Med A Physiol Pathol Clin Med 2003; 50(9):460–465.

40. Gardner SY, Atkins CE, Sams RA, et al. Characterization of the pharmacokinetic and pharmacodynamic properties of the angiotensin-converting enzyme inhibitor, enalapril, in horses. J Vet Intern Med 2004;18(2):231–237.

41. Sleeper MM, McDonnell SM, Ely JJ, Reef VB. Chronic oral therapy with enalapril in normal ponies. J Vet Cardiol 2008;10(2):111–115.

42. Timmermanns PBMWM, Wong PC, Chiu AT, Herblin WF. Nonpeptide angiotensin II receptor antagonists. Trends Pharmacol Sci 1991;12: 55–62.

43. Devereux B, Dahlof B, Gerdts E, et al. Regression of hypertensive left ventricular hypertrophy by losartan compared with atenolol: the Losartan Intervention for Endpoint Reduction in Hypertension (LIFE) trial. Circulation 2004;110(11): 1456–1462.

44. Saygili E, Rana OR, Saygili E, et al. Losartan prevents stretch-induced electrical remodeling in cultured atrial neonatal myocytes. Am J Physiol Heart Circ Physiol 2007;292(6):H2898–H2905.

45. Fogari R, Mugellini A, Destro M, et al. Losartan and prevention of atrial fibrillation recurrence in hypertensive patients. J Cardiovasc Pharmacol 2006;47(1):46–50.

46. Konstam MA, Neaton JD, Poole-Wilson PA, et al. Comparison of losartan and captopril on heart failure-related outcomes and symptoms from the losartan heart failure survival study

47. (ELITE II). Am Heart J 2005; 150(1):123–131.

47. Pitt B, Zannad F, Remme WJ, Cody R, Castaigne A, Perez A, et al. The effect of spironolactone on morbidity and mortality in patients with severe heart failure. Randomized Aldactone Evaluation Study Investigators. N Engl J Med 1999;341(10):709–717.

48. Mill JG, Milanez Mda C, de Resende MM, Gomes Mda G, Leite CM. Spironolactone prevents cardiac collagen proliferation after myocardial infarction in rats. Clin Exp Pharmacol Physiol 2003; 30(10):739–744.

49. Roongsritong C, Sutthiwan P, Bradley J, Simoni J, Power S, Meyerrose GE. Spironolactone improves diastolic function in the elderly. Clin Cardiol 2005;28(10): 484–487.

50. MacDonald KA, Kittleson MD, Kass PH, White SD. Effect of spironolactone on diastolic function and left ventricular mass in Maine Coon cats with familial hypertrophic cardiomyopathy. J Vet Intern Med 2008;22(2):335–341.

51. Yandle TG. Biochemistry of natriuretic peptides. J Intern Med 1994;235:561–576.

52. Falcao LM, Pinto F, Ravara L, van Zwieten PA. BNP and ANP as diagnostic and predictive markers in heart failure with left ventricular systolic dysfunction. J Renin Angiotensin Aldosterone Syst 2004;5(3):121–129.

53. Szafranek A, Jasinski M, Kolowca M, Gemel M, Wos S. Plasma ANP and renin-angiotensin-aldosterone system as new parameters describing the hemodynamics of the circulatory system after implantation of stented or stentless aortic valves. J Heart Valve Dis 2006;15(5):702–708; discussion 709.

54. Hori Y, Tsubaki M, Katou A, Ono Y, Yonezawa T, Li X, et al. Evaluation of NT-pro BNP and CT-ANP as markers of concentric hypertrophy in dogs with a model of compensated aortic stenosis. J Vet Intern Med 2008;22(5): 1118–1123.

55. Asano K, Masuda K, Okumura M, Kadosawa T, Fujinaga T. Plasma

atrial and brain natriuretic peptide levels in dogs with congestive heart failure. J Vet Med Sci 1999;61(5): 523–529.

56. Haggstrom J, Hansson K, Kvart C, Pedersen HD, Vuolteenaho O, Olsson K. Relationship between different natriuretic peptides and severity of naturally acquired mitral regurgitation in dogs with chronic myxomatous valve disease. J Vet Cardiol 2000;2(1):7–16.

57. Gehlen H, Sundermann T, Rohn K, Stadler P. Plasma atrial natriuretic peptide concentration in warmblood horses with heart valve regurgitations. J Vet Cardiol 2007;9(2):99–101.

58. Rosques BP, Beaumont A. Neutral endopeptidase-24.11 inhibitors: from analgesics to antihypertensives. Trends Pharmacol Sci 1990;11:245–249.

59. Northridge DB, Currie PF, Newby DE, McMurray JJ, Ford M, Boon NA, et al. Placebo-controlled comparison of candoxatril, an orally active neutral endopeptidase inhibitor, and captopril in patients with chronic heart failure. Eur J Heart Fail 1999;1(1):67–72.

60. Kentsch M, Otter W, Drummer C, Notges A, Gerzer R, Muller-Esch G. Neutral endopeptidase 24.11 inhibition may not exhibit beneficial haemodynamic effects in patients with congestive heart failure. Eur J Clin Pharmacol 1996;51(3–4):269–272.

61. Campese VM, Lasseter KC, Ferrario CM, Smith WB, Ruddy MC, Grim CE, et al. Omapatrilat versus lisinopril: efficacy and neurohormonal profile in salt-sensitive hypertensive patients. Hypertension 2001;38(6):1342–1348.

62. Klapholz M, Thomas I, Eng C, Iteld BJ, Ponce GA, Niederman AL, et al. Effects of omapatrilat on hemodynamics and safety in patients with heart failure. Am J Cardiol 2001;88(6):657–661.

63. Ferrario CM, Smith RD, Brosnihan B, Chappell MC, Campese VM, Vesterqvist O, et al. Effects of omapatrilat on the renin-angiotensin system in salt-sensitive hypertension. Am J Hypertens 2002;15(6):557–564.

64. Packer M, Califf RM, Konstam MA, Krum H, McMurray JJ, Rouleau JL, et al. Comparison of omapatrilat and enalapril in patients with chronic heart failure: the Omapatrilat Versus Enalapril Randomized Trial of Utility in Reducing Events (OVERTURE). Circulation 2002;106(8):920–926.

65. Moncada S, Palmer RMJ, Higgs EA. Nitric oxide: physiology, pathophysiology, and pharmacology. Pharmacol Rev 1991;43:109–142.

66. Huang PL, Huang Z, Mashimo H, et al. Hypertension in mice lacking the gene for endothelial nitric oxide synthase. Nature 1995;377: 239–242.

67. Davies PF. Flow mediated endothelial mechanotransduction. Physiol Rev 1995;75:519–560.

68. Elliott J, Bryant CE, Soydan J. The role of nitric oxide in the responses of equine digital veins to vasodilator and vasoconstrictor agents. Equine Vet J 1994;26: 378–384.

69. Dusting GJ. Nitric oxide in cardiovascular disorders. J Vasc Res 1995;32:143–161.

70. Sessa WC, Mullane KM. Release of a neutrophil-derived vasoconstrictor agent which augments platelet-induced contractions of blood vessels in vitro. Br J Pharmacol 1990;99: 553–559.

71. Hinckley KA, Fearn S, Howard BR, Henderson IW. Nitric oxide donors as treatment for grass induced acute laminitis in ponies. Equine Vet J 1996;28:17–28.

72. Hoff TK, Hood DM, Wagner IP. Effectiveness of glyceryl trinitrate for enhancing digital submural perfusion in horses. Am J Vet Res 2002;63(5):648–652.

73. Creager MA, Gallagher SJ, Girerd XJ, Coleman SM, Dzau VJ, Cooke JP. L-arginine improves endothelium dependent vasodilatation in hypercholesterolaemic humans. J Clin Invest 1992;90:1248–1253.

74. Yanagisawa M, Kurihara H, Kimura S, et al. A novel potent vasconstrictor peptide produced by vascular endothelial cells. Nature 1988;332:411–415.

75. Opgenorth TJ, Wu-Wong JR, Shiosaki K. Endothelin-converting enzymes. FASEB J 1992;6: 2653–2659.

76. Simonson MS. Endothelins: multifunctional renal peptides. Physiol Rev 1993;73:375–411.

77. Douglas SA, Meek TD, Ohlstein EH. Novel receptor antagonists welcome a new era in endothelin biology. Trends Pharmacol Sci 1994;15:313–316.

78. Benamou AE, Marlin DJ, Callingham BC, Hiley RC, Lekeux R. Spasmogenic action of endothelin-1 on isolated equine pulmonary artery and bronchus. Equine Vet J 2003;35(2):190–196.

79. Katz LM, Marr CM, Elliott J. Characterization and comparison of the responses of equine digital arteries and veins to endothelin-1. Am J Vet Res 2003;64(11): 1438–1443.

80. Keen JA, Hillier C, McGorum BC, Nally JE. Endothelin mediated contraction of equine laminar veins. Equine Vet J 2008;40(5): 488–492.

81. Eades SC, Stokes AM, Johnson PJ, LeBlanc CJ, Ganjam VK, Buff PR, et al. Serial alterations in digital hemodynamics and endothelin-1 immunoreactivity, platelet- neutrophil aggregation, and concentrations of nitric oxide, insulin, and glucose in blood obtained from horses following carbohydrate overload. Am J Vet Res 2007;68(1):87–94.

82. Menzies-Gow NJ, Bailey SR, Stevens K, Katz L, Elliott J, Marr CM. Digital blood flow and plasma endothelin concentration in clinically endotoxemic horses. Am J Vet Res 2005;66(4):630–636.

83. Kalra PR, Moon JC, Coats AJ. Do results of the ENABLE (Endothelin Antagonist Bosentan for Lowering Cardiac Events in Heart Failure) study spell the end for non-selective endothelin antagonism in heart failure? Int J Cardiol 2002;85(2–3):195–197.

84. Kaluski E, Cotter G, Leitman M, Milo-Cotter O, Krakover R, Kobrin I, et al. Clinical and hemodynamic effects of bosentan dose optimization in symptomatic heart failure patients with severe systolic dysfunction, associated with secondary pulmonary hypertension: a multi-center randomized study. Cardiology 2008;109(4):273–280.

85. Packer M, McMurray J, Massie BM, Caspi A, Charlon V, Cohen-Solal A, et al. Clinical effects of endothelin receptor antagonism with bosentan in patients with severe chronic heart failure: results of a pilot study. J Card Fail 2005;11(1): 12–20.

86. Eades SC, Stokes AM, Moore RM. Effects of an endothelin receptor antagonist and nitroglycerin on digital vascular function in horses during the prodromal stages of carbohydrate overload-induced laminitis. Am J Vet Res 2006;67(7): 1204–1211.

Chapter 3

Cardiac responses to exercise and training

David L Evans and Lesley E Young

INTRODUCTION

Heart rate and cardiac output increase quickly at the commencement of exercise, enabling comparatively rapid increases in the rate of oxygen consumption. The 6- to 8-fold increase in heart rate during maximal exercise, coupled with an increase in stroke volume, results in maximal cardiac output during exercise of approximately 300 L/minute, or over 0.6 L/minute/kg in trained horses. This large increase in blood flow to exercising muscle is fundamental to the athletic performance of the horse during intense exercise. This is especially so in events of more than 1 minute duration, which rely mainly on aerobic energy supply.[1] Training results in adaptations that increase the rate of blood flow to skeletal muscle during intense exercise. The main adaptation is an increase in stroke volume. Training also causes changes in the electrocardiogram and echocardiogram.

In this chapter the cardiac responses to exercise and modifications with training will be reviewed. Relationships between cardiac measurements and both fitness assessment and performance prediction will also be discussed.

CARDIAC RESPONSES TO EXERCISE

Heart rate

Heart rate during exercise

Heart rate quickly increases at the commencement of exercise, and reaches a steady state in 2–3 minutes. This increase is associated with increased sympathetic nerve activity and/or catecholamine release.[2] An overshoot of heart rate to levels above the submaximal steady-state heart rate may occur at the commencement of exercise. Thereafter the heart rate gradually decreases to a steady state.[3]

A linear relationship between heart rate and submaximal work effort has been observed in horses trotting, galloping and swimming.[3–8] This relationship is usually defined by use of treadmill or racetrack exercise tests which involve increasing the speed every 1–2 minutes and measuring the heart rate at the completion of exercise at each speed. After a suitable warm up, for example, 3 minutes trotting, the heart rate is stable after 1 minute of further exercise at higher speeds. Heart rates recorded during an exercise test in three groups of Thoroughbred horses are illustrated in Figure 3.1.[8] The figure demonstrates the linear relationship between heart rate and speed of submaximal exercise. At higher speeds, further increases in treadmill speed are not accompanied by an increase in heart rate, and a plateau occurs. The horse is then exercising at its individual maximal heart rate.

The typical relationship between heart rate and speed of exercise enables variables such as V_{200} and V_{HRmax} to be

DOI: 10.1016/B978-0-7020-2817-5.00008-0

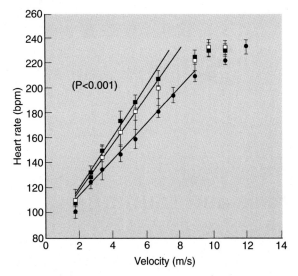

Figure 3.1 Mean heart rate ± SE, as a function of velocity for yearling (■), two-year-old (□) and adult (•) Thoroughbred horses exercising on a treadmill set at 6 degrees; Yearlings: $n = 16$, $y = 93.30 + 19.44x$, $r^2 = 88\%$. Two-year-olds: $n = 12$; $y = 89.85 + 18.05x$, $r^2 = 80\%$. Adults: $n = 14$; $y = 79.99 + 14.60x$, $r^2 = 92\%$.

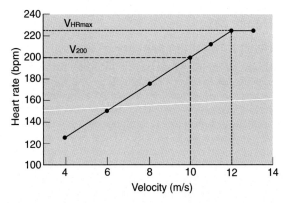

Figure 3.2 Determination of V_{200} and V_{HRmax} from measurements of heart rate at treadmill speeds of 4, 6, 8, 10, 11, 12 and 13 m/s (treadmill slope 10%).[9]

calculated. These measurements have been used to compare different groups of horses, or individual horses with a normal group, or measure changes in the heart rate response to exercise during training or detraining.[9] V_{200} is the velocity which generates a heart rate of 200 beats per minute. V_{HRmax} is the velocity at which the loss of linearity occurs and no further increase in heart rate occurs, despite an increase in velocity. Derivation of these variables is illustrated in Figure 3.2.[9] Some studies have also used V_{140}, the velocity that results in a heart rate of 140 beats per

minute. It has been argued that V_{200} is superior because it approximates the intensity of exercise which results in a blood lactate concentration of 4 mmol/L.[10] However, this argument should not dictate strict adherence to V_{200}. If V_{200} is used to compare the fitness of different horses, the measurement could be very misleading. Two horses could have the same V_{200}, but very different maximal heart rates, and therefore very different velocities at which they reach their maximal heart rates. The V_{200} ignores the cardiac reserve between 200 bpm and maximal HR, and so is best used to measure changes in an individual horse over time, assuming that maximal HR does not change.

The heart rate versus work relationship during treadmill exercise is very reproducible for individual horses at heart rates between 120 and 210 bpm.[5,11] During racetrack exercise, the reproducibility of V_{200} in Standardbred horses measured in a racetrack exercise test was also good.[12] This study also found that V_{200} was not significantly altered by a change of racetrack on which the test was conducted. However, in an individual horse extraneous factors can influence the heart rates during an exercise test. For example, anxiety, the presence of a breathing mask[10] and changes in treadmill exercise testing routine[13] can elevate heart rate during exercise.

The normal heart rate responses to treadmill exercise in Thoroughbred horses have been described.[8,14] Figure 3.1 illustrates the responses in 16 yearling, 12 two-year-old and 14 trained adult Thoroughbreds.[8] The slope of the linear regression of heart rate on m/s in the trained adult horses was significantly less than the slopes for both the untrained two-year-olds and yearlings.

There is a linear relationship between heart rates and oxygen consumption during submaximal exercise (Fig. 3.3A[15]). This relationship is not affected by the slope of the treadmill in the range 0–10%. Likewise, there is a linear relationship between relative heart rate and relative oxygen uptake during submaximal exercise (expressed as percentages of maximal values) (Fig. 3.3B[15]). This close relationship infers that the velocity at which an individual horse attains its maximal oxygen uptake is equivalent to the V_{HRmax}.

The overshoot at the commencement of exercise may be absent if the exercise is at a high intensity. Instead, heart rates may gradually increase to maximal. Overshoot of heart rate occurred at the start of exercise at 50% of V_{O_2max} (maximum oxygen uptake) in Standardbred horses. However, at 100% V_{O_2max}, heart rate gradually increased during a 5 minute period of exercise.[16] The slow increase in heart rate towards the true maximal heart rate in that study may have been related to the absence of a warm up period of exercise.

Heart rates during swimming vary greatly between horses, and are usually in the range 130–180 bpm.[6,17] The mean highest heart rate recorded in nine horses during show jumping were 191 ± 3 bpm.[18] Mean (±s.d.) heart rates during phases A and C of an advanced 3-day event

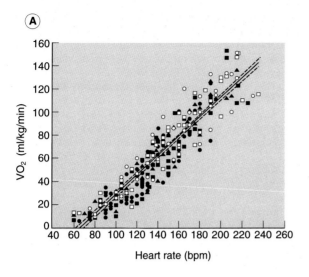

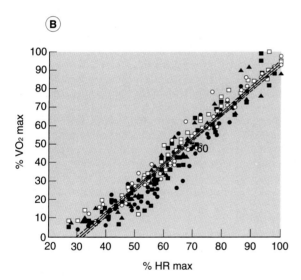

Figure 3.3 Relationships between oxygen uptake (V_{O_2}) and heart rate (HR) (**A**) and between % HRmax and % V_{O_2max} (**B**) in five Thoroughbred racehorses during submaximal treadmill exercise. Results are pooled from exercise tests conducted at 0, 2.5, 5, 7.5 and 10% treadmill inclines.[15] ●, 0%; ■, 2.5%; ▲, 5%; □, 7.5%; ○, 10%. A: $V_{O_2} = 0.833 (HR) - 54.7$, $r^2 = 0.865$. B: % $V_{O_2max} = 1.348$ (% HRmax) $- 41.0$, $r^2 = 0.939$.[15]

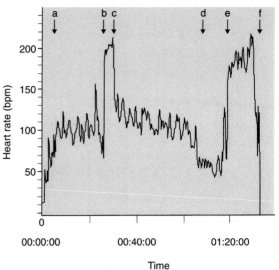

Figure 3.4 Heart rate of a horse competing in an advanced (CCI***) three-day event. [a]Denotes the beginning of phase A, [b]denotes the beginning of phase B, [c]denotes the beginning of phase C, [d]denotes the end of phase C and beginning of 10-minute box, [e]denotes the beginning of phase D and [f]the end of phase D.[19]

were 118 ± 11 and 135 ± 28, respectively. During phases B and D, heart rates were 175 ± 23 and 171 ± 19, respectively. A continuous record of heart rates in a horse competing in the event is illustrated in Figure 3.4.[19]

During prolonged strenuous submaximal exercise at a constant work rate, a gradual increase in heart rate, or "cardiovascular drift" can occur. For example, during 30 minutes of exercise, mean heart rate increased from 154 to 173 bpm.[20] This "drift" was accompanied by increases in minute ventilation and stroke volume, while cardiac output was unchanged. In another study, horses exercising at 55–60% of individual HR$_{max}$ for 60 minutes had minimal changes in heart rate.[21] Heart rate responses during prolonged exercise probably depend on hydration status and the environmental conditions.

The effects of dehydration on heart rate during and after 40 minutes of exercise eliciting approximately 40% of maximal oxygen consumption have been described.[22] Horses were exercised in three conditions; euhydrated, 4 hours after administration of furosemide (1.0 mg/kg i.v.) to induce isotonic dehydration, and after 30 hours without water to induce hypertonic dehydration. The most pronounced heart rate drift occurred in the dehydrated horses. Heart rates after 30 minutes of exercise were significantly higher in the horses dehydrated by treatment with furosemide than in the control, euhydrated condition. During the recovery period heart rates were also higher in both groups of dehydrated horses than in the control horses (Fig. 3.5). This study demonstrated that dehydration results in higher heart rates during and after prolonged submaximal exercise.

Diseases such as chronic obstructive pulmonary disease result in heart rates during submaximal exercise that are significantly higher than those found in normal horses.[23–25]

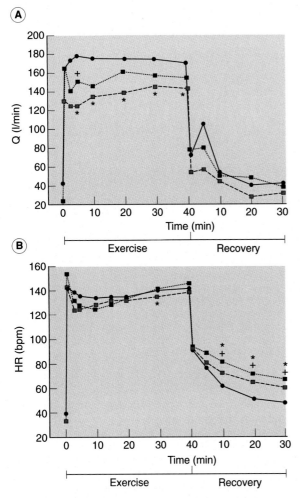

Figure 3.5 Cardiac output Q (**A**) and heart rate HR (**B**) of six horses during exercise at 40% of maximal oxygen uptake for 40 minutes and for 30 minutes after exercise in control conditions (C ●___●), dehydrated by furosemide (FDH ■------■) and by water deprivation (DDH ■........■). *FDH significantly different from C; +DDH significantly different from C[22].

Measurements of heart rate and other cardiorespiratory and metabolic indices during treadmill exercise have also been used to investigate the functional significance of various electrocardiographic findings. This technique was used to illustrate that T wave changes and second degree AV block in the resting electrocardiogram do not result in significantly different heart rates or peak oxygen consumption in Thoroughbred and Standardbred racehorses.[26]

High heart rates during submaximal exercise are also to be expected in horses with diseases which limit stroke volume, such as atrial fibrillation.[27] (AF) When valvular dysfunction, or structural cardiac disease results in cardiac decompensation, affected horses will also have an increased heart rate during exercise, before clinical signs of heart failure are evident at rest.[28]

However, lameness should also be considered as a cause of high heart rates during submaximal exercise tests. Mild unilateral forelimb lameness also causes lower maximal oxygen uptake and more rapid blood lactate accumulation during intense exercise.[29] High heart rates could also be due to anxiety if the horse has not been adequately acclimated to the treadmill test procedures. Field studies of submaximal heart rate could be easier to interpret because the horse is exercising in its usual environment, and should be less subject to the effects of fear or anxiety.

The highest heart rates recorded during racing in 19 Thoroughbreds averaged 223 bpm, with a range of 204–241 beats/minute.[30] Mean peak heart rate in eight yearling Thoroughbreds was approximately 240 beats/minute, compared to 220–230 in 2- to 4-year old horses.[14] Likewise, yearling, two-year-old and adult Thoroughbreds had similar means (229–231 bpm) and ranges (215–254 beats/minute) of peak heart rates during an incremental treadmill exercise test.[8] In a recent retrospective multicentre study, horse age, gender, breed, use and fitness combined with the testing centre itself were shown to affect peak heart rate in 394 horses undergoing standardized treadmill exercise tests.[31] High interindividual variability in heart rates while racing have also been recorded in Standardbreds, ranging from 210 to 238 with a mean of 221 beats/minute.[32] However, in an individual horse, the maximal heart rate is highly repeatable.[11] Further work is required to confirm that the highest (peak) HRs recorded during Thoroughbred and Standardbred races are equal to the maximal HR attainable by the horse.

A new technique has been established for the study of submaximal and maximal heart rates during field gallops in Thoroughbred racehorses. This approach uses simultaneous measurement of velocity with a global positioning system, and heart rates. Derived indices of fitness such as V_{200} and V_{HRmax} during the field gallop on a racetrack have been measured reliably, and have demonstrated increases with training in 2-year-old Thoroughbreds[33] V_{HRmax} has also been correlated with retrospective racing performance in Thoroughbreds.[34]

Heart rate after exercise

(AF)

Heart rate recovery is usually very rapid in the first minute after exercise stops.[3,35–37] It then decreases more gradually towards normal resting values. The rate of heart rate recovery after maximal treadmill exercise is probably independent of training state,[8] although clinical experience suggests that the rate of heart rate recovery does seem to be related to conditioning in a broader range of equine athletes under field conditions. In common with heart rates at rest and during submaximal exercise, heart rates during recovery are also susceptible to rapid fluctuations due to excitement.[35] Heart rates during recovery from the cross country (Phase D) of a 3-day event were not correlated with heart rates during competition.[38]

After prolonged submaximal exercise, recovery heart rates are higher in horses that were dehydrated before exercise.[22] Poorly performing endurance horses have higher postexercise heart rates than the better performers.[39] Horses with heart rates less than 60 beats/minute at 30 minutes post-exercise had less evidence of dehydration and myopathy.[40] Horses with heart rates greater than 65–70 beats/minute at the 30 minute recovery time at the mid-point of an endurance ride were more prone to develop severe dehydration and exhaustion when allowed to continue.[41]

Most studies report that heart rate in resting horses does not decrease after training,[42–45] but decreases do occur during submaximal exercise.[46,47] However, the decrease in heart rate with training is often only 10–20 beats/minute at any submaximal speed.[42] Some studies have also reported that heart rates during submaximal exercise were not significantly different after training.[44,47] In two treadmill training studies which demonstrated significant increases in maximal oxygen consumption, no significant changes were found in heart rate during submaximal exercise.[44,48] Decreasing heart rate during submaximal exercise is therefore an unreliable index of fitness in horses. Perhaps horse excitement, or anxiety, during treadmill exercise tests, renders measurements such as V_{200} less reliable, compared to similar measurements made in the field in a more familiar environment.[33]

The individual HR_{max} is not affected by training, and it is not a useful measure of fitness.[8,47,49] Individual HR_{max} can be affected by the cardiac rhythm abnormality, atrial fibrillation.[28] During atrial fibrillation peak heart rates during exercise are greatly increased compared to during normal sinus rhythm. In clinical cases affected by paroxysmal or sustained atrial fibrillation, heart rates during submaximal exercise can approach 300 beats/minute. As a result of the abnormally high heart rates maximal stroke volume is decreased due to suboptimal ventricular filling, and peak athletic performance is adversely affected. Resolution of the abnormal rhythm after treatment or spontaneous conversion usually results in return to normal individual HR_{max} and previous levels of athleticism.

Postexercise heart rates have shown no significant changes due to training in several studies.[44,45,48] However, heart rates taken within 1–5 minutes of completion of fast work by Thoroughbreds were lower after training

in another study.[47] Analysis of fitness using postexercise heart rates may be limited because of the rapid cardiac deceleration after cessation of exercise and the influence of psychogenic factors at heart rates less than 120 beats/minute.[10]

Heart rate measurements during submaximal treadmill exercise have been expressed relative to treadmill speed in some studies for measurement of fitness. For example, the treadmill velocities which result in heart rates of 140 (V_{140}) or 200 beats/minute (V_{200}) have been used. In an individual horse a decrease in V_{140} or V_{200} indicates that the heart rate is abnormally elevated during submaximal exercise. This decrease could suggest loss of cardiovascular fitness, cardiac or pulmonary disease, or lameness.

Echocardiography has been used to study cardiac function after treadmill exercise.[50] The heart rate recovery appeared to be prolonged after exercise in hot humid conditions (30°C and 80% relative humidity) compared to a recovery after exercise in a cooler environment. Echocardiographic indices of ventricular dimensions and contractile performance were also lower after exercise in hot humid conditions. It was suggested that these responses could reflect a reduction in preload due to the effect of dehydration or the redistribution of blood flow. If echocardiography is used to clinically evaluate cardiac function after exercise as has been suggested[51] the exercise test and environmental conditions must both be strictly standardized.

Stroke volume and cardiac output

Stroke volume in the resting horse is approximately 800–900 mL, or about 2–2.5 mL/kg.[42,43] Stroke volume increases by about 20–50% in the transition from rest to submaximal exercise.[7,46,52,53] It does not change as intensity of exercise increases from approximately 40% V_{O_2max} to 100% V_{O_2max}, despite the limited time available for ventricular filling at high heart rates during exercise.[54] Stroke volumes of 2.4 mL/kg (1250 mL)[54] and 3.8 ± 0.4 mL/kg (approximately 1700 mL)[55] have been reported in fit Thoroughbreds during treadmill exercise at V_{O_2max}. This large difference could reflect biological variation, or differences in the method of measuring oxygen uptake during the exercise test.

Values reported for cardiac output in fit Thoroughbreds during treadmill exercise at V_{O_2max} are 534 ± 54 mL/kg/minute (277 L/minute)[54] and 789 ± 102 mL/kg/minute (355 L/minute).[55]

During tethered swimming at low work loads, stroke volume decreased from 2.06 mL/kg at rest to about 1.5 mL/kg. This response may be related to decreased venous return secondary to the alterations to breathing pattern during swimming.[6]

During prolonged exercise cardiac output is decreased in dehydrated horses, and this limits thermoregulation.[22]

In an experiment in which horses were exercised for 40 minutes while euhydrated, or dehydrated by either withdrawal of water (DDH) or administration of furosemide (FDH), cardiac output was significantly lower in FDH (144.1 ± 8.0 L/minute) and in DDH (156.6 ± 6.9 L/minute) than in euhydrated horses (173.1 ± 6.2 L/minute) after 30 minutes of exercise (see Fig. 3.5). Dehydration resulted in higher temperatures in the middle gluteal muscle and pulmonary artery during exercise, but temperatures in the superficial thoracic vein and at subcutaneous sites on the neck and back were not significantly different. Sweating rates were also similar in control and dehydrated horses, and it was concluded that the impairment of thermoregulation was primarily due to decreased transfer of heat from core to periphery.

CARDIAC RESPONSES TO TRAINING

In human athletes typical adaptations to training include bradycardia, increases in end-diastolic dimension and maximal stroke volume. Maximal cardiac output is increased, largely because of an increase in maximal stroke volume. Heart rate is decreased at rest and during submaximal exercise because of increased parasympathetic tone and the effect of increased stroke volume on reflex sympathetic tone. These cardiac adaptations are coupled with peripheral adaptations in skeletal muscle which increase maximal arteriovenous oxygen content difference during exercise. Peripheral adaptations which increase skeletal muscle oxidative capacity and vascular conductance include increased capillarity and mitochondrial volume density and increased concentrations of oxidative enzymes. The increases in cardiac output and arteriovenous oxygen content difference during maximal exercise result in increased maximal oxygen uptake.[56]

Stroke volume increased in horses after training by approximately 10% during treadmill exercise at 12 km/hour on an 11.5% grade in one study.[46] This response was after 10 weeks trotting training at heart rates of 150 beats/minute. However, the cardiac output during exercise was not changed, reflecting a decrease in heart rate after training. Other treadmill studies have not demonstrated significant changes in stroke volume during submaximal exercise subsequent to treadmill training.[43,46] Variability in results of these studies probably reflects differences in experimental methods and design, and variable responses to different durations and intensities of training.

Changes in maximal oxygen consumption due to training and detraining have been associated with changes in stroke volume. A 23% increase in maximal oxygen consumption was accompanied by a significant increase in stroke volume during maximal exercise.[49] In another study stroke volume during exercise at 100% $V_{O_2 max}$ did not change significantly with training, but decreased significantly by 11% from 1426 ± 50 mL to 1271 ± 68 mL after 6 weeks detraining.[57]

Oxygen pulse (OP) is the ratio of oxygen uptake to heart rate, expressed as millilitres oxygen per beat per kilogram. It has been used as a correlate of stroke volume. For example, a horse exercising with an oxygen uptake of 150 mL oxygen/minute/kg with a HR of 207 beats/minute has an OP of 0.724 mL/beat/kg. An increased peak V_{O_2} after training was associated with an increase in oxygen pulse, but there were no effects of training on respiratory function. The increase in peak V_{O_2} induced by training therefore seems to be mainly due to cardiovascular and haematological changes rather than to ventilatory changes.[58]

The cardiovascular responses to an expanded plasma volume include increased right atrial pressure and stroke volume.[59] Plasma volume in the resting horse increases after training,[60] and this probably accounts for the increased higher mean right atrial pressure and stroke volume found after training.[42] Recent data also showed that right ventricular internal dimensions in diastole, measured using echocardiography, increased in response to commercial race training.[61] Training also caused lower $LVdP/dt_{max}$ at rest and during submaximal exercise.[42]

Trained horses have slightly higher relative heart masses (1.1% of body weight) than untrained horses (0.94%), suggesting that training causes hypertrophy of cardiac muscle.[62] This hypothesis has now been supported by a number of longitudinal and cross-sectional echocardiographic studies that have demonstrated increased calculated LV mass and wall thickness following training and a decrease following detraining.

A longitudinal study of effects of training in 7 2-year-old Thoroughbred racehorses reported that left ventricular internal diameter increased from 11.38 ± 0.58 cm before training to $12.16 \pm 0.7 \pm$ cm after training ($P < 0.001$). Calculated left ventricular mass also increased significantly (mean increase of 33%). Relative wall thickness was also significantly increased in these horses. The responses were independent of changes in body mass.[63] Similar changes in LV dimensions have also been reported for a group of young Standardbred horses.[64] although relative wall thickness was unchanged by training in these horses; a feature that probably reflects the different training methods used. Kriz et al also reported reductions in LV dimensions and indices of cardiac function in Standardbreds at 4 and 12 weeks of a period of detraining[65] and a similar phenomenon has been reported for Thoroughbreds.[62,66]

Absolute and relative internal cardiac dimensions of equine athletes are also affected by race discipline.[67] The observed differences in weight-corrected diastolic left ventricular dimensions LVIDd and SA area of 1 cm (8%) and 16 cm[2] (16%) between race-fit 2-year-old flat horses and seasoned National Hunt steeplechasers were not dissimilar in relative magnitude to the differences between

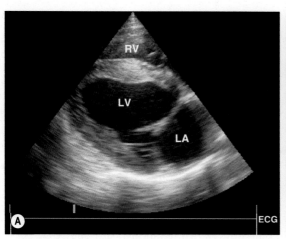
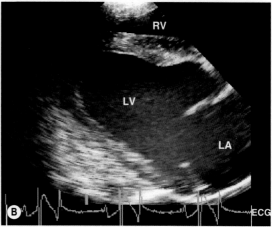

Figure 3.6 (A) A right parasternal long axis four-chamber image from a 4-year-old Arabian gelding previously used for flat racing over distances not exceeding 2.5 miles. **(B)** The same view as in A. A right parasternal long axis four-chamber image from an 11-year-old Arabian endurance horse that competed at international level for the United Kingdom. Note the greatly increased areas of all of its cardiac chambers resulting in a much larger heart in this individual. Increased cardiac chamber volume is a classic adaptation to prolonged endurance exercise.

sedentary humans and competitive athletes.[68] Significant differences in chamber dimensions were consistently present between the long distance steeplechasers and all of the other groups of racehorses studied, except for the hurdlers that compete over similar distances but over lower fences. As left ventricular chamber width increases in response to dynamic exercise and endurance training in both humans[69,70] and horses,[63] these data showed that conditioned racehorses develop a cardiac morphology that is appropriate to the endurance component of their event, adding further weight to the assertion that the endurance component of training and competition also influences cardiac morphology in equine athletes (Fig. 3.6).

Gender also affects cardiac morphology; after adjustment for body weight and age, entire male horses had larger, heavier hearts than female horses at similar levels of fitness.[64,67]

RESTING CARDIAC RHYTHM IN HORSES

Blood pressure homeostasis in the resting horse is controlled by alterations in parasympathetic tone.[2] Increased vagal activity to control arterial pressure results in progressive conduction block at the sinus and atrioventricular node, with the result that a high proportion of normal horses have vagally induced rhythm irregularities at rest,[71,72] the vast majority of which disappear during exercise and are therefore considered physiological. Typical vagal rhythms include sinus bradycardia, sinus arrhythmia, first and second degree atrio-ventricular block and sino-atrial block (see Chapter 15). When any of these dysrhythmias disappear during exercise, they are not implicated in poor performance.[71,73,74] Poor athletic performance can however be associated with atrial fibrillation, complete heart block, and premature atrial and ventricular contractions.[75,76] (AF, AR)

It has been suggested that the resting equine ECG can be used to diagnose abnormal patterns of ventricular repolarization using assessment of the resultant "T" wave and that this is helpful in assessing racehorses with a history of poor performance.[77-79] Proponents of this technique concluded that T-wave abnormalities indicated impaired cardiac function, possibly related to training stress or myocarditis.[78] However, the usefulness of T-wave evaluation for diagnosis of poor performance has been questioned[80] and the technique has largely been discredited. T wave shape changes with training, and is not correlated with poor racing performance.[81]

ATRIOVENTRICULAR VALVE REGURGITATION

Regurgitation at one or more cardiac valves is common in athletic horses and such regurgitation not infrequently results in an audible cardiac murmur.[82] Recent data have shown that the presence of multivalvular regurgitation increases in response to age and athletic training in Thoroughbreds[61,83] and Standardbred racehorses[84] (see Chapter

16). These findings are in agreement with data from human athletes[85,86] and highly trained dogs.[87] It seems increasingly likely that the high prevalence of valvular regurgitation in all athletic species is largely physiological in origin and as such does not imply structural abnormalities of the cardiac valves.[85] Rather, it has been suggested that multivalvular regurgitation in athletes is caused by altered cardiac loading conditions and morphological and functional changes to the valve apparatus invoked by chronic exposure to athletic training. Certainly the prevalence of tricuspid valve regurgitation when assessed by Doppler echocardiographic techniques are very similar in human[85] and equine athletes.[61,83] This assertion is further supported by the relatively low percentage of horses in race training that are affected by cardiac murmurs, or valve regurgitation, that, based on current guidelines,[88,89] might be considered to be "clinically significant" (murmur >grade 3/6). Studies of oxygen pulse (V_{O_2}/HR, mL/beat/kg) or cardiac output in horses with different grades of cardiac murmurs and other suspected cardiac disease might assist with interpretation of clinical significance of murmurs in individual animals. (ET)

ROLE OF THE HEART IN DETERMINING ATHLETIC PERFORMANCE

There has been considerable scientific debate as to whether the cardiac pump or the peripheral utilization of oxygen limits oxygen transport and V_{O_2max} in mammals. Yet in the Thoroughbred industry, it has long been believed that large hearts are associated with racing success. Consequently, electrocardiographic and/or echocardiographic methods have been used over many decades to assess heart size to estimate the likelihood of future racing success. Anecdotes and the historical post mortem records of elite racehorses have always encouraged the practice, despite a lack of convincing scientific evidence in the veterinary literature to support the practice. Eclipse was unbeaten in 26 races and like Phar Lap, the winner of 57 races, his heart after death weighed over 6 kg. This is 20% larger than that of an average racehorse based on post mortem studies.[62] Secretariat, the record-breaking American racehorse, was alleged to have had a heart that weighed over 10 kg, and based on this heart size, it has been suggested that his maximal cardiac output would have exceeded 500 L/minute![90] As discussed previously, the equine cardiovascular system is hugely compliant, with a heart rate range from 20 to 240 beats/minute and a splenic red cell reserve able to double packed cell volume and oxygen delivery during maximal exercise.[91] As Q_{O2} (rate of oxygen transport) is the product of cardiac output and arterial oxygen content (determined from the Fick equation), these adaptations are of huge benefit in optimizing

oxygen transport. Although maximal heart rate is important in determining maximal cardiac output, stroke volume will be determined principally by heart size.[92] In horses, the proportion of skeletal muscle exceeds 50% of lean body weight and the oxidative capacity of equine muscle far exceeds the capacity of the cardiovascular system to deliver oxygen to it.[93] As a result, the stroke volume of the heart should be important in determining aerobic capacity for individuals.[94,95]

Elite human athletes competing in primarily aerobic events have higher maximal oxygen uptake (V_{O_2max}) than normal, nonathletic individuals.[94] In human athletes, there is scientific as well as theoretical evidence to support a link between left ventricular mass and V_{O_2max}.[96,97] It has also been suggested that V_{O_2max} correlates to athletic performance in horses.[98,99] However, there was no relationship between left ventricular size and V_{O_2max} in six Thoroughbreds exercising on a treadmill.[100] However, this and most other studies, focused on flat race Thoroughbreds or Standardbreds that generally run over distances of less than 3200 m (2 miles).

More recently a strong relationship between left ventricular mass and other measurements of cardiac size with V_{O_2max} was reported in a group of 18 Thoroughbred racehorses exercising on a high-speed treadmill.[101] These data showed that V_{O_2max} was significantly correlated with left ventricular (LV) internal diameter in diastole (r = 0.71; P = 0.001), estimated LV mass (r = 0.78; P = 0.0002) and LV short-axis area in diastole (r = 0.69; P = 0.003). When indices of heart size were indexed to body weight the correlation between V_{O_2max} and indices of heart size were LV diastolic diameter (r = 0.57; P = 0.01), LV mass (r = 0.78; P = 0.0002) and LV short-axis area (r = 0.69; P = 0.003) (see Figure 3.7). The distribution of data from these horses also provided further circumstantial evidence of a possible relationship between high V_{O_2max} and long distance performance, as the horses with the highest V_{O_2max} values were both National Hunt horses who had been rated in the top 5% of the population at the peak of their careers, both having won races at the prestigious Cheltenham Festival. The study also included data from a successful sprinter, a colt who had performed successfully over 1000–1200 V_{O_2} m. His heart size indexed to bodyweight and his V_{O_2max} were in the lowest quartile of the present dataset, yet this colt was rated in the top 15% of sprinters.

Whilst a relationship between left ventricular dimensions and V_{O_2max} had been established, whether a similar relationship existed for heart size and athletic performance was still in doubt. However, recent data from a large cross-sectional study of racehorses competing on the flat or over jumps in the United Kingdom[67] did demonstrate a relationship between derived left ventricular mass and published rating (quality) in horses racing over longer distances in jump races (P ≤ 0.001), although the strength of the association with left ventricular mass was less for horses in flat races. Rather, left ventricular ejection fraction

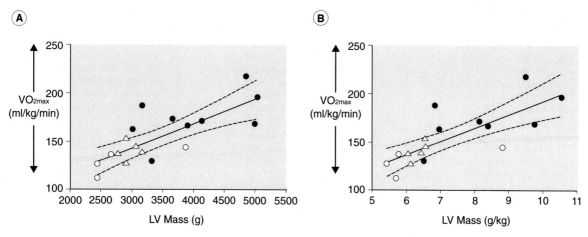

Figure 3.7 The results of fitting a linear model to describe the relationship between V_{O_2max} and LV mass (**A**) and V_{O_2max} and LV mass/kg bodyweight (**B**). The equation of the fitted models, shown as a solid line, are A: $V_{O_2max} = 67.1348 + 0.0249419 \times$ LV mass and B: $V_{O_2max} = 52.9644 + 13.7519 \times$ LV mass/kgBW. ○ = Flat racing TB; ● = research TB, △ = National Hunt TB. The inner bounds show 95.0% confidence limits for the mean V_{O_2max} of many observations at given values of LV mass. The outer bounds show 95.0% prediction limits for new observations. LV mass was determined from an M-mode echocardiograph of the left ventricle at chordal level using the equation in Ref. [106]. TB, Thoroughbred. Reproduced with permission from Young LE, Marlin DJ, Deaton C et al. Heart size estimated by echocardiography correlates with maximal oxygen uptake. Equine Vet J Suppl 2002;34:467–472.

and left ventricular mass combined were positively associated with race rating in older flat race horses running over sprint (<1408 m) and longer distances (>1408 m), explaining 25–35% of overall variation in performance, as well as being closely associated with performance in longer races over jumps (23%). Predicted differences between otherwise equivalent horses with small and large hearts was thus able to explain a significant proportion of the difference between elite and nonelite racehorse performance, thus providing the first direct evidence that cardiac size influenced athletic performance in a group of racehorses. A similar relationship has also been reported for Standardbreds.[64] However, these results conflict with findings in 370 Thoroughbred yearlings, where there was no relationship between echocardiographic measurements of heart size and prospective race performance.[102]

Use of echocardiography to predict future performance of racehorses should nevertheless still be used with caution, because the relative proportion of energy supply from aerobic metabolism probably varies widely. For example, in Thoroughbred races, with a range of 800–3200 m distance, the relative contributions of aerobic energy output could be 40–80%. With the possible exception of horses used for high-level endurance riding, the technique is also likely to have limited value for horses other than those that race, as other skills are likely to be equally or more important influences on their athletic

success than aerobic capacity. Additionally the level of skill required to obtain repeatable images of the equine left ventricle with an echocardiograph for this purpose is high and the confounding effects of gender, fitness, age and body size must always be taken into account. Prediction of maximal cardiac output and maximal oxygen uptake from estimates of stroke volume in a resting horse will also be confounded by variation in maximal heart rates during exercise.

Heart score is the mean of the QRS wave durations (ms) in leads I, II and III, and this measurement was used in several studies for the assessment of cardiac size prior to the use of echocardiography. A study in Thoroughbreds found a high correlation between heart score and cardiac mass, and a moderate but significant correlation between heart score and Thoroughbred race earnings per start.[77] Although these data led to some popularity of the use of heart score as a means of predicting future performance, particularly in Australia, the relationship between heart score and performance was either not reproduced,[81] or the coefficient of determinations for the associations between heart score and racing ability was too low to be of practical value.[103,104] Additionally, heart score was not significantly correlated to V_{O_2max} in 46 racehorses (C. M. King, unpublished data). As well, there are compelling electrophysiological considerations that suggest that the QRS duration is unlikely to accurately reflect cardiac chamber size in horses.[105]

REFERENCES

1. Eaton MD, Evans DL, Hodgson DR, et al. Maximal accumulated oxygen deficit in Thoroughbred racehorses. J Appl Physiol 1995;78:1564–1568.

2. Hamlin RL, Klepinger WL, Gilpin KW, et al. Autonomic control of heart rate in the horse. Am J Physiol 1972;222:976–978.

3. Persson SGB. On blood volume and working capacity in horses. Acta Vet Scand 1967;(Suppl. 19): 1–189.

4. Lindholm A, Saltin B. The physiological and biochemical response of Standardbred horses to exercise of varying speed and duration. Acta Vet Scand 1974; 15:310–324.

5. Ehrlein HJ, Hörnicke H, v Engelhardt W, Tolkmitt G. Die Herzschlagfrequenz während standardisierter Belastüng als Maß fur dieLeistungsfahigkeit von Pferden. Zentralbl Vet med A 1973;20:188–208.

6. Thomas DP, Fregin GF, Gerber NH, et al. Cardio-respiratory adjustments to tethered swimming in the horse. Pflugers Arch 1980;385:65–70.

7. Thomas DP, Fregin GF. Cardiorespiratory and metabolic responses to treadmill exercise in the horse. J Appl Physiol 1981; 50:864–868.

8. Seeherman HJ, Morris EA. Comparison of yearling, two-year-old and adult Thoroughbreds using a standardised exercise test. Equine Vet J 1991;23:175–184.

9. Rose RJ, Hodgson DR. Clinical exercise testing. In: Hodgson DR, Rose RJ, editors. The Athletic Horse. Philadelphia: WB Saunders; 1994. p. 245–257.

10. Persson SGB. Evaluation of exercise tolerance and fitness in the performance horse. In: Snow DH, Persson SGB, Rose RJ, editors. Equine Exercise Physiology. Cambridge: Granta Editions; 1983. p. 441–457.

11. Evans DL, Rose RJ. Determination and repeatability of maximal oxygen consumption and other cardiorespiratory measurements in the exercising horse. Equine Vet J 1988;20:94–98.

12. Dubreucq C, Chatard JC, Courouce A, Avinet B. Reproducibility of a standardised exercise test for Standardbred trotters under field conditions. Equine Vet J 1994;(Suppl. 18): 108–112.

13. King CM, Evans DL, Rose RJ. Acclimation to treadmill exercise. Equine Vet J 1994;(Suppl. 18): 453–456.

14. Rose RJ, Hendrickson DK, Knight PK. Clinical exercise testing in the normal thoroughbred racehorse. Aust Vet J 1990;67:345–348.

15. Eaton MD, Evans DL, Hodgson DR, et al. Effect of treadmill incline and speed on metabolic rate during exercise in thoroughbred horses. J Appl Physiol 1995;79(3):951–957.

16. Evans DL, Rose RJ. Dynamics of cardiorespiratory function in standardbred horses during constant load exercise. J Comp Physiol B 1988;157:791–799.

17. Murakami M, Imahara T, Inui T, Amada A, Senta T, Takagi S. Swimming exercises in horses. Exp Rep Equine Hlth Lab 1976;13:27–49.

18. Art T, Amory H, Desmecht D, Delogne O, Buchet M, Leroy P, Lekeux P. The effect of show jumping on heart rate, blood lactate and other plasma biochemical values. Equine Vet J 1990;(Suppl. 9):78–82.

19. White SL, Williamson LH, Maykuth P, et al. Heart rate and lactate concentration during two different cross country events. Equine Vet J 1995;(Suppl. 18): 463–467.

20. Thomas DP, Fregin GF. Cardiorespiratory drift during exercise in the horse. Equine Vet J 1990;(Suppl. 9):61–65.

21. Hinchcliffe KW, McKeever KH, Schmall, et al. Renal and systemic hemodynamic responses to sustained submaximal exertion in horses. Am J Physiol 1990;258: R1177–R1183.

22. Naylor JR, Bayly WM, Gollnick PD, et al. Effects of dehydration on thermoregulatory responses of horses during low-intensity exercise, J Appl Physiol 1993;75: 994–1001.

23. Littlejohn A, Kruger JM, Bowles F. Exercise studies in horses: 2. The cardiac response to exercise in normal horses and in horses with chronic obstructive pulmonary disease. Equine Vet J 1977;9: 75–83.

24. Littlejohn A, Bowles F, Aschenborn G. Cardio-respiratory adaptations to exercise in riding horses with chronic lung disease. In: Snow DH, Persson SGB, Rose RJ, editors. Equine Exercise Physiology. Cambridge: Granta Editions; 1983. p. 33–45.

25. King CM, Evans DL, Rose RJ. Cardiorespiratory and metabolic responses to exercise in horses with various abnormalities of the upper respiratory tract. Equine Vet J 1994;26:220–225.

26. King CM, Evans DL, Rose RJ. Significance for exercise capacity of some electrocardiographic findings in racehorses. Aust Vet J 1994;71:200–202.

27. Deegen E, Buntenkotter S. Behaviour of the heart rate of horses with auricular fibrillation during exercise and after treatment. Equine Vet J 1976;8: 26–29.

28. Young LE. Diseases of the heart and vessels. In: Hinchcliff KW, Kaneps AJ, Goer RJ, editors. Equine Sports Medicine and Surgery: Basic and Clinical Sciences of the Equine Athlete. Edinburgh: WB Saunders; 2003. p. 728–769.

29. Hinchcliff KW, Geor RJ, Pagan JD. Effects of mild forelimb lameness on exercise performance. Equine Vet J Suppl 2002;36:146–152.

30. Krzywanek H, Wittke G, Bayer A, Borman P. The heart rates of Thoroughbred horses during a race. Equine Vet J 1970;2: 115–117.

31. Vincent TL, Newton JR, Deaton C, Franklin SH, Biddick T, Mc Keever K, et al. A retrospective study of predictive variables for maximal heart rate (HR_{max}) in horses undergoing strenuous treadmill exercise. Equine Vet J Suppl 2006. In Press.

32. Asheim A, Knudsen O, Lindholm A, et al. Heart rates and blood lactate concentrations of Standardbred horses during training and racing. J Am Vet Med Assoc 1970;157:304–312.

33. Vermeulen AD, Evans DL. Measurements of fitness in thoroughbred racehorses using field studies of heart rate and velocity with a global positioning system. Equine Vet J Suppl 2006;36:113–117.

34. Gramkow HL, Evans DL. Correlation of race earnings with velocity at maximal heart rate during a field exercise test in Thoroughbred racehorses. Equine Vet J Suppl 2006;36: 118–122.

35. Banister EW, Purvis AD. Exercise electrocardiography in the horse by radiotelemetry. J Am Vet Med Assoc 1968;152:1004–1008.

36. Hall MC, Steel JD, Stewart GA. Cardiac monitoring during exercise tests in the horse. 2. Heart rate responses to exercise. Aust Vet J 1976;52:1–5.

37. Marsland WP. Heart rate response to submaximal exercise in the Standardbred horse. J Appl Physiol 1968;24:98–101.

38. White SL, Williamson LH, Maykuth PL, et al. Heart rate response and plasma lactate concentrations of horses competing in the cross-country phase of combined training events. Equine Vet J Suppl 1995;20:47.

39. Cardinet GH, Fowler ME, Tyler WS. Heart rates and respiratory rates for evaluating performance in horses during endurance trail ride competition. J Am Vet Med Assoc 1963;143:1303–1309.

40. Rose RJ, Purdue RA, Hensley W. Plasma biochemistry alterations in horses during an endurance ride. Equine Vet J 1977;9: 122–126.

41. Rose RJ. An evaluation of heart rate and respiratory rate recovery for assessment of fitness during endurance rides. In: Persson SGB, Lindholm A, Jeffcott LB, editors. Equine Exercise Physiology. Cambridge: Granta Editions; 1983. p. 505–509.

42. Thomas DP, Fregin GF, Gerber NH, et al. Effects of training on cardiorespiratory function in the horse. Am J Physiol 1983;245: R160–R165.

43. Bayly WM, Gabel AA, Barr SA. Cardiovascular effects of submaximal aerobic training on a treadmill in Standardbred horses, using a standardised exercise test. Am J Vet Res 1983;44:544–553.

44. Milne DW, Gabel AA, Muir WW, Skarda RT. Effects of training on heart rate, cardiac output, and lactic acid in Standardbred horses, using a standardised exercise test. J Equine Med Surg 1977;1:131–135.

45. Skarda RT, Muir WW, Milne DW, et al. Effects of training on resting and postexercise ECG in Standardbred horses, using a standardised exercise test. Am J Vet Res 1976;37:1485–1488.

46. Thornton J, Essén-Gustavsson B, Lindholm A, McMiken D, Persson S. Effects of training and detraining on oxygen uptake, cardiac output, blood gas tensions, pH and lactate concentrations during and after exercise in the horse. In: Snow DH, Persson SGB, Rose RJ, editors. Equine Exercise Physiology. Cambridge: Granta Editions; 1983. p. 470–486.

47. Foreman JH, Bayly WM, Grant BD, et al. Standardized exercise test and daily heart rate responses of Thoroughbreds undergoing conventional race training and detraining. Am J Vet Res 1990; 51:914–920.

48. Rose RJ, Allen JR, Hodgson DR, et al. Responses to submaximal treadmill exercise and training in the horse: changes in haematology, arterial blood gas and acid-base measurements, plasma biochemical values and heart rate. Vet Rec 1983;113: 612–618.

49. Evans DL, Rose RJ. Cardiovascular and respiratory responses to submaximal exercise training in the thoroughbred horse. Pflügers Arch 1988;411: 316–321.

50. Marr CM, Bright JM, Marlin DJ, et al. Pre- and post exercise echocardiography in horses performing treadmill exercise in cool and hot/humid conditions. Equine Vet J Suppl 1999;30:131.

51. Reef VB. Stress echocardiography and its role in performance assessment. Vety Clin North Am Equine Pract 2001;17:179–189.

52. Waugh SL, Fregin GF, Thomas DP, et al. Electromagnetic measurement of cardiac output during exercise in the horse. Am J Vet Res 1980;41:812–815.

53. Weber J-M, Dobson GP, Parkhouse WS, et al. Cardiac output and oxygen consumption in exercising Thoroughbred horses. Am J Physiol 1987;253: R890–R895.

54. Evans DL, Rose RJ. Cardiovascular and respiratory responses to exercise in thoroughbred horses. J Exp Biol 1988;134:397–408.

55. Butler PJ, Woakes AJ, Anderson LS, Roberts CA, Snow DH. The effect of cessation of training on cardiorespiratory variables during exercise. In: Persson SGB, Lindholm A, Jeffcott LB, editors. Equine Exercise Physiology 3. Davis: ICEEP Publications; 1991. p. 71–76.

56. Crawford MH. Physiologic consequences of systematic training. Cardiol Clinics 1992;10: 209–218.

57. Knight PK, Sinha AK, Rose RJ. Effects of training intensity on maximum oxygen uptake. In: Persson SGB, Lindholm A, Jeffcott LB, editors. Equine Exercise Physiology 3. Davis: ICEEP Publications; 1991. p. 77–82.

58. Art T, Lekeux P. Training-induced modifications in cardiorespiratory and ventilatory measurements in Thoroughbred horses. Equine Vet J 1993;25:532.

59. Hopper MK, Pieschl RL Jr, Pelletier NG, Erickson HH.

Cardiopulmonary effects of acute blood volume alteration prior to exercise. In: Persson SGB, Lindholm A, Jeffcott LB, editors. Equine Exercise Physiology 3. Davis: ICEEP Publications; 1991. p. 9–16.

60. McKeever KH, Schurg WA, Jarrett SH, et al. Exercise-training induced hypervolemia in the horse. Med Sci Sports Exerc 1987;19:21–27.

61. Lightfoot G, Jose-Cunelleras E, Rogers K, Newton R, Young LE. An echocardiographic and auscultation study of right heart responses to race training in young national hunt thoroughbreds. Equine Vet J Suppl 2006;36:153–158.

62. Kubo K, Senta T, Osamu, S. Relationship between training and heart in the Thoroughbred racehorse. Exp Rep Equine Hlth Lab 1974;11:87–93.

63. Young LE. Cardiac responses to training in 2-year-old thoroughbreds: an echocardiographic study. Equine Vet J Suppl 1999;30:195.

64. Buhl R, Ersboll AK, Eriksen L, Koch J. Changes over time in echocardiographic measurements in young Standardbred racehorses undergoing training and racing and association with racing performance. J Am Vet Med Assoc 2005;226:1881–1887.

65. Kriz NG, Hodgson DR, Rose RJ. Changes in cardiac dimensions and indices of cardiac function during deconditioning in horses. Am J Vet Res 2000;61(12):1553–1560.

66. Patteson MW. Echocardiographic Studies in Horses. Dissertation, University of Bristol; 1993.

67. Young LE, Rogers K, Wood JL. Left ventricular size and systolic function in Thoroughbred racehorses and their relationships to race performance. J Appl Physiol 2005;99:1278–1285.

68. Maron BJ. Structural features of the athlete heart as defined by echocardiography. J Am Coll Cardiol 1986;7:190–203.

69. Fagard RH. Athlete's heart: a meta-analysis of the echocardiographic experience. Int J Sports Med 1996;17(Suppl. 3):S140–S144.

70. Huonker M, Konig D, Keul J. Assessment of left ventricular dimensions and functions in athletes and sedentary subjects at rest and during exercise using echocardiography, Doppler sonography and radionuclide ventriculography. Int J Sports Med 1996;17(Suppl. 3):S173–S179.

71. Holmes JR, Alps BJ. The effect of exercise on rhythm irregularities in the horse. Vet Rec 1966;78:672.

72. Raekallio M. Long term ECG recording with Holter monitoring in clinically healthy horses. Acta Vet Scand 1992;33:71–75.

73. Bonagura JD. Equine heart disease: an overview. Vet Clin North Am Equine Pract 1985;1:267–274.

74. Marr CM. Treatment of arrhythmias and cardiac failure. In: Robinson NE, editor. Current Therapy in Equine Medicine. Philadelphia: WB Saunders; 1997. p. 250–259.

75. Holmes JR. An investigation of cardiac rhythm using an on-line radiotelemetry/computer link. J Sth Afr Vet Assoc 1974;45:251–261.

76. Hillwig RW. Cardiac arrhythmias in the horse. J Am Vet Med Assoc 1977;170:153–163.

77. Steel JD. Studies on the Electrocardiogram of the Racehorse. Sydney: Australasian Medical Publishing Co.; 1963.

78. Rose RJ, Davis PE. The use of electrocardiography in the diagnosis of poor racing performance in the horse. Aust Vet J 1978;54:51–56.

79. Stewart JH, Rose RJ, Davis PE, Hoffman K. A comparison of electrocardiographic findings in racehorses presented for either routine examination or poor racing performance. In: Snow DH, Persson SGB, Rose RJ, editors. Equine Exercise Physiology. Cambridge: Granta Editions; 1983. p. 135–143.

80. Evans DL. T waves in the equine electrocardiogram: effects of training and implications for race performance. In: Persson SGB, Lindholm A, Jeffcott LB, editors. Equine Exercise Physiology 3. Stockholm: ICEEP Publications; 1991. p. 475–481.

81. Evans DL, Polglaze KE. Relationships between electrocardiographic findings, racing performance and training in Standardbred horses. Aust Vet J 1994;71:375–378.

82. Patteson MW, Cripps PJ. A survey of cardiac auscultatory findings in horses. Equine Vet J 1993;25:409–415.

83. Young LE, Wood JLN. The effects of age and training on murmurs of atrioventricular valvular regurgitation in young Thoroughbreds. Equine Vet J 2000;32:195–199.

84. Buhl R, Ersboll AK, Eriksen L, Koch J. Use of color Doppler echocardiography to assess the development of valvular regurgitation in Standardbred trotters. J Am Vet Med Assoc 2005;227:1630–1635.

85. Douglas PS, Berman GO, O'Toole ML, Hiller WD, Reichek N. Prevalence of multivalvular regurgitation in athletes. Am J Cardiol 1989;64:209–212.

86. Vasconcelos DF, Junqueira Junior LF, Sanchez Osella OF. Doppler echocardiographic comparison of valvular dynamics in bicycling, running, and football athletes, and sedentary subjects. Arq Bras Cardiol 1993;61:161–164.

87. Constable PD, Hinchcliff KW, Olson J, Hamlin RL. Athletic heart syndrome in dogs competing in a long-distance sled race. J Appl Physiol 1994;76:433–438.

88. Reef VB. Heart murmurs in horses: determining their significance with echocardiography. Equine Vet J Suppl 1995;19:71–80.

89. Patteson MW. Equine Cardiology. Oxford: Blackwell Science; 1996.

90. Poole DC, Erikson HH. Heart and Vessels: function during exercise and response to training. In: Hinchcliff KW, Kaneps AJ,

Goer RJ, editors. Equine Sports Medicine and Surgery. Oxford: Elsevier Science; 2004. p. 699–727.

91. McKeever KH, Hinchcliff KW, Reed SM, Robertson JT. Role of decreased plasma volume in hematocrit alterations during incremental treadmill exercise in horses. Am J Physiol 1993;265: R404–R408.

92. Hammond HK, White FC, Bhargava V, Shabetai R. Heart size and maximal cardiac output are limited by the pericardium. Am J Physiol 1992;263: H1675–H1681.

93. Poole DC. Current concepts of oxygen transport during exercise. Equine Compe Exerc Physioly 2004;1:5–22.

94. Wilmore JH, Costill DL. Cardiorespiratory adaptations to training. In: Wilmore JH, Costill DL, editors. Physiology of Sport and Exercise. Campaign, IL: Human Kinetics; 1994. p. 214–238.

95. Saltin B, Strange S. Maximal oxygen uptake: "old" and "new" arguments for a cardiovascular limitation. Med Sci Sport Ex 1992;24:30–37.

96. Al-Hazzaa HM, Chukwuemeka AC. Echocardiographic dimensions and maximal oxygen uptake in elite soccer players. Saudi Med J 2001;22:320–325.

97. Blimkie CJ, Cunningham DA, Nichol PM. Gas transport capacity and echocardiographically determined cardiac size in children. J Appl Physiol 1980;49: 994–999.

98. Harkins JD, Beadle RE, Kamerling SG. The correlation of running ability and physiological variables in thoroughbred racehorses. Equine Vet J 1993;25:53–60.

99. Gauvreau GM, Staempfli H, McCutcheon LJ, Young SS, McDonell WN. Comparison of aerobic capacity between racing standardbred horses. J Appl Physiol 1995;78:1447–1451.

100. Sampson SN, Tucker RL, Bayly WM. Relationship between VO2max, heart score and echocardiographic measurements obtained at rest and immediately following maximal exercise in thoroughbred horses. Equine Vet J Suppl 1999;30:190–194.

101. Young LE, Marlin DJ, Deaton C, Brown-Feltner H, Roberts CA, Wood JLN. Heart size estimated by echocardiography correlates with maximal oxygen uptake. Equine Vet J Suppl 2002;34:467–472.

102. Leadon D, McAllister H, Mullins E, Osborne M. Electrocardiographic and echocardiographic measurements and their relationships in Thoroughbred yearlings to subsequent performance. In: Persson SGB, Lindholm A, Jeffcott LB, editors. Equine Exercise Physiology 3. Davis, CA: ICCEP Publications; 1991. p. 18–22.

103. Leadon DP, Cunningham EP, Mahon GA, et al. Heart score and performance ability in the United Kingdom. Equine Vet J 1982;14:89–90.

104. Nielsen K, Vibe-Petersen G. Relationship between the QRS-duration (heart score) and racing performance in trotters. Equine Vet J 1980;12:81–84.

105. Physick-Sheard PW, Hendren CM. Heart score: physiological basis and confounding variables. In: Snow DH, Persson SGB, Rose RJ, editors. Equine Exercise Physiology 1. Cambridge: Burlington Press; 1998. p. 121–134.

106. Devereux RB, Reichek N. Echocardiographic estimation of ventricular mass in man: anatomic validation of the method. Circulation 1977;55: 613–618.

Cardiac disease and pathology

Mark Bowen

The function of the cardiovascular system depends on both contraction and relaxation in a regular and controlled manner. Due to the integrated nature of the heart, the vasculature, lungs and kidneys, disease of any of these can potentially lead to changes in the other. In the horse, endocardial disease is the predominant form of cardiac disease and myocardial remodelling most commonly occurs as sequel to valvular insufficiencies. Cardiac enlargement and remodelling are however important and contribute to the syndrome of cardiac failure due to excessive chamber enlargement. However, most studies investigating cardiac remodelling relate to human patients with either hypertension or myocardial ischaemia and therefore it may not be appropriate to extrapolate these data to the horse. The purpose of this chapter is to review the mediators of cardiac pathology that are important for the progression of cardiac disease in the horse and relate these to pathological changes in the equine heart.

CARDIAC PATHOLOGICAL EXAMINATION

Most pathological techniques to examine the heart are designed to examine each chamber in isolation, usually opening the chamber along its border with the intra-ventricular septum and displaying its internal surface for examination and determination of weight.[1] While this technique does have several advantages it does not enable the clinician to visualize the heart in the manner to which it has been examined by echocardiography. Therefore, a more clinically orientated approach to gross pathological examination of the heart is recommended.[2] This approach is lesion orientated and therefore should commence by examining the side of the heart which is most affected by disease.

The pericardium should be examined for evidence of pathology, and the pericardial fluid volume should be determined and a sample obtained for cytological and/or bacteriological examination. The left side of the heart is examined by placing metal rods (blunt ended and at least 30 cm in length) through a small hole made in the left atrium and advanced through the mitral valve and rested at the cardiac apex; it is advisable not to place the rod through one of the pulmonary veins as this will not create the correct anatomical view. A second metal rod should be placed through the aortic valve and placed at an angle so that it reaches the same point on the cardiac apex. A large flat knife, such as a 12-inch disposable dissection knife, should then be used to cut alongside these metal guides to create a sagittal section and open the ventricle to mimic a left parasternal view of the left ventricle and left ventricular outflow tract (Fig. 4.1). The right ventricle should be examined in a similar manner by placing a metal rod down through the pulmonary artery and another through the right atrium into the right ventricular apex through the tricuspid valve. Care should be taken to avoid the moderator band within the ventricular lumen (trabeculae septomarginalis). This will mimic the cranially angled right parasternal view of the right ventricle and right ventricular outflow tract.

DOI: 10.1016/B978-0-7020-2817-5.00009-2

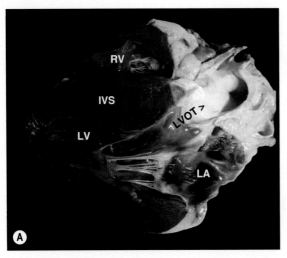
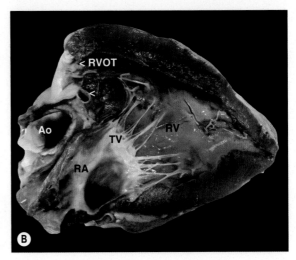

Figure 4.1 Post mortem appearance of equine heart following preparation to mimic imaging planes obtained by echocardiography showing left ventricle (A: right parasternal long axis view of the left ventricle) and right ventricle (B: right ventricular inflow-outflow view) demonstrating left ventricle (LV), left atrium (LA), left ventricular outflow tract (and aorta – LVOT) with arrow pointing towards aortic outflow, intraventricular septum (IVS), right ventricle (RV), right atrium (RA), tricuspid valve (TV), right ventricular outflow tract (RVOT) leading to pulmonary artery (depicted by arrow), aorta (Ao) and coronary artery (arrow head).

The heart should subsequently be examined for evidence of congenital, myocardial, endocardial and valvular pathology. Dimensions can be obtained and ventricular mass can be established; however, changes in myocardial mass can be difficult to interpret since myocardial mass will change in response to eccentric hypertrophy in the trained animal as well as in response to pathological chamber enlargement. In order to take into account changes in body weight it is usual to express changes in left ventricular mass in relation to either body weight or right ventricular mass. There is better correlation between left ventricular mass and right ventricular mass in the normal horse ($r^2 = 0.71$) than between left ventricular mass and body weight ($r^2 = 0.19$) in the normal horse (n = 37; I. M. Bowen, unpublished observations) and the ratio of right ventricle (free wall):left ventricle (including intraventricular septum) in the normal animal is 1:2.81 ± 0.4 (reference range 1:1.98–3.63; n = 37). These figures are based on the weight of myocardial tissue after removal of the atria, pericardium and fat. In interpreting these data it is important to recognize that volume loading, induced by valvular pathology in the horse, creates chamber dilation, rather than thickening of the ventricular wall and in the same study there was no difference in left ventricular mass from horses with mild and moderate aortic insufficiency (n = 17), expressed either as ventricular mass, right ventricle:left ventricle or left ventricle:body weight. Therefore, cardiac dimensions may be a more reliable method of documenting changes in cardiac size than ventricular weights.

PRIMARY MYOCARDIAL PATHOLOGIES (VMD)

Primary myocardial disease occurs rarely in the horse; dilated cardiomyopathies are occasionally reported and are described in Chapter 19. Myocardial fibrosis has been associated with ventricular tachycardia, presumably due to disruption of the cardiac conduction system of the ventricle, but can also be detected as an incidental finding.[3] The gross appearance of these changes are of discolouration within the myocardium, but are rarely specific to a particular disease process (Fig. 4.2).

In most cases a local ischemic event was assumed to be the primary disease process whereas a primary inflammatory aetiology has also been implicated.[4] However, as fibrosis is an end-stage process the primary disease process can be difficult to confirm. In a group of horses microemboli from parasitic lesions were suspected based on statistical associations.[3] In human patients and animal models, fibrosis is associated with myocardial remodelling and this process is described below in more detail. Myocarditis is often a clinical diagnosis based on the presence of ventricular dysrhythmias with no apparent underlying cause, although viral and bacterial causes, including *Streptococcus equi* var *equi*, have been implicated;[1] however, in many cases the primary initiating cause is unknown. (*ET*)

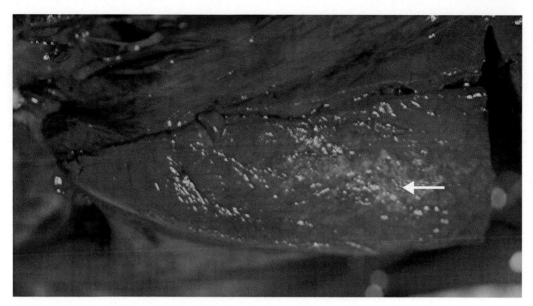

Figure 4.2 Gross post mortem appearance of intraventricular septum showing nonspecific pathology of the myocardium in a 12-month-old colt that presented with lethargy and depression and was found to have multifocal ventricular tachycardia that was resistant to therapy. Histological examination showed a mixed pattern of inflammation, necrosis and fibrosis. No specific aetiology was identified. Picture courtesy of Dr Gayle Hallowell.

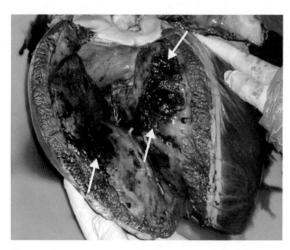

Figure 4.3 Gross post mortem appearance of the left ventricle showing expansive subepicardial haemorrhagic mass in the right ventricular free wall and interventricular septum (arrows) from a 3-year-old Arab mare that was presented with signs of congestive heart failure. Histological examination confirmed the diagnosis of an intramyocardial haemorrhage, with fibrosis and a lymphocytic-plasmacytic infiltrate, although no cause was identified.

Other primary myocardial pathologies are rare, although do occur sporadically (Fig. 4.3) and usually present clinically with cardiac dysrhythmias or signs of low cardiac output (see Chapter 19). (CN)

MYOCARDIAL REMODELLING

In heart disease a range of mediators are produced in order to maintain normal cardiac function and ultimately tissue perfusion as described in Chapter 2. Although the beneficial physiological effects of these mediators are to maintain cardiac function, they also result in remodelling of the myocardium to induce hypertrophy, dilation and fibrosis. In the normal animal the heart can undergo hypertrophy in response to training, resulting in chamber enlargement (dilation) and increases in ventricular wall thickness (eccentric hypertrophy).[5,6] This form of cardiac chamber enlargement can be reversible, nonpathogenic and results in an improvement of cardiac function with a reduction in vascular resistance. It differs from pathological eccentric hypertrophy in terms of the signalling pathways and vascular dynamics. Physiological remodelling is associated with an increase in mitochondria synthesis, increased contractile proteins, and increase in cardiac function without any increase in myocardial collagen content.[7] Further details on cardiac responses to training are discussed in Chapter 3.

Concentric cardiac hypertrophy (increase in ventricular wall thickness with no increase in lumen diameter) is uncommon in the horse and is usually seen in human patients with systemic hypertension but can also occur with animals that have aortic stenosis.[8] Cardiac remodelling is brought about in response to both biomechanical stress and neurohormonal mechanisms. In this form of hypertrophy, it is known that biomechanical stress forces are transferred to the nucleus by cell membrane receptors and cytoskeletal proteins and result in activation of a range of cell signalling pathways. These are mediated by a range of mediators that become upregulated in cardiac failure (see Chapters 2 and 5) and include angiotensin II, aldosterone, endothelin-I and β-adrenoceptor activation.[7] These mediators appear to have a common final pathway leading to activation of gene expression leading to hypertrophy involving calcium-dependent activation of the intracellular enzyme calcineurin.[9]

In the horse, cardiac enlargement is usually seen secondary to valvular insufficiency. (AF, AR, IE, RCT, VMD) This results in volume loading of the cardiac chambers (increased preload) and cardiac dilation. The pathways important in cardiac chamber dilation are different from those in hypertrophy and result in lengthening of the cardiomyocyte.[10] β-Adrenoceptor activation, angiotensin and aldosterone may be important in the genesis of cardiac enlargement in both mitral and aortic valvular regurgitation[11-13] and in the myocardial fibrosis that is reported in aortic valve regurgitation in people. Myocardial fibrosis is a risk factor for subsequent development of congestive heart failure and mortality in human patients with aortic valve regurgitation.[14] Myocardial fibrosis is occasionally reported in horses[3,15] although it has not been investigated extensively. In a study of 14 horses with aortic valve disease, there was no increase in myocardial collagen content (I. M. Bowen, unpublished observations). However, in other species, fibrosis is not consistently associated with increases in collagen content[14] and changes in extracellular matrix may be of importance in the prognosis of equine aortic valve regurgitation.

VALVULAR PATHOLOGY (IE, RCT, VMD)

In few cases, with the exception of infective endocarditis, are the inciting causes of valvular pathology truly understood. Valvular pathology is often described as an ageing related process caused by myxomatous degeneration of the valve. However the factors that initiate and continue

this process are poorly understood. It has been suggested that once valvular regurgitation begins then this sets up a cascade of remodelling and fibrosis of the valve that ultimately leads to thickened degenerate valves.[16] However, the natural history of valvular function and dysfunction is not known in any species. It is, however, clear that the traditional view of cardiac valves as pieces of connective tissue that simply open and close with each cardiac cycle by the kinetics of blood is an oversimplification. Valves are biologically active cell-,[16,17] neurone-,[18,19] and vascular-filled[20] tissues that may have more complex roles than are currently understood. Many of the mediators of valvular pathology have also been described in a variety of species and include the matrix metalloproteinases, collagenases and gelatinases. However, the inciting insult to the valve is not clear.

An important insight into potential causes of valvular degenerative pathologies was the realization that certain drugs can induce valvular disease in human patients taking these drugs. This phenomenon was first described with the appetite suppressant fenfluramine[21] and more recently has included a range of drugs such as MDMA (ecstasy),[22] pergolide and cabergoline.[17,23-27] These drugs' effects are not known to be of any clinical significance to the horse, but they helped to identify pathways of disease that further the understanding of valvular pathologies. All of these drugs have been shown to have direct effects on valvular tissue in vitro on the 5-HT$_{2B}$ receptor on the valve.[22,28] Not only does 5-HT result in changes in proliferation of the valvular interstitial cells and collagen production[29] but it has also been demonstrated to cause regurgitation in vitro.[30] The mechanism by which regurgitation occurs is likely to be due to changes in contractile and relaxant features of the valve, mediated by the contractile nature of the valvular interstitial cells.[17,31-33] The physiological significance of this contractile function of the valve is unknown, although it may play a role in the formation of a competent seal of the valve. Irrespective of the dynamic function of the valve, a range of vasoactive mediators have been shown to manipulate function of the valvular interstitial cells and appear to be important for valvular remodelling in response to load, and may be important in the progressive nature of valvular disease.

REFERENCES

1. Buergelt CD. Equine cardiovascular pathology: an overview. Anim Health Res Rev 2003;4(2):109–129.

2. Fox PR. Principles of Cardiovascular Pathology. Paper presented at the ACVIM Forum, San Antonio, 2008.

3. Cranley JJ, McCullagh KG. Ischaemic myocardial fibrosis and aortic strongylosis in the horse. Equine Vet J 1981;13(1):35–42.

4. Traub-Dargatz JL, Schlipf JW Jr, Boon J, et al. Ventricular tachycardia and myocardial dysfunction in a horse. J Am Vet Med Assoc 1994;205(11):1569–1573.

5. Young LE. Cardiac responses to training in 2-year-old thoroughbreds: an echocardiographic study. Equine Vet J Suppl 1999;30:195–198.

6. Buhl R, Ersboll AK, Eriksen L, Koch J. Changes over time in echocardiographic measurements in young Standardbred racehorses undergoing training and racing and association with racing performance. J Am Vet Med Assoc 2005;226(11):1881–1887.

7. Dorn GW 2nd. The fuzzy logic of physiological cardiac hypertrophy. Hypertension 2007;49(5):962–970.

8. O'Grady MR, Holmberg DL, Miller CW, Cockshutt JR. Canine congenital aortic stenosis: a review of the literature and commentary. Can Vet J 1989;30(10):811–815.

9. Dorn GW 2nd, Force T. Protein kinase cascades in the regulation of cardiac hypertrophy. J Clin Invest 2005;115(3):527–537.

10. Hill JA, Olson EN. Cardiac plasticity. N Engl J Med 2008;358(13):1370–1380.

11. Dell'Italia LJ, The renin-angiotensin system in mitral regurgitation: a typical example of tissue activation. Curr Cardiol Rep 2002;4(2): 97–103.

12. Fielitz, J, Hein S, Mitrovic V, et al. Activation of the cardiac renin-angiotensin system and increased myocardial collagen expression in human aortic valve disease. J Am Coll Cardiol 2001;37(5):1443–1449.

13. Plante E, Lachance D, Champetier S, et al. Benefits of long-term beta-blockade in experimental chronic aortic regurgitation. Am J Physiol Heart Circ Physiol 2008;294(4):H1888–1895.

14. Goldfine SM, Pena M, Magid NM, et al. Myocardial collagen in cardiac hypertrophy resulting from chronic aortic regurgitation. Am J Ther 1998;5(3):139–146.

15. Coudry V, Thibaud D, Riccio B, Audigie F, et al. Myocardial fibrosis in a horse with polymorphic ventricular tachycardia observed during general anesthesia. Can Vet J 2007;48(6):623–626.

16. Else RW, Holmes JR. Cardiac pathology in the horse. 2. Microscopic pathology. Equine Vet J 1972;4(2):57–62.

17. Messier RH, Bass BL, Aly HM Jr., et al. Dual structural and functional phenotypes of the porcine aortic valve interstitial population: characteristics of the leaflet myofibroblast. J Surg Res 1994;57(1):1–21.

18. De Biasi S, Vitellaro Zuccarello L. Intrinsic innervation of porcine semilunar heart valves. Anat Embryol 1982;165(1):71–79.

19. Marron K, Yacoub MH, Polak JM, et al. Innervation of human atrioventricular and arterial valves. Circulation 1996;94(3):368–375.

20. Weind KL, Ellis CG, Boughner DR. The aortic valve blood supply. J Heart Valve Dis 2000;9(1): 1–7; discussion 7–8.

21. Connolly HM, Crary JL, McGoon MD, et al. Valvular heart disease associated with fenfluramine-phentermine. N Engl J Med 1997;337(9):581–588.

22. Setola V, Hufeisen SJ, Grande-Allen KJ, et al. 3,4-methylenedioxymethamphetamine (MDMA, "Ecstasy") induces fenfluramine-like proliferative actions on human cardiac valvular interstitial cells in vitro. Mol Pharmacol 2003;63(6):1223–1229.

23. Pritchett AM, Morrison JF, Edwards WD, et al. Valvular heart disease in patients taking pergolide. Mayo Clin Proc 2002;77(12):1280–1286.

24. Dupuy D, Lesbre JP, Gerard P, et al. Valvular heart disease in patients with Parkinson's disease treated with pergolide: course following treatment modifications. J Neurol 2008;255(7):1045–1048.

25. Zanettini R, Antonini A, Gatto G, et al. Valvular heart disease and the use of dopamine agonists for Parkinson's disease. N Engl J Med 2007;356(1):39–46.

26. Waller EA, Kaplan J. Pergolide-associated valvular heart disease. Compr Ther 2006;32(2):94–101.

27. Scozzafava J, Takahashi J, Johnston W, et al. Valvular heart disease in pergolide-treated Parkinson's disease. Can J Neurol Sci 2006;33(1):111–113.

28. Fitzgerald LW, Burn TC, Brown BS, et al. Possible role of valvular serotonin 5-HT(2B) receptors in the cardiopathy associated with fenfluramine. Mol Pharmacol 2000;57(1):75–81.

29. Hafizi S, Taylor PM, Chester AH, et al. Mitogenic and secretory responses of human valve interstitial cells to vasoactive agents. J Heart Valve Dis 2000;9(3):454–458.

30. Chester AH, Misfeld M, Sievers HH, Yacoub MH. Influence of 5-hydroxytryptamine on aortic valve competence in vitro. J Heart Valve Dis 2001;10(6):822–825; discussion 825–826.

31. Chester AH, Misfeld M, Yacoub MH. Receptor-mediated contraction of aortic valve leaflets. J Heart Valve Dis 2000;9(2): 250–254; discussion 254–255.

32. Misfled M, Chester AH, Sievers H, et al. Contractile Properties of the Different Components of the Aortic Valve. Paper presented at the First Biennial Meeting of The Society for Heart Valve Disease, London, 2001.

33. Bowen IM, Marr CM, Chester AH, et al. In-vitro contraction of the equine aortic valve. J Heart Valve Dis 2004;13(4):593–599.

Chapter | 5 |

Pathophysiology of heart failure

Janice McIntosh Bright

DEFINITIONS

The term *heart disease* refers to any abnormality of the heart; whereas the term *heart failure* refers to a clinical syndrome characterized by congestion and oedema and/or poor peripheral perfusion, either at rest or with exercise. If heart failure is severe enough to produce a marked reduction in cardiac output, systemic hypotension may be present also (cardiogenic shock). However, cardiogenic shock is rare in veterinary patients. *Congestive heart failure* (CHF) is a more specific term that refers to heart failure with congestion of one or more vascular beds. Although heart failure is the result of severe heart disease, heart disease may be present that does not lead to heart failure.

MECHANISMS OF HEART FAILURE

Heart failure is a clinical syndrome that can be caused by a variety of etiologies and mechanisms. The most common haemodynamic mechanism responsible for heart failure in horses is volume overload caused by valvular regurgita-tion or by a left to right shunt. However, myocardial systo-lic failure (reduced contractility) is also recognized in horses and may lead to heart failure. Less commonly heart failure is the result of impaired diastolic function as a result of inadequate cardiac filling in horses with pericar-dial disease.

Regardless of the etiology or mechanism of heart failure, CHF is associated with two primary haemodynamic abnormalities: (1) increased ventricular filling pressures and (2) reduced cardiac output. Increased ventricular filling pressures are responsible for signs of congestion and oedema; whereas reduced cardiac output causes clinical signs of inadequate tissue perfusion. The haemo-dynamic abnormalities and resulting clinical signs that characterize heart failure are illustrated using ventricular function curves in Figure 5.1.

Horses with left-sided failure have increased left ven-tricular filling pressures and subsequently increased left atrial and pulmonary venous pressures leading to pulmo-nary oedema. Thus, clinical signs may include tachypnea, dyspnea, coughing, haemoptysis and the appearance of frothy white or blood-tinged fluid at the nostrils. Horses with right-sided CHF have increased right ventricular filling pressures and subsequently increased right atrial and systemic venous pressures leading to peripheral oedema. Subcutaneous oedema in the dependent areas such as the ventral abdomen, the prepuce and the distal extremities is the most common manifestation of increased right-sided filling pressures. Jugular venous distension and pulsation may also be present. In horses, an increase in left-sided filling pressure frequently stimulates pulmonary vasoconstriction and pulmonary vascular remodelling, changes that result in secondary right-sided heart failure. Thus, in some horses, systemic oedema and jugular distention may be the first clinical signs of chronic left-sided heart disease. Reduced cardiac output causes clinical

DOI: 10.1016/B978-0-7020-2817-5.00010-9

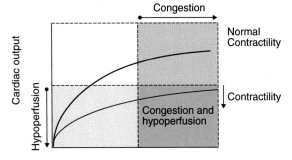

Figure 5.1 A ventricular function curve (Starling curve) from a normal animal (top curve) and from an animal with myocardial systolic failure (bottom curve). The dashed vertical line in the centre represents the upper limit of normal preload (normal ventricular filling pressure). The dashed horizontal line represents the lower limit of normal cardiac output. A horse with valvular regurgitation (volume overload) and normal myocardial contractility is likely to have an operating point on the upper curve and will, therefore, have either no clinical signs or signs of circulatory congestion (oedema). However, a horse with valvular regurgitation and reduced contractility is likely to have an operating point in the lower right quadrant of the graph. Thus, a horse in this situation is quite likely to have clinically apparent oedema in addition to signs of hypoperfusion.

signs referable to poor tissue perfusion, namely fatigue, weakness, exercise intolerance, cold extremities, prolonged capillary refill and hypothermia. With the exception of exercise intolerance and fatigue, these signs are not likely to become apparent until heart failure has become severe. Laboratory evidence of reduced cardiac output includes reduced venous oxygen tension in patients that are not hypoxaemic or anaemic as well as azotaemia and lactic acidosis if cardiac output is markedly decreased. (AF, PC, VMD)

ONSET OF CLINICAL SIGNS OF HEART FAILURE

Because horses are performance animals, exercise intolerance and fatigue are often the first clinical signs of cardiac disease. However, sedentary or unobserved horses with chronic heart failure may present initially with signs of congestion and oedema due to compensatory mechanisms that induce sodium and water retention. Patients with severe chronic heart failure may have signs of congestion and poor perfusion at rest although this is not common.

SECONDARY COMPENSATORY MECHANISMS

In an attempt to maintain circulatory homeostasis in animals with chronic heart failure, the body responds to a reduction in cardiac output by activation of several neuroendocrine compensatory mechanisms. These neuroendocrine systems include stimulation of the sympathetic nervous system, activation of the renin–angiotensin–aldosterone system, enhanced secretion of arginine vasopressin (antidiuretic hormone) and increased circulating levels of endothelin[1,2] (Chapter 2). The overall effects of these compensatory mechanisms are sodium retention, antidiuresis and vasoconstriction. Therefore, these neuroendocrine mechanisms are actually responsible for many clinical manifestations of the heart failure syndrome. Activation of neural and hormonal pathways also contributes to patient mortality by initiating several deleterious, self-perpetuating cycles:

(1) Venoconstriction and the antidiuresis augment the already increased ventricular filling pressures, thereby exacerbating circulatory congestion and increasing extravascular coronary resistance.

(2) Constriction of arterioles together with increased vascular stiffness from accumulation of Na+ and water in blood vessel walls increases outflow impedance which, in turn, reduces stroke volume and increases the myocardial oxygen demand.

The circulatory system is equipped with several counter-regulatory systems that also become activated in patients with CHF, and these counter-regulatory systems reduce or moderate the effects of the compensatory vasoconstrictor, antidiuretic and myocardial growth-promoting systems. Specifically, these systems include secretion of natriuretic peptides, increased production of vasodilating prostaglandins, stimulation of peripheral baroreceptor reflexes and increased myocardial synthesis of endothelium-derived relaxing factors (EDRF),[3] including endothelium-derived nitric oxide.

The prostaglandins PGE_2 and PGI_2 are endogenous vasodilators, and a three- to tenfold increase in circulating levels of these hormones has been documented in people with heart failure.[4] In fact, the magnitude of the elevation of these prostaglandins has been directly correlated to the circulating concentration of angiotensin II, suggesting that the body attempts to maintain circulatory homeostasis by balancing vasoconstrictor and dilator mechanisms. Any change in cardiac performance that increases atrial pressure will be detected by stretch receptors in the walls of the atria and ventricles producing a release of atrial natriuretic peptide (ANP) and brain natriuretic peptide from the atrial and ventricular myocytes, respectively.[5,6] Once released into the circulation, these peptide hormones exert potent direct vasodilator and natriuretic effects on the vasculature and kidneys. ANP and BNP also antagonize the effects of the renin–angiotensin–aldosterone system by suppressing the formation of renin and aldosterone.

Because the body has vasodilator, diuretic and anti-growth mechanisms acting systemically and locally (within the myocardium) to balance deleterious compensatory events, it would seem that circulatory homeostasis would be achieved and maintained. While it is believed that this balance of forces actually does occur in early, subclinical stages of heart failure, the balance of neuroendocrine and local forces apparently becomes disrupted during the development of overt symptomatic CHF.[3,7–10] Very early after the occurrence of a cardiac lesion, circulatory homeostasis is achieved as a result of normally functioning arterial and atrial baroreceptors, secretion of natriuretic peptides, and local production of prostaglandins and nitric oxide. During this early stage of heart failure, cardiac output is normally distributed, there is normal systemic vascular resistance and there is normal sodium balance as long as the patient is at rest. If cardiac function deteriorates, there is a greater decrease in renal perfusion and a greater increase in cardiac work, leading to excessive activation of the vasoconstrictive, antidiuretic and deleterious cardiac remodelling forces. Deleterious positive feedback cycles become initiated. With persistence of cardiac dysfunction and activation of deleterious self-perpetuating events, renal perfusion becomes so severely compromised that natriuretic peptides and prostaglandins become ineffective. Moreover, maladaptive structural changes that characterize ventricular remodelling (myocyte hypertrophy, myocyte necrosis, reparative and replacement fibrosis, apoptosis and myointimal proliferation) result from chronic angiotensin II, aldosterone excess, norepinephrine and, possibly, from cytokine production within the myocardium.[3,11–14] These structural changes further impair cardiac performance.

VENTRICULAR HYPERTROPHY

If cardiac disease is severe enough to cause a significant haemodynamic burden, the heart will hypertrophy in response to the increased workload. Concentric hypertrophy is the response of the myocardium to a chronic pressure overload. Concentric hypertrophy results in an increased wall thickness without ventricular dilation. This form of pathological hypertrophy is uncommon in horses because chronic pressure overload is unusual.

Eccentric hypertrophy is the response of the myocardium to a chronic volume overload and/or loss of contractility. Eccentric hypertrophy is hypertrophy with dilation of the affected chamber(s). This type of hypertrophy is frequently found in horses with valvular regurgitation and is one of the first changes to be noted in horses with significant valvular disease (see Chapter 4).

REFERENCES

1. Mann DL. Mechanisms and models in heart failure: a combinatorial approach. Circulation 1999;100: 999–1008.
2. McMarray J, Pfeffer MA. New therapeutic options in congestive heart failure. Circulation 2002;105: 2099–2227.
3. Dzau VJ. Autocrine and paracrine mechanisms in the pathophysiology of heart failure. Am J Cardiol 1992;70:4C–11C.
4. Dzau VJ, Packer M, Lilly LS. Prostaglandins in severe congestive heart failure. New Engl J Med 1984;310:347–352.
5. de Bold AJ, de Bold ML. Determinants of natriuretic peptide production by the heart: basic and clinical implications. J Invest Med 2005;53:371–377.
6. Pandey KN. Biology of natriuretic peptides and their receptors. Peptides 2005;26:901–932.
7. Packer M. Neurohormonal interactions and adaptations in congestive heart failure. Circulation 1988;77:721–730.
8. Katz AM. Cardiomyopathy of overload: a major determinant of prognosis in congestive heart failure. New Engl J Med 1990;332: 100–110.
9. Treasure CB, Vita JA, Cox DA. Endothelium-dependent dilatation of the coronary microvasculature is impaired in dilated cardiomyopathy. Circulation 1990;81:772–779.
10. Margulies KB, Hildebrand FL, Lerman A, et al. Increased endothelin in experimental heart failure. Circulation 1990;82: 2226–2230.
11. Weber KT, Brilla CG. Pathological hypertrophy and cardiac interstitium. Circulation 1991;83: 1849–1865.
12. Weber KT, Eghbali M. Collagen matrix synthesis and degradation in the development and regression of left ventricular hypertrophy. Cardiovasc Rev Rep 1991;12: 61–69.
13. Kapadia S, Dibbs Z, Kurrelmeyer K, et al. The role of cytokines in the failing human heart. Cardiol Clin 1998;16(4):645–656.
14. Narula J, Hajjar RJ, Dec GW. Apoptosis in the failing heart. Cardiol Clin 1998;16(4):691–710.

Chapter | 6 |

Electrophysiology and arrhythmogenesis

Gunther van Loon and Mark Patteson

CHAPTER CONTENTS

INTRODUCTION

Normal electrical excitation via the specialized conduction pathway within the heart is essential for coordinated myocardial contraction and relaxation. Control of the systemic homeostatic mechanisms alters heart rate in order to maintain an appropriate cardiac output, and may also affect cardiac rhythm. Recording of the depolarization and repolarization of excitable cells is the basis for understanding the electrophysiological properties of the heart which are required for normal cardiac function. Although our understanding of arrhythmogenesis is far from complete, a knowledge of the electrophysiology of cardiac cells is fundamental to an appreciation of the factors which lead to abnormal cardiac rhythm.

RECORDING ELECTRICAL EVENTS IN CELLS

The depolarization process can be detected at different levels by intracellular electrodes, intracardiac electrodes and by electrodes placed on the body surface.[1,2]

Intracellular electrodes have been used to demonstrate the potential difference across the cell membrane, and to record the change in this potential difference which occurs during depolarization and repolarization.[1] Using this method, it is possible to detect differences in transmembrane potentials in specialized tissues, to understand the differences and similarities in the electrophysiological properties of different tissues. Furthermore, it is possible to predict the changes in cell depolarization and repolarization which may result from altered electrolyte levels, drugs and, to some extent, myocardial disease.[1]

A method to obtain an approximation of the transmembrane voltage *in vivo* is to record the monophasic action potential (MAP)[3] (Fig. 6.1). Using a catheter with special electrodes at the tip, introduced transvenously into right atrium or right ventricle, the MAP can be recorded when the catheter tip makes close contact with the myocardium. The orientation of the catheter tip relative to the myocardium is important when interpreting the morphology of MAP recordings.[3] Therefore, it has been suggested that results of contact MAP recordings should only be used to determine action potential duration (APD).[4] Determination of the APD is a useful parameter to study the effect of drugs on cardiac electrophysiological characteristics.

Intracardiac electrodes have also been used to detect the depolarization and repolarization of each tissue in the conduction network and therefore to determine the timing and duration of the activation process. This technique was used to demonstrate the different depolarization processes in different species.[5] Intracardiac electrodes, introduced transvenously, provide a relatively easy way to record atrial and ventricular electrograms in horses (see Chapter 14).

The surface electrocardiogram (ECG) records the potential difference between selected points on the body surface. It allows us to detect changes in the electrical field which is built up around the heart during depolarization and

DOI: 10.1016/B978-0-7020-2817-5.00011-0

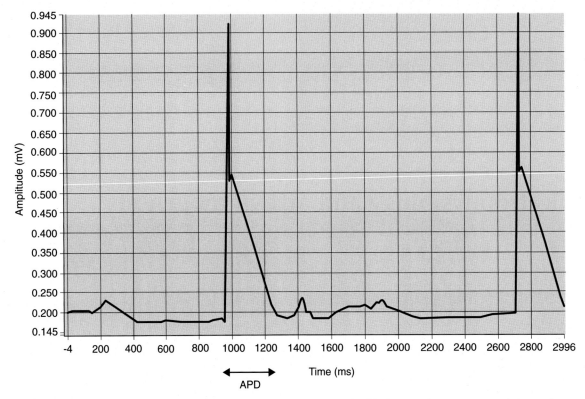

Figure 6.1 A right atrial monophasic action potential (MAP) recording in a healthy horse, using a transvenously inserted catheter, shows the action potential duration (APD).

repolarization. Although the body surface ECG depends on the sum of electrical forces and their conduction to the skin, it does allow clinicians to determine the heart rhythm and, with experience built up over many years of studies, to identify certain disease processes that are associated with specific ECG changes.[6]

CELLULAR PHYSIOLOGY

All myocytes possess the properties of excitability, refractoriness and conductivity.[6] Like nervous tissue, individual cardiac cells exhibit the all-or-none phenomenon – that is once threshold is reached they are completely activated by an action potential. The cells can therefore be described as *excitable*. Once the action potential is initiated, cells cannot be depolarized again until they have returned to the resting potential following repolarization. This property of *refractoriness* ensures that all cardiac cells have a period after activation during which no level of further stimulus will cause an action potential. This prevents heart muscle developing a tetanic spasm, which would prevent relaxation and filling of the chambers, and helps to maintain an organized pattern of depolarization. Myocytes also possess

the ability to *conduct* a stimulus for depolarization to their neighbours. Atrial and ventricular myocytes form two syncytia within which excitation passes from cell to cell through intercalated discs. Other tissues within the heart have specialized conductivity properties so that they conduct the impulse along a network either slowly (atrioventricular node) or rapidly (e.g. Purkinje fibres). While the atrial and ventricular myocytes have *contractile* function, the cells of the specialized conducting network have no contractile protein.

The electrophysiological features of myocytes result from specific properties of the cardiac cell membrane.[1] Like all living cells, the inside of cardiac cells has a negative electrical charge compared to the outside of cells due to an accumulation of negatively charged ions. This voltage difference across the cell membrane is called the transmembrane potential, which is about −80 to −90 mV. All cells have a very high intracellular concentration of potassium and low levels of sodium and calcium. For most cells this situation remains unaltered throughout their lives. However, excitable cells like cardiac cells have tiny pores or channels in the cell membrane. Upon appropriate stimulation, these channels open and close in a predefined way to allow specific ions to move across the cell membrane. This movement of ions results in changes

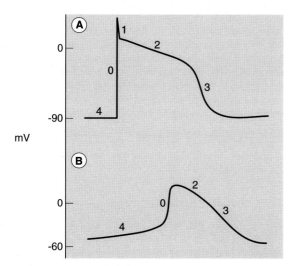

Figure 6.2 Diagrammatic representations of the phases of the action potential in ventricular myocardial cells (**A**) and pacemaker cells (**B**). In the ventricular myocardial cell, the resting potential (–90 mV) is greater than that of the pacemaker cell (–60 mV). The depolarization phase (phase 0) is faster in ventricular cells where it is carried by inward movement of sodium ions compared to the pacemaker cells where it is due to movement of calcium ions. Phase 4 is steepest in pacemaker cells, increasing the rate of automaticity.

in the transmembrane potential, from –90 mV to about +20 mV (depolarization), and finally back to –90 mV (repolarization). A graphical presentation of these changes in transmembrane potential is known as the action potential (Fig. 6.2). The currents, and thus the morphology of the action potential, vary in different tissues and determine the different properties of each specialized cell. Also, changes in extracellular ion concentrations, disease and drugs may influence the action potential of the cells.[1]

The action potential can be divided into five phases, 0–4[1,6] (see Fig. 6.2). However, it is more practical to consider the action potential in terms of three general phases: depolarization, repolarization and resting phase.

Depolarization

Phase 0 represents the depolarization process, and begins once a cell has reached a certain potential (the *threshold potential*), spontaneously in the case of pacemaker cells or as a result of depolarization of adjacent cells in the case of conduction pathway and myocardial cells. The upstroke of the cardiac action potential in atrial and ventricular muscle and His-Purkinje fibres is due to a sudden increase in membrane conductance to Na$^+$, resulting in a massive Na$^+$ influx into the cell. The rate at which the depolarization occurs (slope of phase 0) is a determinant of the conduction velocity for the propagated action potential.

In the slower conducting pacemaker tissues of the sinoatrial (SA) and atrioventricular (AV) nodes, the resting potential of the cell membrane is less negative (around –60 mV) than in nonpacemaker cells. This results in a decreased rate of phase 0 depolarization and relatively slow conduction in pacemaker tissues.[1] In these cells, the contribution of the fast inward current usually carried by sodium is small, and the relatively slow depolarization process is largely due to movement of calcium ions. Consequently, these tissues are relatively sensitive to changes in calcium concentration.[1]

Repolarization

Once a cell is depolarized, it cannot be depolarized again until the cell has first recovered by restoring the initial ion gradients and thus by regaining its polarized state. This recovery process is called the repolarization process and roughly corresponds to phases 1–3 of the action potential. Because during these phases the cell cannot be excited again, this period is called the refractory period and corresponds to the width of the action potential. Consequently, cardiac myocytes do not undergo contraction (i.e. tonic contraction). Although tonic contraction is indeed very important for the normal physiology of skeletal muscle, it would have fatal consequences if it were present in the heart.

The repolarization phase starts with the early rapid repolarization phase (*phase 1*) which shows as a relatively small but sharp drop in potential towards 0 mV, partly owing to inactivation of sodium current or activation of an outward potassium current.

This phase is immediately followed by the plateau phase (*phase 2*) which may last several hundred of milliseconds. During this period, membrane conductance to all ions falls to rather low values, with a complex interaction of ion movements involving sodium, potassium, magnesium and chloride, and in particular an inward L-type calcium current. These channels, especially the latter, interrupt the repolarization process and prolong the action potential. As such, the action potential duration (APD), and therefore the refractory period, is predominantly determined by the balance between the inward and outward currents during the plateau phase, which have a very important role in the generation of some arrhythmias.[7–9]

After the plateau phase, the final rapid repolarization (*phase 3*) takes place due to a series of potassium currents out of the cell. In order to maintain the concentration gradients, sodium is pumped out of the cell in exchange for potassium, resulting in a return of the membrane potential towards the resting level (*phase 4*).[1,6] During this final recovery process, the cardiac myocyte gradually regains excitability. This means that the cell is not excitable during phase 1, phase 2 and the beginning of phase 3, regardless of the magnitude of the stimulating impulse.

This period is called the absolute refractory period (ARP). As the cell repolarizes, it once again becomes excitable. However, there is a period of time during which the cell can only be excited by a large current. This period is known as the relatively refractory period (RRP).[10]

Resting phase or diastolic depolarization

Under normal conditions, membrane potential of atrial and ventricular muscle cells remains steady at around −90 mV throughout diastole (*phase 4*). However, in certain specialized conducting cells or due to leakage of ions across the cell membrane, the resting membrane potential does not remain constant in diastole but gradually depolarizes. This spontaneous diastolic depolarization may reach threshold potential (around −60 mV) by itself and produce an action potential, a characteristic called *automaticity*.[6] The rate of this change in potential is mainly determined by a time-related change in membrane potassium or sodium permeability. It is influenced by autonomic tone, electrolytes, drugs and disease. The steeper the slope of phase 4, the faster the rate of automaticity. Phase 4 is steepest in SA nodal cells. However, the AV node and junctional tissue also have automaticity and will take over as pacemaker if the SA node fails to depolarize. In some disease states, Purkinje tissue may also act as a pacemaker, and abnormal automaticity may occur in other cells.[7,8] The action potentials of a ventricular and pacemaker cell, showing phases 0–4, are shown in Figure 6.2. Compared to the action potential of a ventricular or Purkinje fibre cell, the sinoatrial and atrioventricular nodal cells have a slow depolarization phase (phase 0). This slower depolarization phase occurs because of a lack of rapid sodium channels responsible for the rapid depolarization phase. The sinoatrial and atrioventricular nodes are mainly dependent on the slow calcium channel for depolarization. Because of the slower rate of depolarization, the sinoatrial and atrioventricular nodes conduct electrical pulses slowly. For the atrioventricular node this slow conduction is reflected on the surface ECG as the PR interval.

Innervation of the heart

The cardiovascular system is under the control of both neuronal and humoral components of the autonomic nervous system, acting both on the heart and on the peripheral vasculature.

The heart is innervated by the sympathetic and the parasympathetic nervous system. Parasympathetic fibres are carried in the vagus nerve and their discharge results in a depressed automaticity (slower heart rate), decreased conduction velocity and increased refractory period. This effect is mediated by the release of acetylcholine at nerve endings, which affects the membrane potential of pacemaker cells,[6] particularly in the SA node and, in horses, in the AV node. The sympathetic nervous system acts on the heart via the release of adrenaline and noradrenaline. This results in an increased automaticity, an increased conduction velocity, a shortened refractory period (cells recover more quickly and permit a higher rate of stimulation) and an increased myocardial contractility. The subcellular effect of these hormones is largely due to effects on contractile proteins; however, they also affect transmembrane potentials and alter cardiac rhythm in some circumstances.[8,11]

The conduction process

The conduction process follows a predictable pathway in the normal heart, leading to a coordinated contraction of atrial and then ventricular muscle (Fig. 6.3). An impulse spreads from the SA node, across the atria, to the AV node. Conduction occurs along specialized fibres (internodal tracts); however, the impulse also leads to contraction of atrial muscle. The electrical activity associated with depolarization of this muscle mass results in a sufficiently large electrical field for it to be detected on a body surface ECG as a *P wave* (see Fig. 6.3A). The precise location of impulse formation within the SA node and the pattern of depolarization across the atria can be influenced by heart rate and autonomic tone, which can result in a different configuration of P waves (wandering pacemaker) even though the SA node remains the source of the impulse.[12]

When the impulse reaches the AV junction it finds a barrier to further spread. The specialized cells of the AV node conduct the impulse slowly. Because only a small number of cells are depolarized, no deflection is seen on the surface ECG. This period is represented by the *P–R interval* (see Fig. 6.3B). Conduction through the AV node is profoundly affected by vagal tone in the horse. Even in normal animals, conduction is often sufficiently slowed or reduced in amplitude to result in a marked reduction in the normal rate of conduction (first-degree AV block), or complete abolition of further spread of the impulse (second-degree AV block).[13] (AR, EA)

When the impulse passes through the AV node it is rapidly conducted through the bundle of His and the Purkinje network to the ventricular myocardium. Depolarization of the ventricles is rapid and results in a coordinated contraction. Depolarization of the Purkinje network is not detected on the body surface ECG; however, depolarization of the myocardium results in substantial electrical forces, the net result of which produce the *QRS complex* on the surface ECG (Fig. 6.3C).

Each cell within the heart repolarizes after depolarization. The sum of the repolarization processes within the heart can be detected at the body surface in the same way as the electromotive forces of depolarization. Ventricular

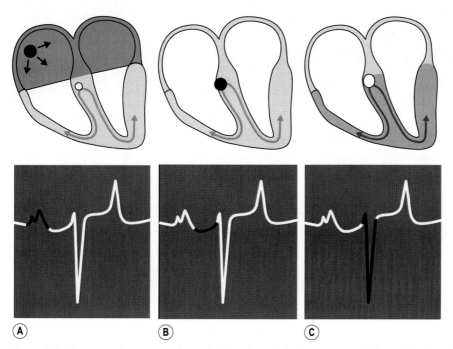

Figure 6.3 Diagrammatic representations of the cardiac conduction system and the relationship of the spread of conduction to the surface ECG. (**A**) Conduction is initiated in the pacemaker within the right atrium and spreads through the atria, represented by the P wave. (**B**) Conduction is delayed at the atrioventricular node, represented by the P–R interval. (**C**) The wave of depolarization is rapidly conducted through the bundle of His and Purkinje network, represented by the QRS complex. Subsequent ventricular repolarization is represented by the T wave.

repolarization is seen as the *T wave*. The change in electrical field caused by atrial repolarization (atrial T wave or Ta wave) may or may not be seen.[6]

In conclusion, deflections on the surface ECG are caused by atrial or ventricular myocardial depolarization. Depolarization of the sinus node or atrioventricular node does not result in any deflection. The slow conduction through the atrioventricular node produces the (flat) PR interval. Identification of the characteristic waveforms allows a clinician to detect when depolarization and repolarization of the atria and ventricles has occurred. The timing of the waves, the relation between the different waves, and the morphology and duration of the complexes and intervals allows deduction of the origin and conduction pathway of the impulse (see Fig. 6.3).

The cardiac electrical field

During the depolarization and repolarization processes, different currents are flowing across the cell membrane at various points, and a potential difference will be present between one part of the cell and another. When current is *flowing*, an external electrical field is set up around the cell, which can be described as acting as a dipole.[6] However, when the cell is depolarized, or repolarized at a resting potential, no electrical field is formed around the cell

because no current is flowing, despite the potential difference between the inside and outside of the cell. Each myocyte forms its own electrical field, but the electrical effects summate to produce an electrical field around the whole heart which, in simplified terms, can then be regarded as a single dipole.[6]

RECORDING OF CARDIAC ELECTRICAL ACTIVITY

The surface ECG

The changes in the electrical field around the heart can be detected by a galvanometer attached to the body surface, which records the potential difference between two electrodes. The link between a positive and negative electrode is called a bipolar lead. An ECG records the potential difference between electrodes placed at various points on the body surface, which reflects the sum of all the electrical fields which are present at any one time. The points at which the ECG electrodes are placed are chosen to represent electrical changes in the heart; however, a number of other factors also affect the potential difference between different areas of the body. The position of the heart

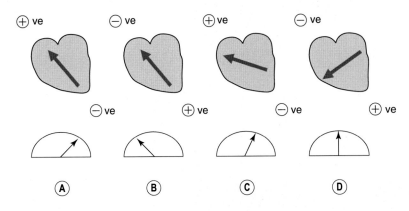

Figure 6.4 Diagrams of vectors of depolarization. (**A**) If current is flowing towards the positive electrode a positive deflection is seen on the ECG. (**B**) If the vector is directed away from the positive electrode a negative deflection is recorded. (**C**) If the current flows along an axis which is oblique to the positive electrode but towards it, a smaller positive deflection is detected. (**D**) If the vector of depolarization is perpendicular to the axis of the electrodes there is no deflection recorded.

within the body, the course of the spread of activation within the heart, the shape of the thorax, the conductivity of tissues between the heart and the electrodes, and the exact location of the body surface electrodes all affect the body surface ECG.[12,13]

The concept of cardiac vector

The surface ECG reflects the combined effects of all the electrical activity of the heart. The sum of the electromotive forces has a direction and magnitude, which is termed the cardiac vector. The ECG voltmeter will have a positive deflection if the net direction of overall activity (vector) is towards the positive electrode of a bipolar lead, and a negative potential if it is away from it (Fig. 6.4). The voltage recorded will be largest when the vector is directly towards the positive electrode. If the direction of the maximum potential difference is at an angle to the lead axis, the deflection will be smaller. If the electrodes are positioned perpendicular to the vector of electromotive force, no potential difference will be detected. The amplitude of the deflection indicates the magnitude of the vector and is proportional to the mass of myocardial tissue which is depolarized.

ECG lead systems

Over the years, a number of lead systems have been developed to record the cardiac electrical field.[6,12,13] (Fig. 6.5). The aim of these systems is to clearly record each of the waveforms and complexes so that the conduction process can be evaluated, and also to gain some information about the direction and magnitude of the cardiac vector. Einthoven's triangle is a lead system that looks at the combined electrical activity which reaches the body surface in the frontal plane, in which the heart is assumed to sit in the centre of a triangle formed by the two forelimbs and the left hind limb.[6] This system, which is commonly used in small animals and humans, can also be used in horses, and provides useful information about

cardiac rhythm and conduction. Other systems have also been designed to accommodate the fact that, in horses, the heart does not sit in the centre of a triangle formed by the limbs. These systems assess the cardiac vector in three dimensions by measuring the electrical field in three semiorthogonal planes.[12,13]

Standard bipolar leads are recorded as follows: lead I is between the left arm electrode (−) and the right arm electrode (+); lead II is between the right arm electrode (−) and the left foot electrode (+) and lead III is between the left arm electrode (−) and the left foot electrode (+). For the augmented unipolar leads the positive exploring electrode (right arm for aV$_R$; left arm for aV$_L$ and left leg for aV$_F$) is compared with the remaining two electrodes (−).

The base-apex lead (see Fig. 6.5) is most frequently used for recording rhythm strips. To record a base-apex lead the left arm electrode (+) is positioned at the cardiac apex, and the right arm electrode (−) is placed two thirds of the way down the right jugular groove or at the top of the right scapular spine. The third electrode is placed at any site remote from the heart. Lead 1 is selected to record the ECG.

For the Y lead the right arm electrode (−) is attached over the *manubrium sterni* and the left arm electrode (+) over the xiphoid process of the sternum. The third electrode is placed at any site remote from the heart. Lead 1 is selected to record the ECG.

Durations of the ECG components in normal horses are listed in Table 6.1.

The ventricular depolarization process

It is very important to realize that the ventricular depolarization process is different in horses compared with human beings and small animals.[5,14,15] In human beings and small animals, the Purkinje network carries the impulse to the subendocardial myocardium, and depolarization then spreads out from the ends of the fibres, through the

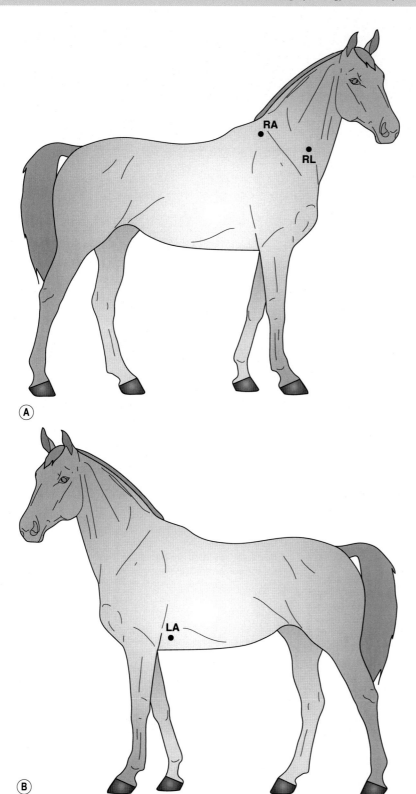

Figure 6.5 Sites for lead placement for obtaining a base-apex electrocardiogram (**A, B**) in a horse. The black circles represent the site of attachment for the electrodes. (**A**) Position of the electrode placement on the right side of the horse for obtaining a base-apex ECG using the electrodes from lead I. RA, right arm; RL, right leg. (**B**) Position of the electrode placement on the left side of the horse for obtaining a base-apex ECG using the electrodes from lead I. LA, left arm.

Table 6.1 Durations of electrocardiographic complexes and intervals in the base-apex lead in normal horses

	DURATION (S)	NO. OF SMALL BOXES (PAPER SPEED 25 MM/S)
P wave	≤0.16	<4
P–R interval	≤0.5	12.5
QRS complex	≤0.14	3.5
Q–T interval	≤0.6	15

myocardium, to the subepicardial layers in a series of wavefronts.[5] Because the left ventricle is the most substantial muscle mass in the normal animal, the sum of the electromotive force is primarily directed towards the left apex, resulting in a large R wave in lead II.[6] The main cardiac vector is altered when there is considerable change in the relative proportions of the left and right ventricles. The changes can be simplified into an average of the cardiac vector in the frontal plane known as the mean electrical axis (MEA).[6] In human beings and small animals, the duration of the QRS complex may be prolonged when the left ventricle is enlarged, because the wavefront takes longer to spread throughout the myocardium.[6] The amplitude of the R wave in lead II may also be increased as a result of the increased muscle mass.[6] However, although ECG changes are relatively specific for enlargement of the left or right ventricles, they are relatively insensitive.

In the horse, the depolarization process differs from that described above because of the very widespread distribution of the Purkinje network.[5,16] The fibres extend throughout the myocardium, and ventricular activation takes place from multiple sites. The electromotive forces therefore tend to cancel each other out and, consequently, no wavefronts are formed. Because the surface ECG represents the sum of the electromotive forces within the heart, the overall effect of the depolarization of most of the left and right ventricles on the ECG is minimal. Most electrical activity seen at the body surface results from depolarization of the basal interventricular septum and part of the left ventricular free-wall.[5] A wavefront spreading towards the heart base is responsible for this last part of ventricular activation, so the cardiac vector is directed dorsally and cranially with respect to the body surface. Frontal plane MEA or the cardiac vector in the orthogonal systems are therefore of very limited value in horses.[17] In addition, the duration of the QRS complex does not depend on the spread of a wavefront across the ventricles, and is therefore not necessarily related to their size.[14] Equine ECGs still give useful information about heart rate and rhythm, but provide very little or no information about the relative or absolute sizes of the ventricles.[17]

Intracavitary electrogram recording

Intracardiac electrograms of right atrium and ventricle can be recorded using a temporary pacing catheter (or permanently implanted lead in case of pacemaker implantation), introduced via the jugular vein, with one or multiple electrodes located at the catheter tip. Once the electrode is entered in the atrium or ventricle, atrial and ventricular electrograms can be recorded. The technique is discussed in more detail in Chapter 14.

CLASSIFICATION AND MECHANISMS OF DYSRHYTHMOGENESIS

Dysrhythmias are classified according to the cardiac structure in which they originate, their rate, and the mechanism responsible for their production. Arrhythmogenesis can be defined either as abnormal impulse generation or as abnormal conduction of the impulse from the SA node.

The mechanism by which arrhythmias are generated is a field of active research in human medicine, and greater understanding of their "electropathogenesis" should help in directing treatment. In general terms, arrhythmias can develop as a result of damage to a few localized cells which act as a focus of abnormal depolarization, or which affect specialized cells within the conduction pathway, or may affect most myocytes.[7,8] Whatever the form of damage (cell death, fibrosis, ischaemia, hypoxia), there are likely to be changes in the membrane properties which govern the electrophysiology of the cells.[1] The active function of the cell membrane in maintaining electrolyte balance inside and outside the cells is reduced, resulting in a reduced negative resting potential, a slow phase 0 depolarization action potential and a reduced duration of the plateau phase.[7,8] The significance of these effects depends on which cells are affected, and any drugs or electrolyte abnormalities which are present at the same time. In addition, the autonomic nervous system may have an effect on normal and abnormal rhythms.

In horses, some arrhythmias are common in normal animals because of the high vagal (parasympathetic) tone in this species.[17] Therefore arrhythmias must also be distinguished as being due to normal variation in autonomic tone ("physiological" arrhythmias), or as arrhythmias which occur because of valvular, myocardial or systemic disease. (AF, AR, EA, SFP, VMD, VT)

Failure of impulse generation

Failure of sinoatrial nodal automaticity, resulting in an insufficient number of impulses emanating from the sinoatrial node, results in bradyarrhythmias. Symptoms occur when the resultant heart rate is insufficient to meet the body's demands. If sinus slowing is profound, subsidiary pacemakers can take over the pacemaker function of the sinus node.

Conduction disturbances

Although it is intuitive that conduction block can cause bradyarrhythmias, conduction abnormalities are also important in the generation of tachyarrhythmias.[7,8,18–23] Conduction disturbances can be functional or structural in origin. In either case, the conduction velocity of the myocardium is affected by the amplitude of the action potential, the rate of phase 0 depolarization, the threshold potential and internal and external electrical conductances.[7,8,18–20] These combine to affect the cable properties of the myocardium, and the electrotonic currents that propagate the impulse, which are the key determinants of conduction velocity. Although these properties are different from the ionic fluxes across the cell membrane that result in the action potential, they are dependent on them.[18–20]

Areas of slow conduction are common where myocytes are affected by disease, electrolyte abnormalities, drugs and toxins. Frequently the slow conduction results in cells being partially depolarized. The action potential of affected ventricular and atrial cells becomes similar to pacemaker cells under such conditions.[20] Once an impulse emerges from an area of slow conduction, normal propagation occurs. This means that there is heterogeneity of myocyte depolarization, and the wavefront effect of a propagating impulse within the atria or ventricles is lost. On occasions an impulse is completely blocked. However, the block may last a short period and later the tissue becomes able to be depolarized once more, or the block may be unidirectional. Unidirectional block is a normal phenomenon at the AV node; however, if it occurs within the atria or ventricles it can lead to the development of re-entry circuits (see below).[7,8,20,21] Slowed conduction can be both physiological and pathological and can result both in bradyarrhythmias and tachyarrhythmias.

Bradyarrhythmias

The SA and AV nodes are the most sensitive areas to (physiological) functional block because the speed of conduction is largely dependent on calcium channel currents.[1] Parasympathetic tone inhibits calcium channel opening and reduces the speed of conduction, while β-adrenergic agonists increase these currents. The release of acetylcholine from parasympathetic nerve endings at the SA node also affects potassium ion channels resulting in hyperpolarization of the tissues, and release of inhibitory factors which reduce the inward pacemaker current and slow conduction.

Functional block resulting in bradyarrhythmias is common in horses because of high vagal tone. If SA node discharge is affected, they result in sinus bradycardia, sinus

block or arrest. The distinction between block and arrest is largely academic because it is unclear whether an impulse is formed but fails to escape from the node or whether its formation is depressed. In horses, increased vagal tone results in a delay in conduction through the AV node much more commonly than it causes sinus bradycardia. A variation in the P–R interval is so common that it is difficult to define first-degree AV block. However, second-degree AV block is found in around 20% of horses, and is probably more common than this in undisturbed animals.[17] It has been shown that when arterial blood pressure reaches a certain level an episode of second-degree AV block may occur.[24] The blocked beat results in a reduction in arterial pressure, followed by a gradual increase in the arterial pressure with each subsequent beat until the same maximum pressure level is reached and second-degree AV block occurs again. This "staircase effect" appears to be a normal homeostatic mechanism to control blood pressure. (AF, AR, EA, RSD, VSD)

Variation in vagal tone can also cause sinus arrhythmia, in which there is a cyclical alteration in sinus rate, or a wandering pacemaker, when the exact site of formation of the impulse in the SA node and/or its conduction through the atria varies, altering P wave morphology. Sinus arrhythmia is not very common at rest, but is frequently found during the recovery period after exercise when there is a change from sympathetic to vagal tone.[17] Extreme postexercise bradycardia and syncope has been reported in a horse and was treated with the implantation of a dual-chamber rate-adaptive pacemaker.[25]

Structural abnormalities affecting conduction through the AV node and major conduction pathways are rare in horses. Third-degree AV block has been reported rarely[26,27] and the precise cause is seldom identified. Bundle branch block is extremely uncommon and may also be difficult to recognize in horses due to their ventricular depolarization pattern.

Tachyarrhythmias

The normal conduction network relies on predictable patterns of depolarization and repolarization, which ensures that the impulse dies out once it reaches the epicardium and that a new sinus impulse is required to cause another ventricular depolarization. This relies on wavefronts meeting in ventricular myocardium and being surrounded by refractory tissue. Localized abnormalities in conduction velocity can result in re-entry mechanisms which are responsible for many supraventricular and ventricular tachyarrhythmias.[7,8,22,23] The development of a re-entry circuit requires areas of slow conduction and unidirectional block (Fig. 6.6). The unidirectional block allows a circuit loop to develop, and slow conduction allows an impulse to take a long time to reach isolated areas of tissue which have had time to cease to be refractory. The area of conduction abnormality will seldom be uniformly spread

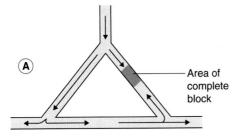

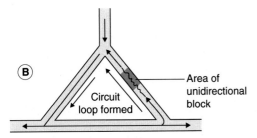

Figure 6.6 A Schmitt/Erlanger diagram of re-entry. (**A**) An area of complete block prevents a circuit loop developing. (**B**) If a portion of myocardium has slow conduction it can be refractory to an initial stimulus, but has become able to be depolarized by the time an impulse is conducted to it via another route (unidirectional block), allowing a re-entry circuit to develop.

through the myocardium. Classically, re-entry pathways can be formed where the Purkinje fibres meet myocardial cells. Branching fibres insert along the length of the myocardial cells, so if an area of unidirectional block exists at a critical site it is possible for an impulse to circle around the anatomical loop (see Fig. 6.6). The same mechanism is thought to occur in many species. This may result in a premature depolarization following a sinus beat, or if the circuit persists it can cause tachycardias. In some cases the formation of the re-entry circuit is dependent on the timing of the initiating impulse. Sinus beats may allow sufficient time for repolarization of all the tissue in the loop and elimination of the area of block; however, a premature depolarization may initiate the re-entry mechanism because some cells are still refractory.[7,8]

A similar form of re-entry can result from a wide variation of states of refractoriness within the atrial or ventricular syncytium, in cells with normal diastolic potentials and rapid rates of depolarization. The properties of unidirectional block and slow conduction in this instance result from an inhomogeneity of refractoriness.[8] When atrial cells in close proximity have different refractory periods, a premature impulse can be conducted through the cells with short different refractory periods, but not through those with a long different refractory period. The impulse can loop round in a circle, so that when it reaches the

original starting point the cells have recovered their excitability and the impulse can be perpetuated.[7,8,21,28–30] The cells in the centre of the circle are continually partially depolarized and fail to generate full action potentials. The larger the syncytium and the greater the variability of refractoriness, the longer the conduction pathway and the more islands of cells with a long refractory period, the greater the chance of such a circus mechanism developing.[7,31,32]

Atrial fibrillation
(AF, VMD)

An example of the circus movement theory is the "electropathogenesis" of atrial fibrillation. An understanding of the mechanisms of atrial fibrillation is a good example of where an understanding of arrhythmogenesis is useful to clinicians and is applied to treatment.

Under normal conditions, each atrial depolarization is generated by the sinus node and conducted towards the atrioventricular node. The period of refractoriness following each depolarization wave prevents the wave from "turning back" towards the sinus node so that it obligatorily ends at the atrioventricular node. Under certain circumstances, important spatial differences in refractoriness occur, creating regions of slow conduction and unidirectional block. These allow the depolarization wave to find a pathway to "loop back", forming a circus (re-entry). Such a re-entry loop (Fig. 6.7) can be drawn as a depolarization wave (black arrow) with a depolarization front (arrow head) that makes a circus movement. At the end of the depolarization wave tissue gradually recovers (grey area) until it has regained full polarization (white area). As such, the white area between head and tail consists of excitable tissue, the "excitable gap". The depolarization wave will continue to turn around as long as the head doesn't hit the tail, i.e. as long as a small excitable gap is present. Whether or not such a re-entry loop "fits" in the atria and continues to turn around, or whether it hits the tail and terminates spontaneously, depends on the substrate, i.e. the atria, and on the size of the loop. Re-entry will persist more easily in large or structurally abnormal (fibrosis) atria and also when the re-entry loop itself is small. The anatomical size or path length (PL) of the loop is defined by the wavelength (WL) of the depolarization wave (length of the arrow) and a small region of excitable tissue (white area), the (spatial) excitable gap (EG). Therefore, PL = WL + EG. The PL of the depolarization wave is the distance the wavefront travels during the refractory period and depends on the conduction velocity (CV) and the duration of the refractory period (RP) of the myocardium. Therefore, WL = CV × RP. The re-entry loop can also be described on a timely based manner. The time it takes for the re-entry loop to make one rotation is the cycle length (CL) which is determined by the refractory period (RP) and a (temporal) excitable period (EP), thus, CL = RP + EP.

Re-entry will persist more easily when the re-entry loop itself is small. A decrease in the size of the loop occurs when CV is slow and/or RP is short (the tissue recovers more quickly).

When only one re-entry loop continuously turns around over a fixed pathway through the atria, it is called *atrial flutter*. The surface ECG shows a saw-toothed pattern, where each undulation represents a rotation of the

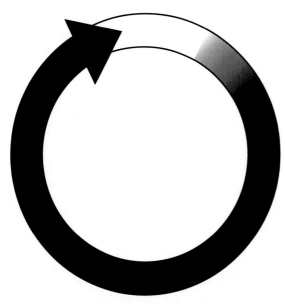

Figure 6.7 Schematic drawing of a re-entry loop. After passing of the depolarization wave front (arrow head), the myocardial tissue is brought in a refractory state (black) for a time equal to the refractory period of that tissue. After that, tissue gradually recovers (grey) until it has regained full excitability (white). The re-entry loop can only propagate when a small area of excitable tissue (excitable gap) precedes the depolarization wave front.

depolarization wave, usually at a rate of 170–250/minute (Fig. 6.8).

During *atrial fibrillation*, multiple atrial re-entry wavelets are present at the same time and meander in a chaotic manner through the atria. Measuring the focal atrial electrical activity usually shows 270–475 depolarizations per minute, which corresponds to an atrial fibrillation cycle length (AFCL) of 220–125 ms (Fig. 6.9). On the one hand some waves might die out because of merging with other waves, meeting refractory tissue or terminating at the atrial borders. On the other hand, new waves will emerge because of fragmentation at anatomical or functional obstacles. As such, there is a continuous variation in the number of waves that coexist in the atria. When the atria contain only a small number of waves, these waves might all terminate at the same time, which means spontaneous conversion to sinus rhythm (paroxysmal atrial fibrillation). When a large number of fibrillation waves are present (due to large atria, slow conduction and/or short refractory period) atrial fibrillation is not likely to convert spontaneously because of the small statistical chance that all waves die out simultaneously (sustained atrial fibrillation). Depending on the reaction to treatment, sustained AF might be further subdivided into permanent AF (can only be terminated with treatment) or persistent AF (cannot be terminated at all despite treatment).[33]

Over the past decades, the multiple re-entry model has been the main mechanism to explain AF in different animal models.[34] However, one observation incompatible with this theory is the response of AF to anti-arrhythmic drugs that block Na+ channels. Such medication is often effective in terminating AF, but should theoretically promote AF because it decreases conduction velocity and thereby decreases wavelength. Recent observations in sheep suggest that single small re-entry circuits or spiral waves, or an ectopic focus, especially in the left atrium, are important to trigger and maintain AF.[35]

Horses are particularly predisposed to the development of atrial fibrillation in normal atrial tissue ("lone" atrial fibrillation) because they have a large syncytium of atrial cells, and because vagal tone results in a relative

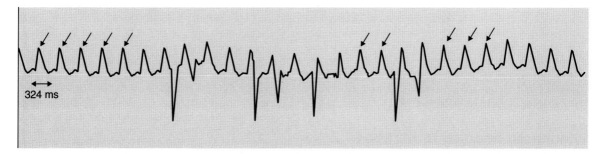

Figure 6.8 In this horse with atrial flutter, saw-toothed flutter waves (arrows) appear at a rate of 185/minute (324-ms interval). Conduction to the ventricle was irregular but ventricular rate was normal.

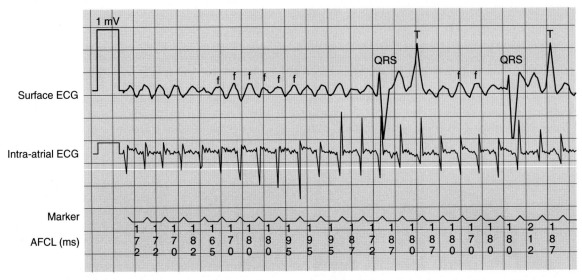

Figure 6.9 Simultaneous recording of the surface ECG (upper trace), with fibrillation waves (f), and the intra-atrial electrogram (middle trace) in a horse with lone atrial fibrillation. On the lower trace markers indicate every intra-atrial depolarization and allow calculation of the instantaneous atrial fibrillation cycle length (AFCL) (ms).

inhomogeneity of refractoriness within the atrium.[36,37] This gives the chance for the re-entry mechanism described above to develop. In other species, and in ponies, atrial fibrillation usually only occurs in the presence of atrial myocardial disease, differences in refractoriness and conduction velocity within different groups of cells, and an increased likelihood of premature depolarizations which could initiate fibrillation. In horses, there is high vagal tone, the atria are relatively large and there are often islands of relatively refractory tissue even within the normal atrium.[37] The effect of atrial size has been illustrated in an experiment in which clamping of the atrial appendage reduced effective atrial mass and resulted in atrial fibrillation converting to sinus rhythm.[38] Also, in horses and ponies, susceptibility to experimentally induced AF has been shown to be related to atrial size.[39,40] The effects of high vagal tone are illustrated by experiments in which atrial fibrillation is maintained in isolated atrial myocardial preparations only in the presence of acetylcholine.[36,41,42] The effects of vagal tone are more marked in some cells than others, resulting in groups of cells with different refractory periods.[36] In life, the marked inhomogeneity of refractoriness of atrial tissue, especially immediately after a premature beat, provides the necessary electrophysiological medium for the development of atrial fibrillation if an initiating premature beat occurs even in the absence of underlying disease.[28,31,37]

Enhanced impulse formation

Ectopic foci arise when cells outside the pacemaker centres develop membrane characteristics which are similar to those of pacemaker cells. This may take the form of abnormal automaticity when there is spontaneous impulse generation from a discrete site, without prior activation of the site, or of triggered rhythms which occur only if activated by one or more impulses from outside the ectopic focus.[7,8,19-21]

Abnormal automaticity

The automaticity of the heart is referred to as the heart's normal pacemaker function and is the result of phase 4 activity which leads to spontaneous depolarization. Usually the SA node is the dominant pacemaker because it has the fastest rate of automaticity. However, other sites within the atria, AV node, junctional tissue, Purkinje fibres or ventricles, which normally have a high negative resting potential (−90 mV), may start showing abnormal acceleration of phase 4 resulting in automatic tachycardia. Such abnormal automaticity occurs in cells with abnormal membrane potentials (around −55 mV).[43] The different membrane potential is due to alteration in the properties of the channels and also affects the relative significance of different ion channels in contributing to the action potential, so that, for example, the inward calcium channel becomes more important.[43] This is a useful base from which to consider treatment to reduce the discharge of these abnormal foci.

Similar to the normal sinus tachycardia, automatic tachycardias often display an increase and decrease in rate when the arrhythmia starts and ends. Also similar to sinus tachycardia, automatic tachycardia often has metabolic causes, such as hypokalaemia, hypomagnesaemia, acid–

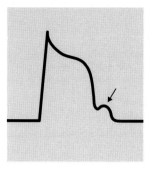

Figure 6.10 Schematic drawing of an early afterdepolarization (arrow) which shows as a "bump" during phase 3 of the action potential.

base disorders, myocardial ischaemia, hypoxemia or a high sympathetic tone.

Triggered activity

Triggered beats occur from a discrete pacemaker site and are subdivided into those caused by early afterdepolarizations (or afterpotentials) and those due to late afterdepolarizations. Early or late afterdepolarizations occur as a "bump" during or after phase 3 of the action potential, respectively (Fig. 6.10), and are caused by excessively large inward currents carried by the Na^+/Ca^{2+} exchanger. If the afterdepolarization is of sufficient amplitude to engage the rapid sodium channels, another action potential can be generated. Triggered activity, like re-entry, can be induced by premature beats or by pacing techniques. Ectopic beats resulting from triggered activity differ from those from abnormal automaticity in that they are often exacerbated by fast heart rates (i.e. they are not overdrive suppressed) and that they can be very irregular and therefore lead to the development of "torsades de pointes" or ventricular fibrillation.[7,8] Digitalis-toxic arrhythmias are thought to be caused by triggered activity.

Specific causes of arrhythmias

Electrolyte abnormalities

Electrolyte abnormalities are an important cause of arrhythmias, and electrolyte levels should be checked in any animal with an unexplained arrhythmia. Horses which are exhausted, or which have severe gastrointestinal or renal disease, are most likely to have significant electrolyte imbalance.[44–47] In particular, abnormal levels of potassium, calcium, sodium and magnesium play an important role in the genesis of arrhythmias.

Hyperkalaemia

An increase in extracellular potassium decreases the amplitude of the action potential and the voltage of the plateau, shortens the plateau duration and accelerates the phase of rapid repolarization. It results in a less negative resting potential, bringing it closer to the threshold potential, which means that the strength of a stimulus needed to reduce the resting membrane potential to the threshold potential will be decreased (the tissue is more excitable). Most importantly, due to the reduced resting membrane potential, the rate of rise of phase 0, and therefore the conduction velocity, will be decreased. The slow depolarization during phase 4, which characterizes automatic cells, is diminished or completely abolished by hyperkalaemia. The effect is more marked in atrial myocytes than in ventricular myocytes and the sinoatrial node.[48,49] Hyperkalaemia might result in cardiac arrest, due to sinus node depression, depression of intra-atrial conduction and/or atrioventricular block, or ventricular fibrillation, due to re-entry because of the slowing of conduction.

Hypokalaemia

Hypokalaemia results in a more negative resting potential. The duration of phase 3 repolarization is increased, increasing the duration of the action potential. Hypokalaemia also results in increased levels of intracellular sodium and calcium. In the clinical setting, hypokalaemia results in a wide spectrum of atrial and ventricular ectopic rhythms. The ectopy is due to enhanced automaticity of latent pacemaker fibers.

The cardiac effects of hypermagnesaemia and hypomagnesaemia mimic those of hyperkalaemia and hypokalaemia, respectively; however, the mechanisms for this have not been clearly described.[49] In humans, magnesium treatment has been reported to prevent early afterdepolarizations induced by quinidine, providing a possible explanation for the demonstrated effectiveness of treatment with magnesium salts for torsades de pointes.[50]

Hypercalcaemia

Hypercalcaemia results in a small increase in QRS duration in human beings,[49] but the effect has not been seen in horses.[51] The duration of phase 2 is prolonged, and this may be reflected by a sinus bradycardia, sinus arrhythmia and AV block. These rhythms may also be due to hypertension during hypercalcaemia. Ventricular arrhythmias develop during marked hypercalcaemia. The cardiac effects of hypercalcaemia are partly dependent on potassium levels.[49]

Hypocalcaemia

Hypocalcaemia may be associated with decreased cardiac function and tachycardia but does not usually produce arrhythmias.

REFERENCES

1. Noble D. The Initiation of the Heart Beat. 2nd ed. Oxford: Oxford University Press; 1979.

2. Fish C. Electrocardiography and vector cardiography. In: Braunwald E, editor. Heart Disease: a Textbook of Cardiovascular Medicine. Philadelphia: WB Saunders; 1988. p. 180–222.

3. Kadish A. What is a monophasic action potential? Cardiovasc Res 2004;63(4):580–581.

4. Kondo M, Nesterenko V, Antzelevitch C. Cellular basis for the monophasic action potential: which electrode is the recording electrode? Cardiovasc Res 2004; 63(4):635–644.

5. Hamlin RL, Smith CR. Categorization of common domestic mammals based upon their ventricular activation process. Ann N Y Acad Sci 1965;127(1): 195–203.

6. Tilley LP. General principles of electrocardiography. In: Tilley LP, editor. Canine and Feline Electrophysiology. Philadelphia: Lea & Febiger; 1985. p. 19–54.

7. Boyden PA, Wit AL. Cellular electrophysiologic basis of cardiac arrhythmias. In: Tilley LP, editor. Canine and Feline Electrophysiology. Philadelphia: Lea & Febiger; 1985. p. 266–277.

8. Dangman KH, Boyden PA. Cellular Mechanisms of Cardiac Arrhythmias. In: Fox PR, editor. Canine and Feline Cardiology. New York: Churchill Livingstone; 1988. p. 269–287.

9. Nattel S. New Ideas about Atrial Fibrillation 50 Years on. Nature 2002;415(6868):219–226.

10. Jalife J, Delmar M, Anumonwo J, Berenfeld O. Basic Cardiac Electrophysiology for the Clinician. Armonk, NY.: Futura; 1999. p. 306.

11. Hamlin RL. Physiology. In: Fox PR, editor. Canine and Feline Cardiology. Churchill Livingstone: New York; 1986.

12. Hamlin RL, Smetzer DL, Smith CR. Analysis of QRS complex recorded through a semi-orthogonal system in the horse. Am JPhysiol 1964; 207:325–333.

13. Holmes JR, Darke PGG. Studies on the development of a new lead system for equine electrocardiography. Equine Vet J 1970;2:12–21.

14. Grauerholz H, Jaeschke G. Problems in Measurement and Estimation of the QRS-Duration in the ECG of the Horse. Berliner und Munchener Tierarztliche Wochenschrift 1986;99(11): 365–369.

15. Muylle E, Oyaert W. Equine electrocardiography: the genesis of the different configurations of the "QRS" complex. Zentralbl Veterinarmed A 1977;24(9): 762–771.

16. Meyling HA, TerBorgh H. The conducting system of the heart in hoofed animals. Cornell Veterinarian 1957;47:419–447.

17. Patteson MW. Equine Cardiology. Oxford: Blackwell Science; 1996. p. 254.

18. Cranefield PF, Wit AL, Hoffman BF. Genesis of Cardiac-Arrhythmias. Circulation 1973; 47(1):190–204.

19. Hoffman BF, Rosen MR. Cellular Mechanisms for Cardiac-Arrhythmias. Circul Res 1981; 49(1):1–15.

20. Zipes DP. Genesis of cardiac arrhythmias: electrophysiological considerations. In: Braunwald E, editor. Heart Disease. Philadelphia: W.B Saunders; 1992. p. 588–627.

21. Waldo AL, Wit AL. Mechanisms of Cardiac-Arrhythmias. Lancet 1993;341(8854):1189–1193.

22. Wit AL, Rosen MR, Hoffman BF. Electrophysiology and Pharmacology of Cardiac-Arrhythmias .2. Relationship of Normal and Abnormal Electrical-Activity of Cardiac Fibers to Genesis of Arrhythmias B Reentry .2. Am Heart J 1974;88(6): 798–806.

23. Wit AL, Rosen MR, Hoffman BF. Electrophysiology and Pharmacology of Cardiac-Arrhythmias .2. Relationship of Normal and Abnormal Electrical-Activity of Cardiac Fibers to Genesis of Arrhythmias-B – Reentry .1. Am Heart J 1974;88(5): 664–670.

24. Miller PJ, Holmes JR. Effect of cardiac arrhythmia on left ventricular and aortic blood pressure parameters in the horse. Res Vet Sci 1983;35(2): 190–199.

25. van Loon G, Fonteyne W, Rottiers H, et al. Implantation of a dual-chamber, rate-adaptive pacemaker in a horse with suspected sick sinus syndrome. Vet Rec 2002;151(20):541–545.

26. van Loon G, Fonteyne W, Rottiers H, et al. Implantation of a programmable atrioventricular pacemaker in a donkey with complete atrioventricular block and syncope. Equine Vet J 1993;25(3):248–251.

27. Reef VB, Clark ES, Oliver JA, et al. Implantation of a permanent transvenous pacing catheter in a horse with complete heart block and syncope. J Am Vet Med Assoc 1986;189(4):449–452.

28. Abildskov JA, Millar K, Burgess MJ. Atrial fibrillation. Am J Cardiol 1971;28(2):263–267.

29. Allessie MA, Bonke FIM, Schopman FJ. Circus Movement in Rabbit Atrial Muscle as a Mechanism of Tachycardia. Circulation Research 1973;33(1):54–62.

30. Allessie MA, Bonke FIM, Schopman FJG. Circus Movement in Rabbit Atrial Muscle as a Mechanism of Tachycardia .3. Leading Circle Concept – New Model of Circus Movement in Cardiac Tissue without Involvement of an Anatomical Obstacle. Circul Res 1977;41(1):9–18.

31. Moe GK, Albildskov JA, Syracuse NY. Atrial fibrillation as a self-sustaining arrhythmia independent of focal discharge. Am Heart J 1959;58(1):59–70.

32. Garrey WE. The nature of fibrillatory contraction of the heart: its relation to tissue mass and form. Am J Physiol 1914;33: 397–414.

33. Allessie MA, Boyden PA, Camm AJ, et al. Pathophysiology and Prevention of Atrial Fibrillation. Circulation 2001;103(5):769–777.

34. Jalife J. Rotors and spiral waves in atrial fibrillation. Journal of Cardiovascular Electrophysiology 2003;14(7):776–780.

35. Comtois P, Kneller J, Nattel S. Of circles and spirals: Bridging the gap between the leading circle and spiral wave concepts of cardiac reentry. Europace 2005;7:S10–S20.

36. Alessi R, Nusynowitz M, Abildskov JA, et al. Non-uniform distribution of vagal effects on the atrial refractory period. Am J Physiol 1958;194:406–410.

37. Bertone JJ, Wingfield WE. Atrial fibrillation in horses. Compendium on Continuing Education for the Practicing Veterinarian 1987;9(7):763–771.

38. Landymore R, Kinley CE. Staple Closure of the Left Atrial Appendage. CanJ Surg 1984;27(2):144–145.

39. van Loon G. Atrial pacing and experimental atrial fibrillation in equines. In: Department of Large Animal Internal Medicine.

Merelbeke: Ghent University; 2001. p. 258.

40. van Loon G, Tavernier R, Duytschaever M, et al. Pacing induced sustained atrial fibrillation in a pony. Can J Vet Res 2000; 64(4):254–258.

41. Burn JH, Vaughan Williams EM, Walker JM. The effects of acetylcholine in the heart-lung preparation including the production of auricular fibrillation. J Physiol 1955;128(2):277–293.

42. Loomis TA, Krop S. Auricular fibrillation induced and maintained in animals by acetylcholine or vagal stimulation. Circul Res 1955;3:390–396.

43. Wit, AL, Rosen MR, Hoffman BF. Electrophysiology and Pharmacology of Cardiac-Arrhythmias. 2. Relationship of Normal and Abnormal Electrical-Activity of Cardiac Fibers to Genesis of Arrhythmias. Am Heart J 1974;88(4):515–524.

44. Cornick JL, Seahorn TL. Cardiac arrhythmias identified in horses with duodenitis/proximal jejunitis: six cases (1985–1988). J Am Vet Med Assoc 1990;197(8):1054–1059.

45. Garber JL, Reef VB, Reimer JM, et al. Postsurgical Ventricular-Tachycardia in a Horse. J Am Vet Med Assoc 1992;201(7):1038–1039.

46. Marr CM, Reef VB. ECG of the month. J Am Vet Med Assoc 1991;198(9):1533–1534.

47. Reimer JM, Reef VB, Sweeney RW. Ventricular arrhythmias in horses: 21 cases (1984–1989). J Am Vet Med Assoc 1992;201(8):1237–1243.

48. Surawicz B. Relationship between electrocardiogram and electrolytes. AmHeart J 1967;73:814–834.

49. Epstein V. Relationship between potassium administration, hyperkalaemia and the electrocardiogram: an experimental study. Equine Vet J 1984;16(5):453–456.

50. Gettes LS. Electrolyte Abnormalities Underlying Lethal and Ventricular Arrhythmias. Circulation 1992; 85(1):70–76.

51. Glazier DB, Littledike ET, Evans RD. Electrocardiographic Changes in Induced Hypocalcemia and Hyper-Calcemia in Horses. J Equine Med Surg 1979;3(10):489–494.

Chapter 7

Pharmacology of drugs used to treat cardiac disease

Abby Sage and Tony D Mogg

DRUGS USED IN THE TREATMENT OF MYOCARDIAL FAILURE

In compensated heart failure due to ineffective myocardial contractility, adaptive mechanisms of the cardiovascular system occur to sustain adequate blood pressure and cardiac output brought about by the sympathetic nervous system, the renin–angiotensin–aldosterone system and by other mediators (see Chapters 2 and 5) that bring about vasoconstriction as well as increases in circulating volume (increased preload), cardiac contractility, cardiac output and heart rate in order to maintain peripheral perfusion. In decompensated heart failure, due to ineffective myocardial contractility, there is little or no further augmentation of stroke volume with increasing filling pressures. Retrograde transmission of increased pressures into the systemic and pulmonic vasculature produces oedema. Vasoconstriction increases afterload, which further decreases cardiac output. Tachycardia from increased sympathetic drive decreases diastolic coronary blood flow. Myocardial hypoxia and excessive ventricular wall stress as a result of increased filling pressure contributes to the decline in stroke volume. The inotropic and chronotropic responses to sympathetic adrenergic stimulation and the increase in work required to pump against the elevated afterload increase myocardial energy expenditure and accelerate the rate of cell death. Oedema of the myocardial tissues produced by fluid retention contributes to poor myocardial function and impairs oxygenation. Oxygenation is also impaired by pulmonary oedema.

The goals in the treatment of heart failure are to decrease fluid retention, decrease afterload, improve contractility of the myocardium and decrease the heart rate. Three main classes of drugs are utilized: (1) vasodilators, (2) diuretics and (3) cardiac glycosides. In addition, iontropic drugs and pressor agents have a role in supporting ventricular function but these drugs are primarily used in supporting cardiac function in patients with circulatory shock or under anaesthesia (see Chapters 20 and 21).

Vasodilators

As cardiac output falls due to ineffective myocardial contractility, activation of the renin–angiotensin–aldosterone system and increase in sympathetic nervous system activity produce venous and arterial vasoconstriction. Excessive increases in preload and afterload cause increased energy expenditure for an already failing heart. Venodilators provide an increase in venous capacitance and decrease ventricular filling pressures, wall stress and preload. Arterial vasodilators provide reduction in afterload, increasing forward stroke volume. Most vasodilators exhibit activity on both arterial and venous vascular beds, although some vasodilators show specificity for certain segments of the vasculature.[1]

© 2010 Elsevier Ltd.
DOI: 10.1016/B978-0-7020-2817-5.00012-2

ANGIOTENSIN-CONVERTING ENZYME INHIBITORS

Mechanism of action

The renin–angiotensin system participates in short- and long-term control of blood pressure, as described in Chapter 2, through production of angiotensin II and aldosterone. Angiotensin II activates AT1 receptors on vascular smooth muscle cells of the precapillary arterioles and postcapillary venules causing vasoconstriction[2] and inactivates bradykinin, a potent vasodilator. It also increases sympathetic tone and vasoconstriction by increasing release of adrenaline and decreasing its reuptake. Angiotensin II opens calcium channels in cardiac myocytes increasing cardiac contractility and increases heart rate by enhancing noradrenergic transmission and facilitating sympathetic tone.[2] Angiotensin II regulates the tone of the efferent arteries of the kidney increasing the filtration fraction and resorption of sodium and water. It also acts directly on the renal tubular epithelial cells to inhibit excretion of sodium and water[2] and acts directly on the adrenal cortex to produce aldosterone.

Angiotensin-converting enzyme inhibitors fall into three categories: (1) those containing a sulfhydryl group that binds to the zinc moiety of angiotensin-converting enzyme (captopril); (2) those containing a carboxyl group that binds to the zinc moiety of angiotensin-converting enzyme (enalapril, lisinopril); and (3) those containing a phosphinic acid group that binds to the zinc moiety of angiotensin-converting enzyme.[3] All angiotensin-converting enzyme inhibitors prevent the conversion of angiotensin I to angiotensin II thereby attenuating the action of angiotensin II. They not only produce vasodilation by decreasing available angiotensin II but by increasing available bradykinin. As a result they inhibit the release of aldosterone from the adrenal cortex and decrease the sodium and water absorption from the kidney, potentiating the effects of diuretics. Angiotensin-converting enzyme inhibitors decrease the heightened stimulation of the sympathetic nervous system decreasing heart rate and vasoconstriction. Pharmacokinetics of angiotensin-converting enzyme inhibitors have undergone preliminary investigation; enalapril is poorly absorbed[4,5] and effective doses have not been established.[5] More recently quinapril has been evaluated in clinical cases using dosages extrapolated from other species and demonstrated changes in stroke volume and cardiac output which may suggest that further investigation of this drug is warranted.[6] (AF, IE, VMD)

Adverse effects

By reducing concentrations of angiotensin II, angiotensin-converting enzyme inhibitors decrease the kidney's ability to autoregulate glomerular filtration fraction. In patients being treated with renin–angiotensin antagonists with marginal cardiac output, low blood pressure or concomitant use of Na^+K^+2Cl symport inhibitors, the glomerular filtration fraction may decline and an increase in serum creatinine concentrations may ensue.[7] A significant decline in blood pressure may occur after an initial dose of angiotensin-converting enzyme inhibitors necessitating initiation of the drug with a low dose. Cough may develop weeks to months after initiation of therapy.[1] Angioedema is a rare side effect in human patients.

Drug interactions

There is no interaction with digoxin. Angiotensin-converting enzyme inhibitors are eliminated by the kidney and caution should be taken in patients with decreased renal function. They are contraindicated in pregnancy due to malformation of the fetal kidneys.

HYDRALAZINE

The mechanism of action of hydralazine is poorly understood. Hydralazine reduces afterload by reducing systemic and pulmonary vascular resistance resulting in increase in forward stroke volume and a decrease in ventricular wall stress.[3] Hydralazine has a direct positive inotropic activity on cardiac myocytes. It has little effect on venous resistance. In human medicine it is combined with an agent with vasodilating capacity such as organic nitrates (isosorbide dinitrate),[3] although these increase the occurrence of side effects such as headache and dizziness in humans. Hydralazine increases renal perfusion by reducing renal vasculature resistance. Hydralazine is useful in patients with marginal renal function that cannot tolerate an angiotensin-converting enzyme inhibitor. Hydralazine is metabolized by the liver. It is available in oral tablets. The recommended dosage in the horse is 0.5–1.5 mg/kg every 12 hours orally.[8]

Diuretics

Diuretics are used in the treatment of heart failure to combat water and sodium retention by the kidneys. Diuretics reduce intravascular volume, ventricular filling pressures (preload) and wall stress. Although they usually do not cause a significant increase in cardiac output, diuretics do ameliorate the symptoms of congestive heart failure and may decrease the rate of progression of cardiac chamber dilatation by reducing ventricular filling pressure.[3] Diuretics should be used intermittently as needed because of the acid-base and electrolyte disturbances that can be attributed to chronic diuretic therapy.

Mechanism of action

Categories of diuretics are based on their molecular pharmacology. The most commonly used diuretic in the horse is frusemide, a Na^+K^+2Cl symport inhibitor, previously referred to as a loop diuretic. Potassium sparing diuretics, which may decrease the risk of digoxin toxicity, fall into two categories, epithelial sodium channel inhibitors (amiloride) and type I mineralocorticoid/glucocorticoid receptor antagonists (spironolactone). Osmotic diuretics, such as mannitol, increase extracellular fluid volume and are contraindicated in decompensated heart failure. Carbonic anhydrase inhibitors (acetazolamide) may induce a metabolic acidosis that may be beneficial in patients with hypochloraemic metabolic alkalosis secondary to prolonged use of a Na^+K^+2Cl symport inhibitor.

Inhibitors of the Na^+K^+2Cl symport

Inhibitors of an ion transport protein, the Na^+K^+2Cl symport, in the thick ascending limb of the loop of Henle were previously known as loop diuretics. They are the only diuretics that are effective alone in moderate to advanced heart failure. The other diuretics act more distally and are less effective because of the enhanced water and solute resorption in proximal nephron segments in heart failure. The Na^+K^+2Cl symport inhibitors may need to be combined with other diuretics in advanced stages of heart failure.[3] Evidence suggests the Na^+K^+2Cl symport inhibitors bind to the chloride binding site but the exact mechanism is unknown.[9] Inhibition of the symporter prevents the renal epithelial cell from absorbing sodium and chloride. Lack of ions in the medullary interstitium reduces its tonicity and decreases the driving force for water resorption in the collecting duct. Excessive sodium and fluid in the distal nephron enhances the secretion of potassium and hydrogen ions. Loop diuretics also inhibit absorption of calcium and magnesium because they are linked to sodium and chloride transport. Frusemide is the most widely used diuretic in this category. Effects of frusemide on the cardiovascular system have been well documented in the normal horse. Decrease in plasma volume, right atrial pressure, stroke volume and cardiac output and an increase in systemic vascular resistance occur acutely following administration. These rapid haemodynamic actions of loop diuretics are attenuated in studied human patients with chronic congestive heart failure.[3] Chronic use of frusemide may induce hypokalaemia, hypochloraemic alkalosis, hyponatraemia and hypomagnesaemia. These electrolyte disturbances increase the risk for development of digoxin toxicity in patients treated with both drugs. Frusemide should be used intermittently to control the symptoms of heart failure. Horses treated with long-term digoxin and frusemide should have serum electrolyte concentrations monitored routinely. Supplementation with the appropriate electrolyte or change of diuretic is warranted if electrolyte disturbances are detected. The dosage of frusemide in the horse is 1 mg/kg IV, IM as needed, usually twice daily.[10] Continuous rate infusions have been evaluated in the horse and cause more profound diuresis in the first 8 hours of treatment using a loading dose of 0.12 mg/kg followed by an infusion of 0.12 mg/kg/hour.[11] This may be useful for initial stabilization of horses presenting with acute congestive heart failure, although there is no improvement in diuresis after the first 8 hours of treatment over conventional intravenous medication every 8 hours.[11] The oral bioavailability of frusemide is poor and highly variable[12] and therefore intramuscular administration is recommended for ongoing therapy. (PH, VMD)

Potassium-sparing diuretics

Potassium-sparing diuretics are divided into two categories based on their molecular pharmacology. Diuretics, such as amiloride, inhibit sodium selective channels in the late distal convoluted tubule and the cortical collecting duct. The other category of potassium sparing diuretics are inhibitors of type I mineralocorticoid/glucocorticoid receptors and act as an aldosterone antagonist, such as spironolactone. Neither of these diuretics is sufficient alone in advanced heart failure although they may affect cardiac remodelling as discussed in Chapter 2. Care should be taken when using these diuretics with ACE inhibitors or in patients with reduced renal function, which may increase the serum potassium concentration. Potassium-sparing diuretics also cause less magnesium wasting than the Na^+K^+2Cl symport inhibitors. Pharmacokinetics and dosage for the potassium-sparing diuretics have not been established in the horse.

Inhibitors of the $Na^+ Cl^-$ symporter

Thiazide diuretics inhibit the sodium/chloride symporter in the renal epithelial cell in the distal convoluted tubule increasing loss of sodium, chloride and water into the urine. Excessive sodium and fluid in the distal nephron enhances the secretion of potassium and hydrogen ions. Alone, these diuretics are only useful in mild heart failure. However, when combined with loop diuretics, they exhibit synergism which may be useful in patients resistant to loop diuretics. Pharmacokinetics and dosage for the thiazide diuretics have not been established in the horse.

Cardiac glycosides (AF, VT)

Cardiac glycosides occur naturally in a variety of plants and as venom in some toad species. Digitalis glycosides are those cardiac glycosides that are derived from *Digitalis* species of plants. *Digitalis* species include *Digitalis purpurea* (foxglove plant), and *Digitalis lanata* (digitoxin and digoxin).[1] Cardiac glycosides have a chemical structure consisting of a steroid nucleus with an unsaturated lactone at the C17 position and one or more glycosidic residues at C3.[1] Digoxin is the most commonly used cardiac glycoside in the horse. It is relatively inexpensive, easy to administer and the pharmacokinetics have been established. Pharmacokinetics and dosage have not been established for digitoxin in the horse.

Mechanism of action

Positive inotropic effect, inhibition of Na⁺K⁺ATPase

Positive inotropic effect, inhibition of Na$^+$K$^+$ATPase

Depolarization of the cardiac myocyte occurs when fast sodium channels open producing phase 0 of the action potential.[13] The depolarization of the cell activates L-type calcium channels which are voltage sensitive and found on the cell membrane.[1,3] Calcium enters the cell producing the slow inward current, phase 2 of the cardiac action potential. This influx of calcium into the cell causes a release of calcium from the sarcoplasmic reticulum, an intracellular compartment. As the myocyte undergoes repolarization and relaxation, calcium is removed from the cell by a Ca^{2+}ATPase that sequesters the calcium back into the sarcoplasmic reticulum. Also, a Ca^{2+}ATPase and a Na^+Ca^{2+} exchanger in the sarcolemmal membrane remove calcium from the cytoplasm.[1,3] The calcium within the cell is exchanged for the sodium outside the cell. The difference in sodium concentration from inside the cell to outside the cell drives the Na^+Ca^{2+} exchanger; if the sodium concentration within the cell is high, the exchange of calcium for sodium will be diminished.

Normally there is a large concentration gradient of sodium, most being outside the cell, which is maintained by the Na^+K^+ATPase pump exchanging intracellular sodium for extracellular potassium. Cardiac glycosides bind to and inhibit the Na^+K^+ATPase causing sodium to accumulate inside the cell. The increased amount of sodium inside the cell prevents the Na^+Ca^{2+} exchanger from working efficiently and calcium is not pumped from the cell. The extra calcium within the cell is then taken up by the sarcoplasmic reticulum. This allows for more calcium to be released from the sarcoplasmic reticulum during contraction. The excess calcium binds to the sarcomere and increases the velocity and extent of sarcomere shortening increasing contractility.[3] The alpha subunit of the Na^+K^+ATPase, the binding site for cardiac glycosides, is present on the extracytoplasmic side of the cell membrane.[3] Excessive extracellular potassium decreases the binding affinity of cardiac glycosides for Na^+K^+ATPase by promoting dephosphorylation which is an initial step in the translocation of the enzyme into the cytosol.[1] Therefore, increased extracellular potassium will reverse some manifestations of digitalis toxicity.

Regulation of sympathetic nervous system activity

In human patients in heart failure, an increase in sympathetic nervous activity may in part be due to insensitivity to the arterial baroreflex.[1] The rise in blood pressure does not cause a decrease in sympathetic tone as it would in the normal heart. This insensitivity also contributes to sustained levels of noradrenaline, renin and vasopressin.[1] Cardiac glycosides appear to decrease sympathetic nervous system activity by a centrally mediated effect and enhance baroreceptor sensitivity in patients with heart failure. Ferguson et al[14] demonstrated in patients with moderate to severe heart failure given a cardiac glycoside, a decrease in heart rate and increased forearm blood flow and cardiac index. In addition, a simultaneous decrease in skeletal muscle sympathetic nervous system activity occurred, suggesting an overall decrease in centrally mediated sympathetic activity. The decrease in sympathetic nervous system activity and the increase in vagal tone will decrease automaticity and increase the diastolic resting membrane potential in the atrial and atrioventricular nodal tissue. The effective refractory period is prolonged and atrioventricular nodal conduction velocity is decreased.[1] Because myocardial perfusion occurs in diastole, a decrease in heart rate will decrease myocardial ischaemia. A decrease in heart rate will also improve stroke volume by allowing more time for ventricular filling, and decrease myocardial oxygen consumption.

Pharmacokinetics

Digoxin is available as oral tablets, elixir and intravenous formulations. Because there is considerable variability in the systemic availability of oral formulations of digoxin on the market, the same product should be used consistently during maintenance therapy.[3] Digoxin should not be given intramuscularly as it causes local irritation and is absorbed erratically.[3] Pharmacokinetic studies of digoxin have been performed in the normal horse and in horses in congestive heart failure.[15-20] Digoxin is eliminated by glomerular filtration and tubular secretion.[3] In patients with decreased kidney function or those on diuretics or sympathomimetic agents with increased renal clearance, the dosage of the drug should be adjusted. Because of its large volume of distribution, digoxin cannot be removed by peritoneal dialysis.[3] Digoxin is stored in the skeletal muscle, not fat, so dosage should be calculated on lean body mass. Digoxin has been shown to cross the placenta in humans.[3] In the horse, 20–40% of digoxin in the plasma is protein bound.[15]

Bioavailability of oral digoxin is approximately 20%.[17,19,20] Time to peak serum concentration is 1–2 hours after oral administration.[16,19,20] A second rise in serum concentration occurs 4–8 hours later most likely due to enterohepatic recycling of the drug, slowed absorption or delayed availability of partially dissolved tablets.[17,20] There is considerable variation in the serum concentration of digoxin following oral administration in individual animals.[17,19] The reported range for the biological half-life of digoxin in the horse is 17–23 hours.[15,17,19] Without loading doses, the serum concentration of digoxin reaches a steady state in the horse within 3.5 days for 12 hour dosing interval.[19] The dosage for intravenous maintenance is 2.2 µg/kg every 12 hours and for oral maintenance is 11 µg/kg every 12 hours.[20] An initial maintenance dose (2.2 µg/kg IV) given intravenously will result in achievement of therapeutic concentration more rapidly than oral administration for a portion of the dosing interval. Larger loading doses will increase the chance of toxicity.[20] The therapeutic plasma concentration of digoxin is between 0.5 and 2.0 ng/mL.[17]

Therapeutic drug monitoring and adverse effects

 VT)

Because there is a narrow safety margin between the therapeutic and toxic levels of digoxin and because digoxin interacts with many commonly used medications, digitalis toxicity may occur during treatment. The initial signs of digoxin toxicity are anorexia, colic and diarrhoea due to alterations in sympathetic tone. Cardiac dysrhythmias are a common and potentially life-threatening result of digitalis intoxication. Close monitoring of the clinical response and plasma digoxin concentration must be performed in treated horses to avoid toxicity. The level at which clinical symptoms of toxicity show a rapid increase in prevalence is above 2.0 ng/mL. Some patients may show signs of toxicity within the "therapeutic" range. Serum levels should be taken 3.5 days after initiation of therapy since individual animals vary in their response.[19,20] Serum samples should be taken at the time of peak and trough concentrations, 2 and 12 hours, respectively, after the last dose is administered.[20]

There are many drugs that may potentially interact with digoxin; H₂ blockers, bran and albuterol may decrease the blood concentration of digoxin[1] while propafenone, quinidine, verapamil, erythromycin, omeprazole, phenylbutazone and tetracycline may increase serum concentrations of digoxin.[1,10] Hypoproteinaemia may decrease protein binding thereby increasing the unbound, metabolically active, concentration of the drug. Hypokalaemia, hypomagnesaemia and hypocalcaemia make the patient more sensitive to the toxic effects of digoxin. Hyperkalaemia decreases the binding affinity for digoxin and decreases the sensitivity to toxic effects, although it may exacerbate digoxin-induced conduction disorders and result in high-grade atrioventricular nodal block.[3]

Digoxin toxicity produces an increase in sympathetic tone and progressive inhibition of the Na⁺K⁺ATPase. The inhibition of Na⁺K⁺ATPase leads to a loss of cardiac cellular potential and excessive accumulation of intracellular calcium that alters cardiac conduction.[10] Ectopic beats of atrioventricular junctional or ventricular origin, first-degree atrioventricular block and an excessively slow ventricular response to atrial fibrillation are the most common dysrhythmias in humans.[1]

In the case of digoxin toxicity, digoxin therapy should be immediately discontinued. Serum electrolyte and digoxin concentrations and acid-base status should be determined. Treatment for fluid, electrolyte and acid-base disturbances should be instituted. Even if the serum concentration of potassium is in the normal range, potassium can be administered to animals with life-threatening dysrhythmias, unless high-degree atrioventricular block is present. Hypomagnesaemia, hypokalaemia and hypocalcaemia make the patient more susceptible to toxic effects and should be corrected. Lignocaine or phenytoin may be used for worsening ventricular dysrhythmias that cause the patient to be haemodynamically unstable.[21] Care should be taken with quinidine administration as it will increase unbound digoxin levels. If symptomatic, sinus bradycardia, sinoatrial arrest and 3rd degree atrioventricular block usually respond to the administration of atropine.[1] Antidigoxin immunotherapy is available for humans, but is prohibitively expensive for equine patients.

Calcium channel blockers

In human heart failure patients with systolic dysfunction, calcium channel antagonists may worsen symptoms and increase mortality.[3] The mechanism for the adverse effects is unclear. Calcium channel antagonists may result in an increase in the negative inotropy. Continued research into "second generation" calcium channel blockers is ongoing.

Phosphodiesterase inhibitors

Of the phosphodiesterase inhibitors only theophylline and caffeine have been studied in the horse. Phosphodiesterase isoenzyme subclass specific inhibitors used in human medicine include amrinone and milrinone. Phosphodiesterase inhibitors increase intracellular concentrations of cAMP that causes positive chronotropy and inotropy in cardiac cells and relaxation of bronchial smooth muscle cells. They are only useful in the short-term support of circulation in advanced heart failure. Sildenafil, a phosphodiesterase subtype 5 inhibitor, has also been proposed as a treatment for persistent pulmonary hypertension in the neonatal human patient[22,23] and may have a role in the management of foals with perinatal asphyxia syndrome. (PH)

Adrenergic and dopaminergic agonists

Dobutamine

Dobutamine is useful for short-term circulatory support of patients with acute heart failure. Due to the development of tolerance and lack of an enteral formulation, dobutamine is not appropriate for long-term therapy. Lower doses of dobutamine (1–10 µg/kg/minute IV infusion) stimulate β$_1$-adrenergic receptor subtypes producing a positive inotropic effect. Dobutamine does not activate dopaminergic receptors and does not increase renal blood flow selectively. Dobutamine is used to support blood pressure during anaesthesia (see Chapter 20) and in hypotensive foals. It may be more appropriate to use it in conjunction with the pressor agent noradrenaline in this setting.[24]

Dopamine

Actions of dopamine are often quoted to be based on the infusion rate. At low infusion rates (1–3 µg/kg/minute), dopamine stimulates dopaminergic pre- and postsynaptic receptors in the peripheral vasculature and renal proximal tubular cells of some species resulting in vasodilation of splanchnic and renal arterial beds causing an increase in renal perfusion. At intermediate infusion rates (3–5 µg/kg/minute) dopamine stimulates β$_1$-adrenergic receptors in the heart resulting in positive inotropy and chronotropy. Infusion rates of 5–20 µg/kg/minute stimulate α-adrenergic receptors causing peripheral vasoconstriction.[25] There is considerable controversy about the use of dopamine for improving renal perfusion in patients with acute renal failure,[26] and variability in the selectivity means that it is rarely indicated to support cardiac function in heart failure in the horse. Other drugs with more predictable pressor and inotropic effects are usually recommended in the horse for the treatment of hypovolaemic and endotoxic shock.

DRUGS USED IN THE TREATMENT OF CARDIAC DYSRHYTHMIAS

The Vaughan Williams classification of antiarrhythmic drugs categorizes the drugs according to the ion channels or adrenoceptors they block. Class I includes drugs that block the fast inward sodium channels of myocardial cells. There are three subcategories. Class IA consists of drugs that decrease myocardial conduction velocity, increase the refractoriness of myocardial cells and prolong the QRS and QT intervals. Quinidine and procainamide belong to this group. Class IB contain drugs (lignocaine and phenytoin) that shorten the action potential. Class IC drugs slow conduction and mildly prolong refractoriness. Propafenone is an example of this class. Class II drugs block β-adrenergic receptors. Propranolol and timolol are examples. Class III contains drugs that block potassium channels and prolong repolarization. Amiodarone and bretylium are in this category. Class IV include verapamil and diltiazem and are slow calcium channel blockers. Dosage regimens for drugs used to treat dysrhythmias in horses are listed in Table 7.1 and further details of the clinical indications for use of these drugs are discussed in Chapter 13. It is important to recognize that there are limited data to support dosage regimens for many antidysrhythmic drugs and the reader is advised to consult recent literature for modifications and recommendations made after the time of publication of this text.

Class I antiarrhythmic drugs

Quinidine

Mechanism of action

 ACF, AF, VT)

Class IA antiarrhythmics include quinidine and procainamide. Quinidine is the drug most frequently used to treat cardiac dysrhythmias and the most well studied of the antiarrhythmics in the horse and is derived from the bark of the cinchona tree. Quinidine blocks the sodium channels and multiple cardiac potassium currents, decreasing automaticity of Purkinje fibres and ectopic pacemakers by decreasing the slope of phase 4 of the cardiac action potential, shifting the threshold voltage towards zero. It prolongs the duration of the action potential and the effective refractory period. The prolongation of the effective refractory period has been assumed to be responsible for its effect in terminating atrial fibrillation and other re-entry arrhythmias. For example, in atrial fibrillation the refractory period of all atrial cells is increased so there are fewer areas of tissue at different stages of the action potential (and therefore at different levels of refractoriness) and so fewer islands of refractory tissue, which are the basis for the re-entry mechanism, can exist. However, more recent experimental research in a goat model of atrial fibrillation has shown that quinidine did not result in lengthening of the refractory period but rather in a widening of the excitable gap.[27] In addition, sodium channel blockade results in conduction slowing, which should theoretically promote atrial fibrillation. These findings have led to a new model to explain atrial fibrillation, the spiral wave concept. In this model one or more spiral waves are supposed to circle around (re-entry) and serve as a continuous source to maintain atrial fibrillation. According to this model, administration of class I drugs would have an antiarrhythmic action by altering the rotation of the spiral wave.[28,29] Optical mapping in isolated

Table 7.1 Indications and doses of antidysrhythmic drugs used in horses

DRUG	INDICATIONS	DOSE
Amiodarone	VT, AF	5 mg/kg/hour for 1 hour then 0.83 mg/kg/hour for 23 hours*
Atropine	Sinus bradycardia, AV block	0.005–0.01 mg/kg IV
Bretylium tosylate	Life-threatening VT, ventricular fibrillation	3–5 mg/kg IV, can repeat up to 10 mg/kg*
Digoxin	SVT	0.0022 mg/kg IV bid 0.011 mg/kg PO bid
Diltiazem	SVT	0.125 mg/kg IV over 2 minutes repeated every 12 minutes*
Dopamine	Advanced and complete AV block	3–5 µg/kg/minute
Adrenaline (epinephrine)	Sinus bradycardia	0.01 mg/kg IV
Flecainide	AF	4.1 mg/kg q 2 hours for a maximum of 4–6 doses then q 4–6 hours* DO NOT USE INTRAVENOUSLY
Isoproterenol	Advanced and complete AV block	0.05–0.2 µg/kg/minute CRI
Lignocaine	VT	0.02–0.05 mg/kg/minutes; 0.25–0.5 mg/kg IV slowly, can repeat in 5–10 minutes Or loading bolus of 1.3 mg/kg IV over 5 minutes followed by CRI at 0.05 mg/kg/minute
Magnesium sulphate	VT	2.2–4.4 mg/kg IV slowly, can repeat in 5 minutes to total dose of 55 mg/kg total*
Phenytoin	Digoxin toxicity, supraventricular and ventricular arrhythmias	7.5–8.8 mg/kg iv single bolus Loading dose 20 mg/kg PO, bid then modify to keep plasma [phenytoin] = 5–10 mg/L
Procainamide	VT, AF, supraventricular and ventricular arrhythmias	1 mg/kg/minute IV to total dose of 20 mg/kg 25–35 mg/kg PO tid
Propafenone	VT, AF, supraventricular and ventricular arrhythmias	0.5–1 mg/kg in 5% dextrose IV over 5–8 minutes 2 mg/kg PO tid*
Propanolol	VT and SVT	0.03–0.1 mg/kg IV 0.38–0.78 mg/kg PO tid
Quinidine gluconate	VT, AF	0.5–2.2 mg/kg IV q 10 minutes to total dose 12 mg/kg
Quinidine sulphate	AF	22 mg/kg via nasogastric tube until converted, toxic or plasma [quindine] = 3–5 mg/L, usually 4–6 doses, then q 6 hours until converted or toxic
Verapamil	SVT	0.025–0.05 mg/kg IV q 30 minutes to total dose 0.2 mg/kg*

*Note there are limited data to support these dosage regimens and the reader is advised to also consult recent literature for modifications and recommendations made after the time of publication of this text.

AF, atrial fibrillation; CRI continuous rate infusion; SVT, supraventricular tachycardia; VT, ventricular tachycardia.

perfused preparations of equine atria suggested that atrial fibrillation, produced in vitro by a rapid pacing protocol, results from spatial variations in the action potential durations and diastolic intervals.[30] These changes produce regions of conduction block and Wenckebach conduction with the atrium. Multiple conduction frequencies are present due to regions of conduction block. Quinidine terminates the in vitro atrial fibrillation by increasing the effective refractory period, thereby decreasing the maximal dominant frequency and increasing the spatial homogeneity of frequencies present within the atrium.

Quinidine has an anticholinergic effect and α-adrenergic blockade. α-Adrenergic receptor block causes vasodilation, a decrease in peripheral vascular resistance and hypotension. Reflex stimulation of the sympathetic nervous system and the vagolytic properties increases sinus nodal discharge rate and produces tachycardia. Improvement in atrioventricular nodal conduction will increase the heart rate in atrial flutter or fibrillation. By blocking the sodium channels, quinidine has a direct myocardial depressant effect resulting in decreased inotropy.[31]

Pharmacokinetics

Quinidine is available as quinidine sulfate for oral administration and quinidine gluconate for intravenous administration. Quinidine should not be given intramuscularly due to tissue necrosis. Pharmacokinetics have been established for oral quinidine sulfate and intravenous quinidine gluconate in the horse. Oral administration of 22 mg/kg of quinidine sulfate to an adult horse yields 50% absorption and a peak plasma concentration of 1.5 µg/mL in 2 hours. The therapeutic range of plasma concentration of quinidine is 2–5 µg/mL.[32] The average half life of intravenously administered quinidine is 6.5 hours (range 4–12 hours).[32] Approximately 80% of plasma quinidine is protein bound, especially to the α1-acid glycoprotein, the expression of which increases in heart failure. Quinidine undergoes both hepatic and renal excretion and is metabolized by the P450 cytochrome system. Plasma quinidine may be increased in patients with hepatic or renal disease or congestive heart failure.

Indications

Quinidine is the drug of choice for pharmacological conversion of atrial fibrillation. Quinidine sulfate is given via nasogastric tube at a dosage of 22 mg/kg every 2 hours until therapeutic concentrations are achieved (usually 4–5 doses) or signs of toxicity occur (see Table 7.1). If conversion has not been achieved after four doses, plasma quinidine concentrations should be determined prior to the next dose to determine if a fifth dose should be given. If plasma quinidine concentrations cannot be determined or if the concentration is in the therapeutic range, the interval of dosing should be increased to every 6 hours. Quinidine

may be administered every 6 hours until signs of toxicity are seen or conversion is achieved. Plasma quinidine concentrations should be determined daily to prevent toxicity. Digoxin can be combined into this protocol at a dosage of 0.011 mg/kg orally once a day. This is often initiated on the second day of therapy. Plasma digoxin concentrations should be monitored daily because quinidine and digoxin competitively bind with plasma proteins. Digitalization of horses with decreased myocardial function is recommended prior to treatment with quinidine. Diltiazem has also been used in combination with quinidine sulfate in order to control ventricular rate and limit the occurrence of ventricular dysrhythmias.[33]

Quinidine may also be used for treatment of frequent supraventricular and ventricular premature complexes and sustained supraventricular and ventricular tachydysrhythmias. The intravenous dosage of quinidine gluconate is 2.2 mg/kg bolus every 10 minutes to a total of 8.8–11 mg/kg. Intravenous infusion rate for quinidine gluconate is 0.7–3.0 mg/kg per hour[34] (see Table 7.1).

Adverse effects

The plasma concentration of quinidine that is associated with toxic signs is just above the therapeutic range. Care must be taken to monitor plasma concentrations of quinidine. Prolongation of the QRS complex by 10–20% is seen when quinidine levels are in the therapeutic range.[35] An increase in duration of the QRS greater than 25% indicates quinidine toxicity. Gastrointestinal signs of quinidine toxicity are anorexia, flatulence, colic and diarrhoea. Neurological signs include ataxia, bizarre behaviour and seizures. Depression and nasal oedema are common findings although this latter sign rarely necessitates a nasotracheal tube or tracheotomy. Urticaria is an uncommon side effect. Hypotension, as a result of α1-adrenoceptor blockade may lead to weakness and sometimes to collapse. Laminitis is a potential complication, but its incidence is insignificant in horses receiving oral quinidine therapy with no structural cardiovascular disease.[10] Most signs of quinidine toxicity will resolve when the drug levels diminish. Life-threatening dysrhythmias that develop are supraventricular and ventricular tachycardia or torsades de pointes. Quinidine toxicity is treated with removal of the drug or increasing the dosing interval. For more life-threatening toxic side effects sodium bicarbonate (0.5–1.0 mEq/kg IV) will increase the amount of quinidine bound to albumin decreasing the amount of available free drug.[10] Drugs that induce hepatic enzymes such as phenobarbital or phenytoin can shorten the duration of quinidine's action by increasing its rate of elimination. Supraventricular tachycardia secondary to quinidine toxicity is treated with digoxin. Ventricular tachycardia and torsades de pointes are treated with intravenous infusion of magnesium sulfate (55.5 mg/kg diluted in saline and given over 20 minutes).

Drug interactions

Quinidine may elevate serum digoxin concentration by decreasing the renal clearance, volume of distribution and affinity of tissue receptors to digoxin.[36]

Procainamide

Mechanism of action

Procainamide exerts electrophysiological effects similar to those of quinidine but procainamide does not have the anticholinergic effects or cause α-adrenergic blockade. Procainamide blocks sodium channels and also has an effect on potassium channels and so prolongs the effective refractory period, decreases automaticity and slows conduction. Procainamide is eliminated by hepatic metabolism and renal excretion. It is metabolized to *N*-acetyl procainamide (NAPA), by conjugation by *N*-acetyl transferase. NAPA lacks the sodium channel blocking activity of procainamide and acts as a potassium channel blocker, prolonging the action potential duration and the effective refractory period. NAPA is more slowly eliminated by the kidney than the parent drug; therefore, the dosage should be adjusted in patients with renal failure to prevent potentially life-threatening concentrations of procainamide and NAPA. The half lives of procainamide (administered IV over 10 minutes) and NAPA are 3.49 ± 0.61 hours and 6.31 ± 1.49 hours, respectively.[31] Procainamide can be administered by intravenous infusion (1 mg/kg/minute IV to a total of 20 mg/kg) or orally (25–35 mg/kg every 8 hours, see Table 7.1).

Adverse effects

(ACF, VT)

Procainamide can depress myocardial contractility in high doses. Although it does not exert α-adrenergic blockade it may result in vasodilation due to sympatholytic effects on the brain and spinal cord.[13] Torsades de pointes has been reported in humans when NAPA concentrations exceeded 30 μg/mL. Procainamide can be proarrhythmic resulting in ventricular tachydysrhythmias.

Drug interactions

Procainamide does not increase digoxin concentration.

Lignocaine

Mechanism of action

(ACF, VT)

Lignocaine (lidocaine) is a class IB antiarrhythmic. It blocks sodium channels and shortens the action potential. Lignocaine decreases cardiac excitability, cardiac impulse conduction and abnormal automaticity and eliminates large disparities in myocardial refractoriness. Lignocaine decreases automaticity in the ventricular myocardium by decreasing the slope of phase 4 of the cardiac action potential and increasing the threshold for excitability. It does not affect normal sinus nodal automaticity. Part of its effect may be to inhibit cardiac sympathetic nervous system activity.[13] Heart rate, arterial blood pressure, cardiac contractility and cardiac output are minimally affected following intravenous doses of lignocaine.[10] Lignocaine is not effective against atrial dysrhythmias.

Pharmacokinetics

Lignocaine is most effective when administered by the intravenous route through bolus or infusion. The half life for lignocaine following intravenous administration is very short due to active hepatic metabolism.[10] Oral administration of lignocaine is subject to first-pass elimination by the liver and produces high concentrations of potentially toxic metabolites. Intramuscular administration has resulted in sporadic absorption patterns, low plasma lignocaine concentrations and poor antiarrhythmic efficacy.[10] Because of the propensity to cause seizures at a dose greater than or equal to 1.5 mg/kg the dose should be administered in 0.5 mg/kg boluses with 5 minutes between doses.[10] Alternatively, continuous rate infusions can be given at a rate of 0.05 mg/kg/minute after a loading bolus of 1.3 mg/kg given over 5 minutes[37] (see Table 7.1). The therapeutic range of plasma concentrations is 1.5–5.0 μg/mL.[31]

Adverse effects

Lignocaine may induce neurological signs including seizures in horses following rapid intravenous administration. Nervous signs include agitation, excitement, sweating, tachycardia and seizures. Nervous signs usually resolve as the lignocaine concentration decreases. Seizures can be treated with diazepam (0.2 mg/kg IV). Because lignocaine is metabolized by the liver, diseases of the liver and congestive heart failure may prolong the duration of action of lignocaine and predispose to toxicity.[10] Beta-adrenoceptor blockers can decrease hepatic blood flow and increase serum lignocaine concentrations.[13] In congestive heart failure, the central volume of distribution is decreased so the total dose should be decreased.[35] Lignocaine does not have a significant effect on haemodynamics.

Phenytoin

Mechanism of action

Phenytoin is an anticonvulsant and has been used to treat a variety of muscle disorders in the horse. Because of its ability to block sodium channels in the heart, it is used to suppress ventricular dysrhythmias due to digitalis intoxication in humans. Phenytoin effectively abolishes abnormal automaticity caused by digoxin toxicity in humans[13] and has been used for this purpose in the horse.[21] Phenytoin decreases the action potential duration more than it shortens the effective refractory period, increasing the ratio of effective refractory period to action potential duration. Phenytoin can cause depolarized cells to repolarize by increasing potassium conductance The rate of rise of action potentials initiated early in the relative refractory period is increased as is membrane responsiveness, possibly reducing the chance for impaired conduction and block. In digitalis toxicity in humans, phenytoin may reduce the traffic in cardiac sympathetic nerves. It undergoes extensive first pass hepatic metabolism. Phenytoin administered orally was used to successfully treat ventricular extrasystoles and ventricular tachycardia in seven horses that were refractory to other antiarrhythmic therapies.[38] In all cases ventricular extrasystoles or ventricular tachycardia was reduced or abolished within 2–6 hours after the first dose of phenytoin. Normal sinus rhythm was attained within four doses of phenytoin in all cases.

Pharmacokinetics

Therapeutic concentrations are 10–20 µg/mL in humans. The dosage for phenytoin in the horse is 10–22 mg/kg orally every 12 hours (see Table 7.1).

Propafenone

Mechanism of action

(VT)

Propafenone is a class IC sodium channel blocker. Propafenone decreases excitability and suppresses spontaneous automaticity and triggered activity. Effects on action potential vary with the species. It suppresses sinus nodal automaticity. Propafenone is used in the treatment of sustained supraventricular and ventricular tachycardia and ventricular premature complexes in humans. Propafenone was unsuccessful in converting horses with naturally occurring and experimentally induced atrial fibrillation when administered as an intravenous bolus followed by an intravenous infusion lasting 2 hours.[39]

Adverse effects

High doses produce negative inotropy. Patients with decreased left ventricular function may have a worsening of symptoms. Propafenone also acts as a beta-adrenergic antagonist and may produce sinus bradycardia and bronchospasm.

Pharmacokinetics

Pharmacokinetics have not been established in horses. Dosages for intravenous and oral use in the horse that

have been extrapolated from human dosages are 0.5–1 mg/kg in 5% dextrose slowly IV over 5–8 minutes and 2 mg/kg every 8 hours orally.[8] In humans maximum therapeutic effects occur at serum concentrations of 0.2–1.5 µg/mL. Elimination is by hepatic and renal routes.

Drug interactions

Quinidine may inhibit metabolism of propafenone. Propafenone increases the plasma level of warfarin and digoxin.

Flecainide

Flecainide is a class IC sodium channel blocker that prolongs the cardiac action potential. It has been used to treat atrial fibrillation in humans with lone atrial fibrillation using both intravenous and oral administration.[40] The pharmacokinetics of flecainide have been established in the horse.[41,42] It was ineffective when used intravenously in chronic atrial fibrillation.[43,44] Furthermore, potential life-threatening ventricular dysrhythmias were seen in some horses.[44] Therefore, intravenous flecainide cannot be recommended for the treatment of atrial fibrillation. However, a protocol for oral administration of flecainide has been used successfully in an experimental AF model,[41] and at the current time, in one naturally occurring case[45] (see Table 7.1). Collapse and sudden death was associated with the administration of oral flecainide in two horses with naturally occurring atrial fibrillation.[46] Both horses had been treated with multiple oral doses of quinidine sulphate, with the last dose only 12–24 hours prior to beginning treatment with flecainide. These adverse effects may have been the result of quinidine-induced inhibition of flecainide metabolism or the combined proarrhythmic effects of quinidine and flecainide.

Class II antiarrhythmics drugs

Propranolol

Mechanism of action

(AF)

β-Blockers competitively inhibit catecholamine binding at β-adrenergic receptors. Propranolol blocks sodium channels and is a non-specific β-adrenoceptor blocking agent, although most of its effects are due to β_1 blockade. It slows spontaneous automaticity in the sinus node or in the Purkinje fibres that are being stimulated by adrenergic tone. The P–R interval lengthens, atrioventricular nodal conduction is slowed, and the effective and functional refractory periods are increased. Propranolol may be used for the control of supraventricular and ventricular tachydysrhythmias and may be useful in treating digoxin-induced dysrhythmias such as atrial tachycardia, nonparoxysmal atrioventricular junctional tachycardia, premature ventricular complexes or ventricular tachycardia. Therapeutic concentrations of propranolol slows the heart rate and decreases cardiac contractility. It is rapidly metabolized by the liver and oral bioavailability is low due to the first pass effect in horses.[31] Caution should be used when administered to animals with clinical signs of congestive heart failure or impaired hepatic blood flow.[10]

Dosage

Dosage should be titrated to individual response to therapy such as a reduction in heart rate. The initial intravenous dose should not exceed 0.1 mg/kg slowly over 1 minute. Single IV doses >0.3 mg/kg can cause bradycardia, hypotension and muscular weakness in horses with heart disease.[10] (see Table 7.1). Pharmacokinetic studies of propranolol in horses indicate that therapy 3–4 times a day is required to maintain therapeutic plasma concentrations.[10]

Adverse effects

Propranolol exerts negative inotropic effects and can precipitate or worsen heart failure. Due to the role of β_2-adrenoceptors in maintaining bronchial smooth tone, nonselective effects of propranolol may worsen bronchospasm of recurrent airway disease. The prevailing sympathetic tone determines the pharmacological response to propranolol and accounts for the variability in response to the drug.

Class III antiarrhythmic drugs

Amiodarone

 AF)

Amiodarone has been evaluated for the treatment of atrial fibrillation in the horse using a continuous rate infusion. The pharmacokinetics have been determined and show poor oral bioavailability and that the drug is excreted mainly in urine.[47,48] Although the drug has shown some promise for treatment of naturally occurring atrial fibrillation,[49,50] and ventricular dysrhythmias[51] in the horse, side effects, including diarrhoea, have been reported.[50] It was used successfully in one horse with ventricular tachycardia given 5 mg/kg/hour for 1 hour then 0.83 mg/kg/hour for 23 hours but further work is needed to refine the optimal dosage protocols. A regimen of amiodarone and quinidine sulphate was found to be no more efficacious in the treatment of atrial fibrillation than quinidine sulphate alone.[52]

Bretylium

Bretylium is used in human patients with life-threatening ventricular tachydysrhythmias that have not responded to other drug therapies. Bretylium has been reported in humans to treat ventricular fibrillation. Bretylium is a quaternary ammonium compound that prolongs cardiac action potentials, most likely through inhibition of potassium channels. In addition, it increases the refractoriness of normal atrial and ventricular myocardium and Purkinje fibres, suppressing re-entry. Bretylium interferes with the release and reuptake of noradrenaline by sympathetic neurones. Hypotension may result due to blocking the efferent limb of the baroreceptor reflex. Pharmacokinetics and dosage in the horse have not been established.

Other antiarrhythmic drugs

Magnesium sulphate

Magnesium sulphate is a physiological calcium channel blocker. In humans it is used to treat supraventricular and ventricular dysrhythmias and is effective even in patients with normal serum magnesium concentrations. It has been used in the treatment of ventricular tachycardia and torsades de pointes in the horse.[8] It is given by intravenous infusion at 55.5 mg/kg diluted in saline over 20 minutes.

REFERENCES

1. Kelly RA, Smith TW. Pharmacological treatment of heart failure. In: Hardman JG, Limbird LE, Molinoff PB, et al, editors. Goodman and Gilman's The Pharmacological Basis of Therapeutics, 9th ed. New York: McGraw-Hill; 1996. p. 809–839.

2. Jackson EK, Garrison JC. Renin and angiotensin. In: Hardman JG, Limbird LE, Molinoff PB, et al, editors. Goodman and Gilman's The Pharmacological Basis of Therapeutics, 9th ed. New York: McGraw-Hill; 1996. p. 733–758.

3. Kelly RA, Smith TW. Drugs used in the treatment of heart failure. In: Braunwald E, editor. Heart Disease: A Textbook of Cardiovascular Medicine, 5th ed. Philadelphia: W.B Saunders; 1997. p. 471–491.

4. Gardner SY, et al. Characterization of the pharmacokinetic and pharmacodynamic properties of the angiotensin-converting enzyme inhibitor, enalapril, in horses. J Vet Intern Med 2004;18(2):231–237.

5. Sleeper MM, McDonnell SM, Ely JJ, et al. Chronic oral therapy with

enalapril in normal ponies. J Vet Cardiol 2008;10(2):111–115.

6. Gehlen H, Vieht JC, Stadler P. Effects of the ACE inhibitor quinapril on echocardiographic variables in horses with mitral valve insufficiency. J Vet Med A Physiol Pathol Clin Med 2003;50(9):460–465.

7. Mandal AK, Markert RJ, Saklayen MG, et al. Diuretics potentiate angiotensin converting enzyme inhibitor-induced acute renal failure. Clin Nephrol 1994;42: 170–174.

8. Marr CM, Reimer JM. The cardiovascular system. In: Higgins AJ, Wright IM, editors. The Equine Manual. Philadelphia: WB Saunders; 1995. p. 381–408.

9. Jackson EK. Diuretics. In: Hardman JG, Limbird LE, Molinoff PB, et al, editors. Goodman and Gilman's The Pharmacological Basis of Therapeutics, 9th ed. New York: McGraw-Hill; 1996. p. 685–715.

10. Muir WM, McGuirk SM. Pharmacology and pharmacokinetics of drugs used to treat cardiac disease in the horse. Vet Clin N Am: Eq Pract 1985;1: 353–370.

11. Johansson AM, Gardner SY, Levine JF, et al. Furosemide continuous rate infusion in the horse: evaluation of enhanced efficacy and reduced side effects. J Vet Intern Med 2003;17(6):887–895.

12. Johansson AM, Gardner SY, Levine JF, et al. Pharmacokinetics and pharmacodynamics of furosemide after oral administration to horses. J Vet Intern Med 2004;18(5): 739–743.

13. Zipes DP. Management of cardiac arrhythmias: pharmacological, electrical and surgical techniques. In: Braunwald E, editor. Heart Disease: A Textbook of Cardiovascular Medicine, 5th ed. Philadelphia: WB Saunders; 1997. p. 593–639.

14. Ferguson DW, Berg WJ, Sanders JS, et al. Sympathoinhibitory responses to digitalis glycosides in heart failure patients. Circulation 1989;80:65–77.

15. Francfort P, Schatzmann HJ. Pharmacological experiments as a basis for the administration of digoxin in the horse. Res Vet Sci 1976;20:84–89.

16. Perdersoli WM, Belmonte AA, Purohit RC, et al. Pharmacokinetics of digoxin in the horse. J Eq Med Surg 1978;2:384–388.

17. Button C, Gross DR, Johnston JT, et al. Digoxin pharmacokinetics, bioavailability, efficacy, and dosage regimens in the horse. Am J Vet Res 1980;41:1388–1395.

18. Pedersoli WM, Ravis WR, Belmonte AA, et al. Pharmacokinetics of a single, orally administered dose of digoxin in horses. Am J Vet Res 1981;42:1412–1414.

19. Brumbaugh GW, Thomas WP, Enos LR, et al. A phamacokinetic study of digoxin in the horse. J Vet Pharmacol Therap 1983;6: 163–172.

20. Sweeney RW, Reef VB, Reimer JM. Pharmacokinetics of digoxin administered to horses with congestive heart failure. Am J Vet Res 1993;54:1108–1111.

21. Wijnberg ID, van der Kolk JH, Hiddink EG. Use of phenytoin to treat digitalis-induced cardiac arrhythmias in a miniature Shetland pony. Vet Rec 1999; 144(10):259–261.

22. Baquero H, Soliz A, Neira F, et al. Oral sildenafil in infants with persistent pulmonary hypertension of the newborn: a pilot randomized blinded study. Pediatrics 2006;117(4):1077–1083.

23. Binns-Loveman KM, Kaplowitz MR, Fike CD. Sildenafil and an early stage of chronic hypoxia-induced pulmonary hypertension in newborn piglets. Pediatr Pulmonol 2005;40(1):72–80.

24. Hollis AR, Ousey JC, Palmer L, et al. Effects of norepinephrine and a combined norepinephrine and dobutamine infusion on systemic hemodynamics and indices of renal function in normotensive neonatal thoroughbred foals. J Vet Intern Med 2006;20(6): 1437–1442.

25. Vaala WE, Marr CM, Maxson AD, et al. Perinatology. In: Higgins AJ, Wright IM, editors. The Equine Manual. Philadelphia: WB Saunders; 1995. p. 637–723.

26. Denton MD, Chertow GM, Brady HR. "Renal-dose" dopamine for the treatment of acute renal failure: scientific rationale, experimental studies and clinical trials. Kidney Int 1996;50(1):4–14.

27. Allessie MA, Wijffels MC, Dorland R. Mechanisms of pharmacologic cardioversion of atrial fibrillation by Class I drugs. J Cardiovasc Electrophysiol 1998;9(8 Suppl): S69–S77.

28. Comtois P, Kneller J, Nattel S. Of circles and spirals: bridging the gap between the leading circle and spiral wave concepts of cardiac reentry. Europace 2005;7:S10-S20.

29. Jalife J. Rotors and spiral waves in atrial fibrillation. J Cardiovasc Electrophysiol 2003;14(7): 776–780.

30. Fenton F, Cherry EM, Kornreich BG. Termination of equine atrial fibrillation by quinidine: an optical mapping study. J Vet Cardiol 2008;10(2):87–109.

31. Baggot JD. The pharmacological basis of cardiac drug selection for use in horses. Eq Vet J Suppl 1995;19:97–100.

32. McGuirk SM, Muir WW, Sams RA. Pharmacokinetic analysis of intravenously and orally administered quinidine in horses. Am J Vet Res 1981;42:938–942. 19.

33. Schwarzwald CC, Hamlin RL, Bonagura JD, et al. Atrial, SA nodal, and AV nodal electrophysiology in standing horses: normal findings and electrophysiologic effects of quinidine and diltiazem. J Vet Intern Med 2007;21(1):166–175.

34. Marr CM. Treatment of cardiac arrhythmias and cardiac failure. In: Robinson NE, editor. Current Therapy in Equine Medicine, 4th ed. Philadelphia: W. B. Saunders; 1997. p. 250–254.

35. Roden DM. Antiarrhythmic drugs. In: Hardman JG, Limbird LE, Molinoff PB, et al, editors. Goodman and Gilman's The Pharmacological Basis of Therapeutics, 9th ed. New York: McGraw-Hill; 1996. p. 839–874.

36. Parraga ME, Kittleson MD, Drake CM. Quinidine administration increases steady state serum digoxin concentration in horses. Eq Vet J Suppl 1995;19:114–119.

37. Dickey EJ, McKenzie HC 3rd, Brown KA, et al. Serum concentrations of lidocaine and its metabolites after prolonged infusion in healthy horses. Equine Vet J 2008;40(4):348–352.

38. Wijnberg ID, Ververs FF. Phenytoin sodium as a treatment for ventricular dysrhythmia in horses. J Vet Intern Med 2004;18(3): 350–353.

39. De Clercq D, van Loon G, Tavernier R, Verbesselt R, Deprez P. Use of propafenone for conversion of chronic atrial fibrillation in horses. Am J Vet Res 2009;70(2): 223–227.

40. Alp NJ, Bell JA, Shahi M. Randomised double blind trial of oral versus intravenous flecainide for the cardioversion of acute atrial fibrillation. Heart 2000;84(1): 37–40.

41. Ohmura H, Hiraga A, Aida H, et al. Determination of oral dosage and pharmacokinetic analysis of flecainide in horses. J Vet Med Sci 2001;63(5):511–514.

42. Ohmura H, Hiraga A, Aida H, et al. Safe and efficacious dosage of flecainide acetate for treating equine atrial fibrillation. J Vet Med Sci 2000;62(7):711–715.

43. Birettoni F, Porciello F, Rishniw M, et al. Treatment of chronic atrial fibrillation in the horse with flecainide: personal observation. Vet Res Commun 2007;31 (Suppl 1):273–275.

44. van Loon G, Blissitt KJ, Keen JA, et al. Use of intravenous flecainide in horses with naturally-occurring atrial fibrillation. Equine Vet J 2004;36(7):609–614.

45. Risberg AI, McGuirk SM. Successful conversion of equine atrial fibrillation using oral flecainide. J Vet Intern Med 2006;20(1): 207–209.

46. Robinson S, Feary DJ. Sudden death following oral administration of flecainide to horses with naturally occuring atrial fibrillation. Aust Equine Vet 2008;27:49–51.

47. De Clercq D, Baert K, Croubels S, et al. Evaluation of the pharmacokinetics and bioavailability of intravenously and orally administered amiodarone in horses. Am J Vet Res 2006;67(3):448–454.

48. Trachsel D, Tschudi P, Portier CJ, et al. Pharmacokinetics and pharmacodynamic effects of amiodarone in plasma of ponies after single intravenous administration. Toxicol Appl Pharmacol 2004;195(1): 113–125.

49. De Clercq D, van Loon G, Baert K, et al. Intravenous amiodarone treatment in horses with chronic atrial fibrillation. Vet J 2006;172(1):129–134.

50. De Clercq D, van Loon G, Baert K, et al. Effects of an adapted intravenous amiodarone treatment protocol in horses with atrial fibrillation. Equine Vet J 2007;39(4):344–349.

51. De Clercq D, van Loon G, Baert K, et al. Treatment with amiodarone of refractory ventricular tachycardia in a horse. J Vet Intern Med 2007;21(4):878–880.

52. Imhasly A, Tschuid PR, Gerber C. Combined amiodarone and chinidine sulfate show no advantage over chinidine sulfate alone in equine atrial fibrillation. Pferdeheilkunde 2008;24(5): 693–698.

Section | 2 |

Diagnostic methods

Chapter | 8 |

Auscultation

Karen Blissitt

INTRODUCTION

Despite the lack of gross changes to the tricuspid valve at post mortem examination,[1] Stockman, an Edinburgh pathologist, believed tricuspid regurgitation (TR) to be the commonest affliction of the horse.[2] This diagnosis made solely by auscultation has been supported by more recent epidemiological studies using Doppler echocardiography.[3] However, despite the increased availability of this more sensitive diagnostic technique, auscultation remains the principal means to evaluate the equine heart.[4] Opinions differ as to the accuracy of auscultation when used to diagnose cardiac murmurs. Young and Wood[3] reported 100% specificity for the diagnosis of mitral regurgitation (MR) and TR whereas Naylor and others[5] reported poor accuracy for the diagnosis of a recording of a cardiac murmur; accuracies of 29, 33 and 53% were reported for second year veterinary students, general practitioners and diplomates of a European or American College of internal medicine, respectively. The accuracy of diagnosis was shown to be significantly influenced by training with only diplomates being able to reliably differentiate systolic from diastolic murmurs, although the ability to hear the physical properties of the murmur remained unchanged. However, other authors also believe that a high degree of accuracy can be achieved for the diagnosis of most murmurs in the living animal[4,6] and agree that Doppler echocardiography, by increasing our knowledge of the origin of many types of murmur,[3,6] has improved teaching and learning, further improving the accuracy of diagnosis by auscultation. This chapter aims to improve diagnostic skill by describing how to differentiate the common cardiac murmurs in horses. Recordings of a variety of cardiac murmurs are presented in the case studies included with this book. However, it must be remembered that the challenge in diagnosis is not in hearing and diagnosing the cause of a cardiac murmur on a recording but in finding and accurately localizing the origin of a murmur in a live animal. With a thorough understanding of normal cardiac physiology, accuracy in diagnosis can be achieved, providing auscultation is undertaken in a quiet environment and sufficient time and thought is put into the examination. A thorough systematic physical examination before reaching for a stethoscope will help in identifying the significance of any cardiac murmurs and prevent such murmurs from being overlooked.

AETIOLOGY OF CARDIAC MURMURS

A murmur is a series of auditory vibrations[7] occurring during a normally silent period of the cardiac cycle.[8] Murmurs have been attributed to the presence of turbulent blood flow,[9,10] periodic wake fluctuations[11] or to eddy and vortex formation causing vibration of solid structures.[12,13] Murmurs can be associated with congenital cardiac abnormalities,[14] and often develop as a result of valvular dysfunction,[15] but they are also present in a large number of clinically normal horses.[3,16,17,18]

Turbulent flow occurs when blood flows at high velocity in wide tubes[19] and has been recorded in the aorta of clinically normal horses during ventricular systole and in the left ventricle during rapid filling.[20] Murmurs during ventricular ejection and filling are audible in up to 50% and 15% of normal horses, respectively.[16] The intensity of these physiological flow murmurs varies and tends to increase with excitement.[17] In disease states, e.g. MR and aortic regurgitation (AR) where there is an increase in the blood flow velocities during rapid ventricular filling and ventricular ejection, respectively, flow murmurs may become audible.[21] Turbulent flow is also present during increased flow states, e.g. anaemia and exercise.[10]

Turbulent jets with eddies and vortices at their boundaries are produced when blood flows through narrow orifices into wide channels, as occurs during valvular regurgitation.[13] Sound is also thought to be produced by jets directly striking vessel or chamber walls.[13]

IDENTIFICATION OF NORMAL HEART SOUNDS (EA)

It is necessary to identify the normal sounds to accurately time and therefore diagnose the cause of cardiac murmurs. Low-frequency sounds are easily palpated and the low frequency components of the first, second and third heart sounds can be palpated in the left cardiac area of slim athletic horses. Palpation of the left cardiac area before auscultation will help the examiner to concentrate on the heart rate and rhythm, the identification of the heart sounds and any abnormal vibrations before being distracted by the presence of cardiac murmurs.

The first (S1) and second (S2) heart sound can be heard at the level of the apex beat and mark the beginning and end of systole, respectively. The first sound is a relatively long sound compared to S2 and occurs at the onset of ventricular ejection. It is caused by the initial movement of the ventricle, the abrupt arrest of intracardiac blood flow as the atrioventricular (AV) valves tense, and the early part of ejection.[16,22] The second heart sound, which is shorter and higher pitched than S1, is caused by the change in direction of blood flow in the aorta and pulmonary trunk at the end of systole, closing the aortic and pulmonary valves.[16] In athletic horses with low resting heart rates, two components of S2 (of pulmonic and aortic origin) can often be distinguished when the stethoscope is positioned over the pulmonary valve area. However, two separate sounds can only be heard if they are separated by more than 30 ms,[23] which only occurs at low

heart rates. There is marked variation between individual clinicians in their ability to distinguish sounds that are close together; however, this does not influence their ability to accurately diagnose the cause of cardiac murmurs. Very marked separation or differences in intensity of the two components of S2 may occur in disease states, e.g. pulmonary hypertension.

The third heart sound (S3) is commonly heard in Thoroughbred-type horses. It occurs at the end of the active relaxation of the ventricle and is associated with the abrupt checking of the outward movement of the ventricular walls.[22] It can be differentiated from a split S2 by the different location in which it is heard and its timing. The third heart sound is commonly heard at or slightly caudal and dorsal to the apex beat, whereas a split S2 is heard cranially over the pulmonary valve area. The two components of S2 are temporally very close together and of similar frequency whereas S2 and S3 are more widely separated with S3 being of lower frequency (Fig. 8.1). The intensity of S3 is often increased in horses with atrial fibrillation and in those with very severe MR.[24] (AF, RCT, VMD)

The fourth heart sound (S4) is associated with the transient closure of the AV valves following the atrial contraction and the sudden checking of the distended ventricle.[16] It is commonly heard in Thoroughbred-type horses closely preceding S1 (see Fig. 8.1) but is heard less commonly in ponies. An earlier group of vibrations associated with the atrial contractions and AV blood flow is not normally audible at the thoracic wall. A split S1, where the two sounds are of similar frequencies, is less commonly heard and is due to separation of the sounds originating from

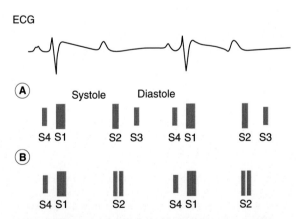

Figure 8.1 (**A**) Timing of heart sounds commonly audible over the apex beat in resting horses. S1 and S2 are of higher frequency than S4 and S3 and are therefore heard more clearly. (**B**) Timing of heart sounds commonly audible over the pulmonary valve area in resting Thoroughbred horses. In this location S3 is not usually audible, S4 may or may not be audible, and S2 may be split.

the left and right ventricle. This is most commonly identified in horses with atrial fibrillation where the atrial contraction and S4 is absent. This can cause difficulties in diagnosis as the split S1 can be mistakenly identified as S4 and S1.

The choice of stethoscope will not limit the cardiac examination as much as the amount of care and thought taken using it; however, various factors should be considered. Higher frequency sounds (e.g. S1 and S2, and AV valve regurgitation) are damped by a large volume of air between the chest and the ear piece.[7] Thicker and shorter tubing decreases the audibility of extraneous noise; therefore, short stethoscopes 10–12 inches (25–30 cm) are advantageous.[7] The diaphragm of the stethoscope damps out lower frequency sound whereas the bell of the stethoscope is more suitable for detecting these sounds (e.g. S3 and S4, and diastolic murmurs). Cardiovascular sounds and murmurs are usually in the range 20–1000 Hz but the human ear is most sensitive within the range 1000–4000 Hz. Due to the decreased sensitivity of the human ear to low frequency sounds these must be of greater amplitude to reach the threshold of audibility of a sound of higher frequency.[25] Sensor-based electronic stethoscopes are now available which allow the operator to increase the amplitude of detected sounds and to select the frequency range over which they wish to listen. A frequency range of 20–420 Hz has been set by one manufacturer to correspond to the "bell" of the stethoscope for the detection of most heart sounds and murmurs, whereas 350–1900 Hz is used to represent the diaphragm mode to detect higher frequency sounds (high frequency murmurs, clicks, ejection sounds and lung sounds). Sensor-based stethoscopes allow data to be stored digitally and replayed or analysed at a later date.

IDENTIFICATION OF MURMURS

The differentiation of the various cardiac murmurs in horses can be difficult: especially the systolic murmurs that are the most common, and can arise from a number of sites.[26,27] In addition to the high prevalence of physiological flow murmurs in horses,[17,18,26] MR and TR have been shown to develop in Standardbred[28] and Thoroughbred racehorses in response to training with up to 30% of normal young Thoroughbred racehorses affected.[3] Reduced athletic performance is also common in racehorses but it is important to recognize that cardiac murmurs are often an incidental finding in these horses.[29] Recently there has been extensive research on the relationship of cardiac murmurs to performance;[30] murmurs of AV regurgitation are not necessarily associated with performance limitations and this is discussed in more detail in Chapter 16.

Cardiac murmurs are classified and diagnosed based on the following criteria: location, timing, quality, radiation and intensity.

Location

(EA)

The point of maximum intensity (PMI) of a cardiac murmur is generally located over the site of turbulence,[7] and gives an indication of the origin of the murmur.[4,8,31,32] As most cardiac murmurs in horses originate from the cardiac valves, it is important to be able to relate the PMI of any murmur to the location of the cardiac valves. The apex beat, which can be palpated over the left thoracic wall at the level of the olecranon process, locates the PMI of sounds originating at the mitral valve (mitral valve area) and a murmur of MR will be heard most clearly at this location.[4,8]

Once the apex beat is located the other valve areas can be identified from changes in the intensity of the heart sounds. The first heart sound is heard most clearly over the apex beat, whereas S2 is heard most clearly dorsal and cranial to the apex beat. This is the site to which sounds originating at the aortic valve most commonly radiate. Sounds originating from the pulmonary valve are audible cranial and ventral to the aortic valve area with the stethoscope pushed cranial beneath the triceps mass. The pulmonary valve area can be identified more precisely in horses where a split S2 can be heard (see Fig. 8.1).

Sounds originating from the tricuspid valve are audible over the right hemithorax, cranial to the location of the apex beat palpated on the left side of the chest. It is helpful to localize valve areas from the apex beat, rather than by identifying specific intercostal spaces in relation to the olecranon process, as horses vary in the placement of the forelimbs. If auscultation is always commenced by placing the stethoscope immediately behind the triceps mass, this will result in too caudal a placement in most cobs, the heart sounds will appear quieter and murmurs may be missed. This is especially true when auscultating the right side of the thorax. In some horses it is necessary to place the stethoscope well forward under the triceps mass or position the right forelimb cranial to hear the sounds and murmurs associated with the tricuspid valve.

Although the mitral, aortic, pulmonic and tricuspid valve areas are the main areas for cardiac auscultation, auscultation should not be limited to these areas. The stethoscope should be kept in contact with the thoracic wall as it is moved between the valve areas, as this decreases the chances of missing audible sounds and murmurs. Radiation of murmurs will be influenced by thoracic conformation, chamber enlargement and the direction of abnormal blood flow.

Timing

(EA)

The causes of cardiac murmurs can be further differentiated from their timing within the cardiac cycle.[22,32] Murmurs may be systolic (AF, IE, RCT, RSD, SFP, VMD, VSD), diastolic (AF, AR, CCD, IE, RSD) or continuous (AF). Once the stethoscope is located over the apex beat it should be moved around until S1 is heard most clearly. The clinician should then listen to the rate and rhythm, identify the heart sounds present and then listen to systole (the period between S1 and S2) and diastole (the period between S2 and S1) for the presence of cardiac murmurs.[33] This process should then be repeated as the stethoscope is moved over the other valve areas. The underlying heart rhythm can then be identified and superimposed on the murmur to confirm timing. If it is still difficult to differentiate systole from diastole due to the heart sounds being obscured by a murmur, it is helpful to remember that diastole is longer than systole therefore a very long murmur is more often diastolic (see Fig. 8.1). If the heart sounds are obscured by a murmur such that systole and diastole cannot be identified, it is helpful to find a location where the heart sounds can still be heard and the murmur is less prominent or to palpate the arterial pulses while asculating the heart: a systolic murmur will be coincident with the pulse whereas a diastolic murmur alternates with the pulse. The heart rate and the regularity of the underlying rhythm should always be recorded as this will help in appreciating the significance of any cardiac murmur. A horse in congestive cardiac failure will have an increased heart rate 60–70 beats per minute. Disturbances in cardiac rhythm are discussed more fully in Chapter 13.

Systolic murmurs result as blood regurgitates through incompetent AV (mitral and tricuspid) valves or as blood is ejected through the semilunar (aortic and pulmonic) valves. MR and TR are common causes of systolic murmurs in adult horses.[16–18,26–28,30] Systolic ejection murmurs occur when there is increased flow through the semilunar valves, obstruction to ventricular outflow (valve stenosis), valvular damage without stenosis or dilatation of the vessel beyond the valve.[34] Systolic ejection murmurs have been recorded over the aorta and pulmonary artery in clinically normal horses. Aortic and pulmonic stenosis, although common in man[7] and dogs,[35] have been rarely reported in horses.[4] Pulmonic stenosis has been reported in foals with multiple cardiac abnormalities related to tetralogy of Fallot[36,37] but hardly ever presents as an isolated finding.[38,39]

Due to variations in terminology, there is confusion in the veterinary literature as to the incidence of aortic stenosis in horses. Congenital stenosis of the aortic valve is a rare occurrence.[16,40–43] However, acquired stenosis may develop in cases of endocarditis[4,42] and a relative stenosis can occur due to increased blood flow through the valve,

in cases with severe AR.[21] Confirmed reports of aortic stenosis causing obstruction to blood flow are rare.[44]

Diastolic murmurs can be divided into three categories: atrial systolic murmurs (presystolic) occurring between S4 and S1, ventricular filling murmurs occurring between S2 and S3, and regurgitant murmurs from the aortic and pulmonary valves.[34] Presystolic murmurs and ventricular filling murmurs are audible in clinically normal horses.[16,17,18,26–28] Stenosis of the AV valves is extremely rare; therefore, the most likely cause of a diastolic murmur extending beyond the third heart sound is incompetence or regurgitation of the semilunar valves – most likely the aortic valve.

Continuous murmurs start in systole and extend through S2 into diastole.[8] They result from aortopulmonary, aortocardiac or arteriovenous connections or from flow disturbances in arteries and veins. The most common aortopulmonary connection is the patent ductus arteriosus although in adult horses, a murmur audible throughout systole and diastole is more likely to be due to a combination of two or more separate murmurs. (ACF)

Differentiation of the timing within systole and diastole can further aid diagnosis. Ejection murmurs are early to mid systolic and end before S2,[16,34] whereas regurgitant murmurs may occur at any time during systole (early, mid, late) and may extend beyond S2. This can be easily understood by reference to the pressure changes in the heart and great vessels during the cardiac cycle (Fig. 8.2), although there is some confusion in the terminology used to describe these murmurs. The term pansystolic describes a murmur which begins with or replaces S1, continues throughout systole and ends beyond S2, whereas the term holosystolic describes a murmur which starts at the end of S1 and continues to the start of S2, although some authors use the terms interchangeably.[25] Murmurs that last throughout systole and extend beyond S2 are likely to be of greater clinical significance than those murmurs which occupy only part of systole[45] and it is helpful to reserve the term pansystolic to describe these longer murmurs as this represents clinically important information.

Diastolic murmurs associated with ventricular filling end with S3, which marks the end of rapid filling caused by active relaxation of the ventricle, whereas the murmur of AR is often present throughout diastole[15,46] (Fig. 8.3). In order to differentiate these murmurs and the presystolic murmur, it is necessary to be able to identify the normal heart sounds and be aware of the normal timing of these sounds, so that murmurs can be diagnosed in horses in which S3 and S4 are not readily audible.

Frequency

(EA)

Most murmurs are noisy and are composed of a broad range of frequencies; however some, termed musical, have

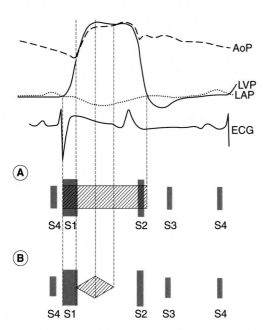

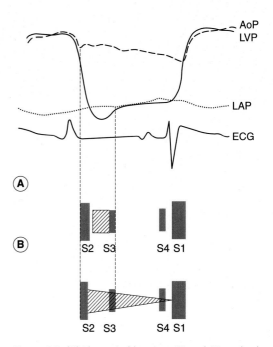

Figure 8.2 (**A**) Ventricular pressure (LVP) exceeds atrial pressure (LAP) from the onset of S1 until after S2. Therefore the murmur of mitral regurgitation can start with S1 and may continue until after S2 (pansystolic). (**B**) Ventricular pressure (LVP) exceeds aortic pressure (AoP) during the first two-thirds of ejection. In the last third forward flow is maintained by the momentum imparted to the column of blood. Therefore, the ejection murmur occurs in the first two-thirds of systole, when blood flow is fastest, and ends before S2.

Figure 8.3 (**A**) The period between S2 and S3 marks the rapid filling of the ventricle when the pressure gradient between the atrium (LAP) and ventricle (LVP) is greatest. A murmur caused by ventricular filling may be audible in normal horses at this time. (**B**) The murmur of aortic regurgitation starts with S2 as the aortic valve closes. Aortic pressure (AoP) remains higher than ventricular pressure throughout diastole until the start of ventricular systole. Therefore, the murmur of aortic regurgitation may continue throughout this period.

a pure tone being composed of harmonic frequencies.[47] Many terms are used to describe cardiac murmurs although these are not used in a consistent manner.[48] The terms musical, buzzing, honking and blowing are used most consistently[48]; musical, buzzing and honking are used to describe harmonic murmurs with a peak dominant frequency. Low-frequency harmonic murmurs are described as buzzing whereas higher frequency harmonic murmurs are described as musical. The term honking was used to describe harmonic murmurs of very short duration although an alternative and possibly less confusing approach would be to describe these murmurs as short musical or buzzing murmurs. The term blowing was predominantly used to describe noisy murmurs without harmonics. However, as any murmur not described as musical or buzzing can be assumed to have no harmonic frequencies the use of the term blowing is probably unnecessary.

The frequency or pitch of a murmur may aid diagnosis of the underlying cause.[8,32] The diastolic murmur of AR is often musical,[15] whereas the diastolic murmur associated with ventricular filling in healthy young horses often presents as a high-pitched squeak.[49] (AR)

Radiation

The direction in which a murmur radiates over the body surface also helps in localizing the site of origin.[22] The murmur caused by a membranous ventricular septal defect (VSD) is audible over the right hemithorax at the level of the tricuspid valve. It can be differentiated from the murmur of TR because it radiates cranially and ventrally towards the sternal border. Murmurs of AR tend to radiate to the left hemithorax at the aortic valve level; however, when the degree of valvular dysfunction increases, the murmur is also audible over the right hemithorax. (AR, VSD)

The area over which a murmur radiates also gives an indication of its likely significance.[50] Therefore, once a murmur has been identified, the stethoscope should be moved around the thoracic wall to determine the extent of its radiation. The more widely the murmur radiates the more clinically significant the lesion is likely to be. However, this information must be used in conjunction with knowledge of the murmur's frequency. If a murmur has harmonic frequencies, i.e. it is musical or buzzing, radiation will not be related to severity.[25] Musical or buzzing murmurs can be heard over a very large area and yet be of limited clinical significance.

Intensity

Murmurs may also be differentiated by characteristic variations in their intensity.[8,32] The murmur of AR decreases in intensity throughout diastole (see Fig. 8.3) and may increase in intensity immediately following S4.[15,46] Systolic ejection murmurs often increase in intensity, reaching a crescendo in mid-systole, and then decrease,[16,34] whereas regurgitant murmurs are usually of constant intensity[22] and are described as band shaped[8] (see Fig. 8.2). The intensity of heart murmurs is graded using either a grade 1–6 system[33] or a 1–5 system.[22] Grade 4–5/5 and 5–6/6 murmurs are associated with a palpable precordial thrill and are thought always to be associated with significant cardiovascular dysfunction.[51] Precordial thrills are palpable manifestations of loud harsh murmurs of low frequency[7] and it is these murmurs that are more likely to be associated with significant cardiovascular disease in horses.

The significance of the intensity of a murmur is debatable. Some authors have suggested that innocent murmurs in healthy horses are always grade 3/5 or less.[8,51] However, not all serious valvular lesions cause loud murmurs and not all loud murmurs arise from serious valvular lesions.[50] This is supported by the use of colour flow Doppler echocardiography which has confirmed grade 4/6 ejection murmurs in a small number of normal horses. The intensity of a murmur is governed by the quantity and velocity of blood flow across the sound-producing area,[7] the distance from the stethoscope and the ease of transmission of the sound through the various tissues between the stethoscope and the origin of the murmur. High-frequency musical murmurs tend to be more easily audible than low-frequency noisy murmurs for a given degree of valvular dysfunction.[52] Restrictive VSDs which are of no clinical significance may give rise to a loud murmur, whereas loud murmurs of MR and TR are usually associated with marked valvular dysfunction. (VSD) A study in human patients has shown that the audibility of regurgitant murmurs is highly dependent on the severity of regurgitation; mild regurgitation detected by Doppler echocardiography was associated with quieter murmurs that were only audible in 10–40% of cases whereas severe regurgitation caused murmurs that were audible in 86–100% of cases.[52] Murmurs of severe MR and TR, however, will reduce in intensity as the heart goes into failure. Therefore, it is important to make an accurate diagnosis of the cause of a particular murmur before using the intensity as an indication of severity. It must be noted that with the exception of musical or buzzing murmurs, the radiation of a particular murmur often gives a greater indication of severity than the intensity alone.

DIAGNOSIS OF SPECIFIC MURMURS

Left-sided systolic murmurs

(AF, CCD, IE, RCT, RSD, SFP, VMD)

The most common causes of left-sided systolic murmurs in adult horses are normal ventricular ejection and MR. It is often important to differentiate these two murmurs, as the former is not indicative of valvular disease, whereas a murmur of MR may be associated with valvular dysfunction although this may or may not be progressive and it may or may not impact on the horse's general health and athletic capacity.

Aortic stenosis is very rare in horses (see section on Timing above) and can effectively be ignored in the differential diagnosis of a systolic murmur in adult horses. MR can range in its severity from clinically insignificant to life threatening. It is the most common cause of cardiac failure in horses. However, the progression of the disease in mild to moderate cases of regurgitation, and the underlying pathology, is not fully understood. Difficulty in the diagnosis of systolic murmurs has been reported in humans,[54] and a left-sided systolic murmur is the most common reason for referral for further diagnosis using echocardiography in horses.

Differentiation of mitral regurgitation and functional ejection murmurs

(EA)

Functional ejection murmurs are caused by disturbed blood flow[20] and can be heard over the aorta and pulmonary artery during systole.[16] They occur in clinically normal horses, the earliest report describing them in 66% of normal horses.[55] Later studies have supported this observation.[3,16] They can usually be differentiated from murmurs of MR using the methods described above. The PMI of functional ejection murmurs is over the aortic or pulmonary valve, whereas that of MR is over the apex beat. Problems in diagnosis arise when the PMI of the murmur lies between the aortic valve area and the apex beat or when loud ejection murmurs radiate to the cardiac apex.[34] This is especially true in horses with colic, which commonly have loud systolic ejection murmurs that extend to the cardiac apex. These are not associated with cardiac pathology and disappear as the horse recovers. Similarly MR murmurs may radiate dorsally towards the aortic valve, making differentiation difficult. In these cases diagnosis can be aided by attempting to alter the intensity of the functional murmur. Functional murmurs have been shown to change in character following exercise, some disappearing and some becoming more accentuated.[16,56] Some ejection murmurs only become apparent during exercise or excitement.[16] Most often functional murmurs tend to increase in intensity if the horse is turned quickly in the loose box, or stopped abruptly after a brief trot. After more prolonged exercise more appropriate to the animal's fitness, many functional murmurs disappear. By changing the intensity of the functional murmur it is usually possible to locate the PMI more accurately. Horses with a systolic murmur in which the PMI is located between the two sites are often found to have a functional murmur and mild MR. Functional murmurs never have a precordial thrill.

The timing of the murmur can also be used to differentiate functional ejection murmurs from the murmur of MR. Ventricular pressure is higher than atrial pressure from the onset of the S1 until after S2 (see Fig. 8.2). Therefore, regurgitation may occur throughout this period. Ejection, however, can only start when the ventricular pressure exceeds arterial pressure at the end of S1 and always ends before the S2 arising from that side of the heart.[47] The functional ejection murmur is caused by disturbed high-velocity blood flow in the early part of ejection. Figure 8.4 shows that the velocity of aortic flow increases in the first third of ejection, decreases in the second third and then

forward flow is maintained only by the momentum imparted to the column of blood. Therefore, ejection murmurs are only audible in early to mid-systole and do not extend to S2. Classically, ejection murmurs are described as crescendo-decrescendo. They increase in intensity as the velocity of flow increases in the first third of systole and then decrease in intensity in the second third. A systolic murmur over the left hemithorax that continues to S2 is most likely to be caused by MR (Fig. 8.5). In small animals where valvular stenosis is a differential in the diagnosis of systolic murmurs, this assumption cannot be made. Although a murmur of valvular stenosis will end before the S2 originating from the valve on that side, it may continue up to or beyond the S2 component originating from the other semilunar valve giving the impression that the murmur continues to S2.[47]

Unfortunately regurgitant murmurs do not always continue throughout systole. Depending on the cause, murmurs of MR may be early, mid-, late, pan (ending after S2) or holosystolic (ending at the start of S2) (see Fig. 8.5). MR may be caused by rupture of the chordae tendineae of the valve,[57,58] thickening and rounding of the valve leaflets,[59] papillary muscle dysfunction,[59] dilatation of the mitral valve annulus,[59] congenital abnormalities,[60] infective endocarditis (rare)[61] or associated with no obvious underlying pathology. Murmurs associated with a major chordal rupture usually continue throughout systole

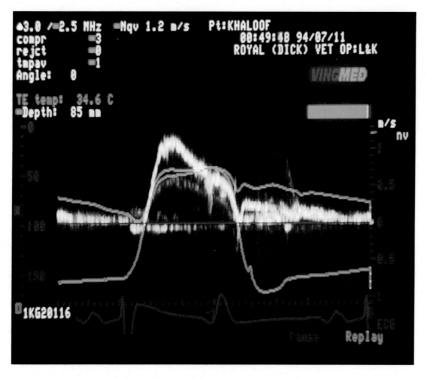

Figure 8.4 Transoesophageal Doppler echocardiograph showing the velocity of blood flow in the aorta (gold signal). Velocity is on the y-axis (right) in m/s. Time is on the x-axis. The ECG is at the bottom of the image (purple trace). Flow in the aorta is not recorded until the left ventricular pressure (blue trace) exceeds aortic pressure (green trace). The velocity of flow then increases rapidly in the first third of systole to approximately 1.2 ms. The blood decelerates in the second third of systole to approximately 0.6 m/s. In the last third of systole when aortic pressure is greater than left ventricular pressure, forward flow is maintained by the momentum imparted to the column of blood.

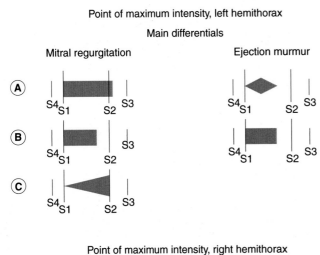

Point of maximum intensity, left hemithorax

Main differentials

Mitral regurgitation   Ejection murmur

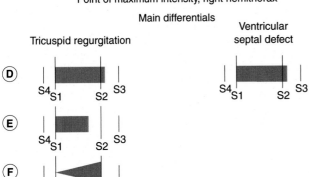

Point of maximum intensity, right hemithorax

Main differentials

Tricuspid regurgitation   Ventricular septal defect

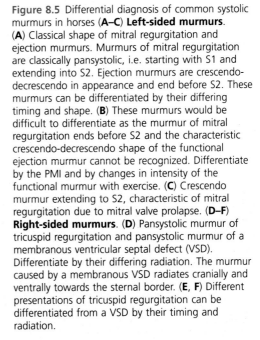

Figure 8.5 Differential diagnosis of common systolic murmurs in horses (**A–C**) **Left-sided murmurs**. (**A**) Classical shape of mitral regurgitation and ejection murmurs. Murmurs of mitral regurgitation are classically pansystolic, i.e. starting with S1 and extending into S2. Ejection murmurs are crescendo-decrescendo in appearance and end before S2. These murmurs can be differentiated by their differing timing and shape. (**B**) These murmurs would be difficult to differentiate as the murmur of mitral regurgitation ends before S2 and the characteristic crescendo-decrescendo shape of the functional ejection murmur cannot be recognized. Differentiate by the PMI and by changes in intensity of the functional murmur with exercise. (**C**) Crescendo murmur extending to S2, characteristic of mitral regurgitation due to mitral valve prolapse. (**D–F**) **Right-sided murmurs**. (**D**) Pansystolic murmur of tricuspid regurgitation and pansystolic murmur of a membranous ventricular septal defect (VSD). Differentiate by their differing radiation. The murmur caused by a membranous VSD radiates cranially and ventrally towards the sternal border. (**E**, **F**) Different presentations of tricuspid regurgitation can be differentiated from a VSD by their timing and radiation.

and end after S2. Whilst the timing and intensity of the regurgitant murmur may give an indication of the underlying cause further tests are required for a definitive diagnosis of the cause of the valvular regurgitation (see Chapters 9 and 16). (AF, RCT)

Murmurs of MR are most commonly band or plateau shaped, being of constant intensity throughout, or crescendo, increasing in intensity throughout. (SFP) Crescendo murmurs are thought to be due to mitral valve prolapse, the valve being competent during the start of systole, but prolapsing into the left atrium at the end of systole (see Fig. 8.5). These murmurs are relatively easy to diagnose due to this characteristic sound, the PMI and the fact that they continue to S2. Murmurs of MR that are limited to early or mid-systole are difficult to differentiate from the functional ejection murmur; however, in these cases the severity of MR is usually mild.

If the murmur of MR is not buzzing, severity can be assessed from the intensity and the area of auscultation of the murmur. Generally, for regurgitant murmurs the louder the murmur the more severe the valvular dysfunc-

tion. However, as the heart goes into failure, left atrial pressure rises, the pressure gradient across the mitral valve is reduced and the intensity of the sound decreases. In these cases the severity of the condition can be diagnosed by the area of radiation, which may include a large area of the thorax and other clinical signs of heart failure. An indication of the severity of MR can also be gained from the intensity of S3 and the presence of an early diastolic filling murmur. (RCT, VMD) In cases of severe MR S3 can be exaggerated and a pronounced flow murmur is often heard between S2 and S3, due to the increased inflow into the left ventricle during diastole.[24,32,58,59] In these cases the loud S3 can be confused with S2 and timing of the murmur can be difficult. It may help to listen to the heart sounds over the right hemithorax where the systolic and diastolic periods may be easier to identify before trying to superimpose the left-sided murmurs onto this rhythm. However, it must be remembered that functional early diastolic murmurs may coexist with mild MR, therefore this should not be used in isolation from other clinical findings. Although it has been reported that murmurs of MR can in some cases be heard on the right side of the thorax,[58] most often a right-sided murmur is due to coexisting TR.

Right-sided systolic murmurs (AF, CCD, EA, RSD, VMD, VSD)

The two systolic murmurs most commonly heard over the right hemithorax are those caused by a membranous VSD and TR (see Fig. 8.5). The VSD is the commonest congenital heart defect in horses,[14] while the murmur of TR is the most common murmur identified in National Hunt[3,17] and other racehorses. As horses with a small VSD often continue to perform normally,[62] this murmur may be detected as an incidental finding in adult horses. The murmurs of a membranous VSD and TR can be differentiated by their differing radiation. The systolic murmur associated with a VSD radiates ventral towards the sternal border, whereas the murmur of TR tends to radiate concentrically from its PMI over the tricuspid valve. Murmurs of TR are not normally heard cranially on the left side of the chest as has been previously suggested.[63] However in the very rare event of severe right ventricular dilatation associated with primary right-sided heart failure, this may occur.

Further evidence of the presence of a VSD is an associated systolic ejection murmur over the left hemithorax at the level of the pulmonary valve.[14] This is the murmur of relative pulmonic stenosis, caused by the increased flow of blood out of the right ventricle.

Murmurs associated with VSDs located in the muscular septum do not necessarily radiate in a cranial and ventral direction. However, the murmur will sound different from that caused by TR. In cases where the VSD is so large that the left and right ventricular pressures tend to equalize, there may be no murmur, as the flow across the VSD will be minimal. These cases are likely to have ventricular dilatation and the only murmurs present are likely to result from tricuspid and MR that has developed secondary to dilatation of the mitral and tricuspid valve annuli.

A less common form of VSD occurs in the infundibular septum beneath the pulmonary valve.[4] This is a rare condition that results in a harsh systolic ejection murmur over the left hemithorax at the level of the pulmonary valve. The murmur sounds like the murmur you would expect from pulmonic stenosis. However, as pulmonic stenosis occurs only rarely as an isolated finding,[38,39] this would be an unlikely differential in an adult horse. Echocardiography enables a definitive diagnosis to be made.

The severity of a VSD cannot be assessed from the intensity of the murmur, whereas colour flow Doppler studies have confirmed that the severity of TR does relate to the intensity of the murmur.[64] The severity of TR can also be inferred from the area over which the murmur can be heard and by the presence of a loud filling murmur or S3.

However, as stated for left-sided murmurs, a functional filling murmur may coexist with very mild TR. The best indication of the significance of TR is gained from observation of the jugular groove. With the head elevated, jugular pulsations extending above the lower third of the jugular groove are indicative of elevated right atrial pressure. If this is associated with a loud systolic murmur audible over a large area, the degree of TR is likely to be severe.

The causes of TR are similar to those described for MR, although rupture of the chordae tendineae, thickening of the valve leaflets and endocarditis are less common (see Chapter 16).[1] In most horses TR is not associated with any gross abnormality of the valve apparatus.

Diastolic murmurs (AF, AR, CCD, EA, IE, RSD)

Atrial systolic murmurs (occurring between S4 and S1) and ventricular filling murmurs (occurring between S2 and S3) have been reported in clinically healthy horses.[16,49] Ventricular filling murmurs also occur in association with severe MR due to the increased volume of blood flowing back into the left ventricle. Mitral and tricuspid stenoses are a recognized cause of diastolic murmurs in man,[7] but occur rarely in horses,[22,26] although they have been reported in foals as part of complex congenital disorders.[37]

AR is a common condition in horses, especially in older animals,[41,42,65] caused by thickening and distortion of the valve leaflets.[1,46] Pulmonic regurgitation (PR) can occur in horses but is rarely associated with an obvious murmur.[42]

Differentiation of the various diastolic murmurs (Fig. 8.6)

Early diastolic murmur (AF, EA)

The early diastolic filling murmur which occurs in normal horses can be differentiated from other diastolic murmurs by its timing and frequency. It occurs between S2 and S3, during the rapid filling phase of the left ventricle.[49] As S3 is not audible in all horses it is helpful to be aware of the normal rhythm of the heart sounds, so that the timing of this early diastolic murmur can be determined. The murmur often presents as a distinct squeak coincident with S3 (see Fig. 8.6A), although in some horses it is a longer sound,[40] beginning shortly after S2[22] and extending to S3[16] (see Fig. 8.6B). The squeak at S3 appears to be associated with the abrupt end of the active relaxation of the ventricle, whereas the soft murmur may be associated with the disturbed flow in the left ventricle during rapid filling.[20] As active relaxation and the velocity of ventricular filling vary with changes in sympathetic tone, so the murmur also varies. Similar to murmurs associated with

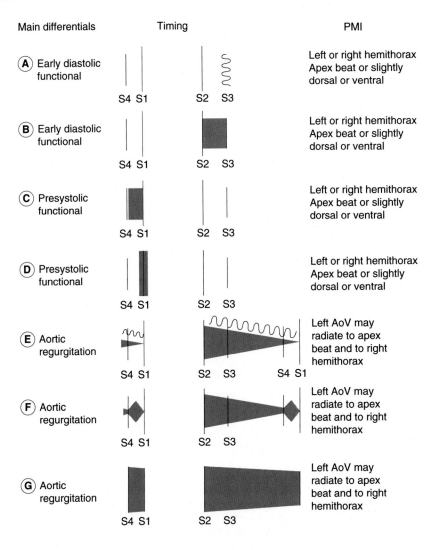

Main differentials — **Timing** — **PMI**

(A) Early diastolic functional
S4 S1 S2 S3
Left or right hemithorax Apex beat or slightly dorsal or ventral

(B) Early diastolic functional
S4 S1 S2 S3
Left or right hemithorax Apex beat or slightly dorsal or ventral

(C) Presystolic functional
S4 S1 S2 S3
Left or right hemithorax Apex beat or slightly dorsal or ventral

(D) Presystolic functional
S4 S1 S2 S3
Left or right hemithorax Apex beat or slightly dorsal or ventral

(E) Aortic regurgitation
S4 S1 S2 S3 S4 S1
Left AoV may radiate to apex beat and to right hemithorax

(F) Aortic regurgitation
S4 S1 S2 S3
Left AoV may radiate to apex beat and to right hemithorax

(G) Aortic regurgitation
S4 S1 S2 S3
Left AoV may radiate to apex beat and to right hemithorax

Figure 8.6 Differential diagnosis of common diastolic murmurs in horses. Diastolic murmurs can be differentiated by their timing. When a musical murmur is associated with S3 it can present as a squeak or a whoo sound. (**A**, **B**) Functional murmurs associated with ventricular filling. (**C**, **D**) Functional presystolic murmur commonly heard in National Hunt horses. (**E**, **F**) The murmur of aortic regurgitation is classically a musical decrescendo murmur that may increase in intensity following S4 (**F**). (**G**) Unusual presentation of an aortic regurgitation murmur. The murmur is coarse and obliterates the heart sounds and could be confused with a pansystolic murmur of mitral regurgitation. Differentiate by the length of diastole which is much longer than systole. Also palpate the pulses and auscultate the heart away from the murmur so that the heart sounds can be heard and the timing established.

ventricular ejection, early diastolic filling murmurs may disappear or increase in intensity with changes in sympathetic tone. They also vary in intensity in resting horses with normal variations in cycle length. These murmurs can be heard on either side of the thorax usually slightly dorsal to the mitral and tricuspid valve area, but can be heard ventrally.[4] These are heard very commonly in racing Thoroughbreds.[3,17]

Presystolic murmurs

Atrial systolic murmurs (presystolic murmurs) occur between S4 and S1[16] (see Fig. 8.6C, D). They are also heard in clinically healthy horses[22,40,42] and, as for the early diastolic murmur, can be differentiated by their timing within the cardiac cycle. These murmurs can be detected on both sides of the thorax, more commonly on the right, and are often very coarse. In many horses they start just

before and merge into S1. It has been suggested that this sound is associated with blood flow through the AV orifice during atrial systole,[16] but may be associated with presystolic regurgitation through the AV valves. When heard over the right hemithorax, the length and intensity of the presystolic murmur varies with breathing.

Aortic regurgitation
(AR, IE, RSD)

The murmur of AR can be identified by its PMI, timing, frequency and its characteristic decrescendo quality. The murmur is heard more intensely over the left side of the thorax at the level of the aortic valve. However, when the murmur increases in intensity it also becomes audible over the right side of the thorax. The murmur characteristically decreases in intensity throughout diastole (see Fig.

8.6E), but may increase again immediately following S4[15,46] (see Fig. 8.6F) due to distortion of the aortic valve during atrial systole.[15]

The murmur is often musical[15] and this makes diagnosis relatively easy. However, in some horses the murmur is noisy with no fundamental frequency and is similar in quality to a systolic regurgitant murmur. If these noisy diastolic murmurs are sufficiently loud to occlude the heart sounds, misdiagnosis often occurs (see Fig. 8.6G). In these cases the murmur can be recognized as diastolic by its length; diastole lasting longer than systole and because it alternates in its timing with the arterial pulse.

The musical quality of AR murmurs results from vibrations of the aortic root, aortic valve, interventricular septum or anterior mitral valve leaflet caused by the regurgitant blood flow. In these cases the severity of the regurgitation cannot be determined from the intensity of the murmur or area of radiation of the murmur,[53] as the loud buzzing or musical murmur radiates over a greater area and is heard more clearly than the softer noisy decrescendo murmur of the regurgitant flow. Severity may be assessed from palpation of the arterial pulses which have a wide pulse difference and can be described as bounding or hyperkinetic.[66] The increased preload and enhanced stroke volume present in those horses with more advanced disease may also cause a loud ejection murmur. Horses with AR should be monitored regularly for the development of left ventricular dilatation and MR secondary to dilatation of the mitral valve annulus; however, as mild MR is a common finding it may occur as an incidental finding in horses with AR. AR caused by thickening and fibrosis of the aortic valve leaflets is most common in older horses (see Chapter 16).[1] If a loud murmur of AR is detected in a younger horse (<10 years), the clinician should investigate causes of early valvular dysfunction. This may be caused by prolapse of the aortic valve leaflet into a membranous VSD,[62] which may or may not be patent, or a congenital abnormality of the aortic valve[67] (see Chapter 16).

Pulmonic regurgitation

PR is a common echocardiographic finding in horses, although it is not usually associated with a murmur. This is possibly due to the lower pressure gradient between the pulmonary artery and right ventricle, compared with that found on the left side of the heart. However, in horses with pulmonary hypertension, a diastolic murmur may be audible combined with a loud S2.

Continuous murmurs

(ACF, EA)

In neonates, the most common cause of a continuous murmur is the patent ductus arteriosus. The murmur is caused by blood flowing from the aorta to the pulmonary artery during systole and diastole and is audible over the left hemithorax at the aortic and pulmonary valve areas. The diastolic component of the murmur usually disappears within 24 hours of birth as the ductus closes. However, the systolic component may remain for up to 4 days. Murmurs present after this time are considered to be abnormal.[42] Persistence of the ductus arteriosus in mature horses is very rare. In these cases the murmur may only be present in systole, either because the ductus is effectively closed in diastole or due to pulmonary hypertension limiting diastolic flow.[68]

A murmur present in systole and diastole in adult horses is more likely to comprise two separate murmurs although a continuous murmur can present in older horses with aortocardiac fistulas.[69] These latter murmurs are audible over the right hemithorax as blood flows through the fistula in systole and diastole from the aorta to the right ventricle or right atrium. More rarely the fistula opens into the left ventricle or dissects into the septal myocardium. Murmurs associated with aortocardiac fistulas may be referred to the left hemithorax and if there is increased flow through the pulmonary valve the systolic component of the murmur will be increased.

Murmurs associated with congenital abnormalities
(CCD, VSD)

Developmental abnormalities range from simple isolated defects, such as persistence of the foramen ovale, to more complex multiple defects such as tetralogy of Fallot.[36,37] An attempt can be made to separate these complex murmurs into their component parts by application of the basic principles outlined above for the diagnosis of systolic and diastolic murmurs. However, in these cases the list of differentials has to be expanded to include valvular stenoses. Confirmation of diagnosis is best gained by two-dimensional echocardiography (see Chapters 9 and 15).

Other noises

Pericardial friction rubs

Friction rubs are coarse scratching sounds produced as the inflamed pericardium and epicardium slide over one another and can be present even when there is considerable pericardial effusion.[7] They can occur whenever the heart moves within the pericardium and therefore may be audible during atrial contraction (between S4 and S1), during ventricular contraction (between S1 and S2) and during ventricular relaxation (between S2 and S3). This causes a triphasic pericardial friction rub. However, the sounds may not be present during every phase of the cardiac cycle and may therefore be monophasic or biphasic. Friction rubs, although in phase with the cardiac cycle, sound as though they are extracardiac in origin.

Systolic clicks

In human medicine midsystolic clicks are associated with mitral and, more rarely, tricuspid valve prolapse.[7] This is also thought to be the case in horses[70] although clicks can also occur at the onset of systole. In the veterinary literature systolic clicks have been reported to occur in normal horses[8] associated with minor abnormalities of the chordae tendineae[71] and aortic dilatation.[32] Systolic clicks are rare, are often clearly audible to the rider and tend to occur briefly after periods of fast work or tachycardia. Their clinical significance remains unclear and will be dependent on the underlying cause.

REFERENCES

1. Else RW, Holmes JR. Cardiac pathology in the horse: (1) Gross pathology. Equine Vet J 1972;4: 1–7.

2. Stockman S. Contribution to the study of heart disease in the horse. J Comp Pathol 1894;7:138–160.

3. Young LE, Wood JLN. The effects of age and training on murmurs of atrioventricular valvular regurgitation in young Thoroughbreds. Equine Vet J 2000;32:195–199.

4. Bonagura JD. Clinical evaluation and management of heart disease. Equine Vet Educ 1990;2:31–37.

5. Naylor JM, Yadernuck LM, Oharr JW. An assessment of the ability of diplomates, practitioners, and students to describe and interpret recordings of heart murmurs and arrhythmia. J Vet Int Med 2001;15: 507–515.

6. Blissitt KJ, Bonagura JD. Colour flow Doppler echocardiography in horses with cardiac murmurs. Equine Vet J 1995;(Suppl 19): 82–85.

7. Braunwald E. Heart Disease, 4th ed. Philadelphia: WB Saunders; 1989.

8. Reef VB. Evaluation of the equine cardiovascular system. Vet Clin North Am Equine Pract 1985;1: 275–288.

9. Rushmer RF. Cardiovascular Dynamics, 3rd ed. Philadelphia: WB Saunders; 1992.

10. Sabbah HN, Stein PD. Turbulent blood flow in humans: its primary role in the production of ejection murmurs. Circ Res 1976;38: 513–525.

11. Bruns DL. A general theory of the causes of murmurs in the cardiovascular system. Am J Med 1959;27:360–374.

12. McDonald DA. Murmurs in relation to turbulence and eddy formation in the circulation. Circulation 1957;16:278–281.

13. Rushmer RF, Morgan C. Meaning of murmurs. Am J Cardiol 1968; 21:722–730.

14. Reef VB. Cardiovascular disease in the equine neonate. Vet Clin North Am Equine Pract 1985;1:117–129.

15. Smetzer DL, Bishop S, Smith CR. Diastolic murmur of aortic insufficiency. Am Heart J 1966;72: 489–497.

16. Patterson DF, Detweiler DK, Glendenning SA. Heart sounds and murmurs of the normal horse. Ann NY Acad Sci 1965;127: 242–305.

17. Patteson MW, Cripps PJ. A survey of cardiac auscultatory findings in horses. Equine Vet J 1993;25: 409–415.

18. Kriz NG, Hodgson DR, Rose RJ. Prevalence and clinical importance of heart murmurs in racehorses. J Am Vet Med Assoc 2000;216: 1441–1445.

19. Reynolds O. An experimental investigation of the circumstances which determine whether the motion of water shall be direct or sinuous, and the law of resistance in parallel channels. Philos Trans R Soc 1883;174:935–982.

20. Nerem RM, Rumberger JA, Gross DR, Hamlin RL, Geiger GL. Hot-film anemometer velocity measurements of arterial blood flow in horses. Circ Res 1974;34: 193–203.

21. Brown CM, Holmes JR. Phonocardiography in the horse: 2. The relationship of the external phonocardiogram to intracardiac pressure and sound. Equine Vet J 1979;11:183–186.

22. Detweiler DK, Patterson DF. The cardiovascular system. In: Catcott EJ, Smithcors JF editors. Equine Medicine and Surgery. Wheaten, IL: American Veterinary Publications; 1972. p. 277–347.

23. Welker FH, Muir WW. An investigation of the second heart sound in the normal horse. Equine Vet J 1990;22:403–407.

24. Reef VB, Bain FT, Spencer PA. Severe mitral regurgitation in horses: clinical, echocardiographic and pathological findings. Equine Vet J 1998;30:18–27.

25. Alexander RW, Schlant RC, Foster V. Hurst's The Heart, Vol 1, 9th ed. New York: McGraw-Hill; 1998.

26. Glendinning SA. Significance of clinical abnormalities of the heart in soundness. Equine Vet J 1972;4: 21–30.

27. Reef VB. Heart murmurs in horses: determining their significance with echocardiography. Equine Vet J 1995;(Suppl 19):71–81.

28. Buhl R, Ersbøll AK, Eriksen L, Koch J. Use of color Doppler echocardiography to assess the development of valvular regurgitation in Standardbred trotters. J Am Vet Med Assoc 2005;227:1630–1635.

29. Martin BB Jr, Reef VB, Parente EJ, Sage AD. Causes of poor

performance of horses during training, racing, or showing: 348 cases (1992–1996). J AmVet Med Assoc 2000;216(4):554–558.

30. Young LE, Rogers K, Wood JL. Heart murmurs and valvular regurgitation in thoroughbred racehorses: epidemiology and associations with athletic performance. J Vet Intern Med 2008;22:418–426.

31. Levick JR. An Introduction to Cardiovascular Physiology, 2nd ed. Oxford: Butterworth-Heinemann; 1981.

32. Littlewort MCG. The clinical auscultation of the equine heart. Vet Rec 1962;74:1247–1259.

33. Levine SA, Harvey WP. Clinical Examination of the Heart. Philadelphia: WB Saunders; 1950. p. 51.

34. Leatham A. Auscultation of the heart. Lancet 1958;ii:757–766.

35. Olivier NB. Congenital heart disease in dogs. In: Fox PR, editor. Canine and Feline Cardiology. New York: Churchill Livingstone; 1988. p. 365,370.

36. Reynolds DJ, Nicholl TK. Tetralogy of Fallot and cranial mesenteric arteritis in a foal. Equine Vet J 1978;10:185–187.

37. Bayly WM, Reed SM, Leathers CW, et al. Multiple congenital heart anomalies in five Arabian foals. J Am Vet Med Assoc 1982;181: 684–689.

38. Hinchcliff KW, Adams WM. Critical pulmonary stenosis in a newborn foal. Equine Vet J 1991;23: 318–320.

39. Gehlen H, Bubeck K, Stadler P. Valvular pulmonic stenosis with normal aortic root and intact ventricular and atrial septa in an Arabian horse. Equine Vet Educ 2001;13:286–288.

40. Muylle E, Oyaert W. Auscultatie van het hart bij het paard. Vlaams Diergeneesk Tijdschr 1980;49: 167–177.

41. Glazier DB. The examination of the equine heart – some physiological and pathophysiological aspects. Vet Update 1984;1:28–36.

42. Reef VB. Heart murmurs, irregularities and other cardiac abnormalities. In: Brown CM, editors. Problems in Equine

Medicine. Philadelphia: Lea and Febiger; 1989. p. 122–137.

43. Holmes JR, Else RW. Cardiac pathology in the horse. (3) Clinical correlations. Equine Vet J 1972;4: 195–203.

44. Holmes JR. Equine phonocardiography. Med Biol Illustration 1966;16:16–25.

45. Holmes JR. Prognosis of equine cardiac conditions. Equine Vet J 1977;9:181–182.

46. Bishop SP, Cole CR, Smetzer DL. Functional and morphologic pathology of equine aortic insufficiency. Pathol Vet 1966;3: 137–158.

47. Humphries JO, Criley JM. Comparison of heart sounds and murmurs in man and animals. Ann N Y Acad Sci 1965 127:341–353.

48. Naylor JM, Wolker RE, Pharr JW. An assessment of the terminology used by diplomates and students to describe the character of equine mitral and aortic valve regurgitant murmurs: correlations with the physical properties of the sounds. J Vet Int Med 2003;17:332–336.

49. Glendinning SA. A distinctive diastolic murmur observed in healthy young horses. Vet Rec 1964;76:341–342.

50. Brown CM. Acquired cardiovascular disease. Vet Clin North Am Equine Pract 1985;1: 371–382.

51. Fregin GF. The Purchase Examination: The Cardiovascular System Proceedings of the 24th Annual Convention of the American Association of Equine Practitioners, St Louis, MO: Stouffer's Riverfront Towers; 1978. p. 583–590.

52. Rahko PS. Prevalence of regurgitant murmurs in patients with valvular regurgitation detected by Doppler echocardiography. Ann Intern Med 1989;111:466–472.

53. Patteson MW. Echocardiographic evaluation of horses with aortic regurgitation. Equine Vet Educ 1994;6:159–166.

54. Hoffmann A, Burckhardt D. Evaluation of systolic murmurs by Doppler ultrasonography. Br Heart J 1983;50:337–342.

55. Niemetz E. Über das funktionelle systolishe geräusch an der

pulmonalis bei pferden. Wien Tierarztl Monatsschr 1924;11: 321–327.

56. Perevezentsev VV. K voprosu o diagnostike funktsional'nykh serdechnykh shumov u loshadei. Vet Bull 1944;14:245(abstract).

57. Brown CM, Bell TG, Paradis MR, Breeze RG. Rupture of the mitral chordae tendineae in two horses. J Am Vet Med Assoc 1983;182: 281–283.

58. Holmes JR, Miller PJ. Three cases of ruptured mitral valve chordae in the horse. Equine Vet J 1984;16: 125–135.

59. Miller PJ, Holmes JR. Observations on seven cases of mitral insufficiency in the horse. Equine Vet J 1985;17:181–190.

60. Rooney JR, Franks WC. Congenital cardiac anomalies in horses. Path Vet 1964;1:454–464.

61. Buergelt CD, Cooley AJ, Hines SA, Pipers FS. Endocarditis in six horses. Vet Pathol 1985;22:333–337.

62. Reef VB. Evaluation of ventricular septal defects in horses using two-dimensional and Doppler echocardiography. Equine Vet J Suppl 1995;19:86–96.

63. Holmes JR. Equine Cardiology, Vol 3. Bristol: Langford; 1987.

64. Long KJ. Echocardiographic Study of Valvular and Ventricular Function in Horses. Unpublished PhD thesis, University of Edinburgh, 1993.

65. Bonagura JD. Equine heart disease: an overview. Vet Clin North Am Equine Pract 1985;1:267–274.

66. Young LE. Diseases of the heart and vessels. In: Hinchcliff KW, Kaneps AJ, Geor RJ, Bayly W, editors. Equine Sports Medicine and Surgery. Edinburgh: WB Saunders; 2004. p. 750.

67. Clark ES, Reef VB, Sweeney CR, Lichtensteiger C. Aortic valve insufficiency in a one-year-old colt. J Am Vet Med Assoc 1987;191: 841–844.

68. Buergelt C-D, Carmichael JA, Tashjian RJ, Das KM. Spontaneous rupture of the left pulmonary artery in a horse with patent ductus arteriosus. J Am Vet Med Assoc 1970;157:313–320.

69. Marr CM, Reef VB, Brazil TJ, et al. Aorto-cardiac fistulas in seven horses. Vet Radiol Ultrasound 1998;39(1):22–31.

70. Marr CM, Reef VB. Disturbances of blood flow. In: Kobluk CN, Ames TR, Geor RJ, editors. The Horse: Diseases and Clinical Management. Philadelphia: WB Saunders; 1995. p. 165.

71. Patteson MW. Equine Cardiology. Oxford: Blackwell Science; 1995.

Chapter | 9 |

Echocardiography

Celia M Marr and Mark Patteson

CHAPTER CONTENTS

INTRODUCTION

Echocardiography, including two-dimensional (2DE), M-mode and various Doppler modalities, have revolutionized equine cardiology. These technologies provide a better understanding of the normal physiology of the equine heart and an improved ability to diagnose and assess the severity of many forms of heart disease.[1] A clear understanding of the principles of echocardiography, the technical ability to produce standard and consistent images and knowledge of common echocardiographic findings in normal and diseased animals are essential for the successful clinical use of echocardiography.

PHYSICS AND PRINCIPLES

Two-dimensional and M-mode echocardiography

(ET)

The heart is an excellent subject for imaging with ultrasound because blood within the cardiac chambers is relatively anechoic and therefore appears black, outlining the echogenic valves and chamber walls. However, ultrasound does not easily pass through air or bone; therefore the heart must be imaged through the "acoustic windows" which are found where the heart is in direct contact with the chest wall. In horses the sternum prevents imaging from the ventrum, furthermore the heart is positioned with the apex on the sternum and the base apex axis almost perpendicular to it. This restricts equine echocardiographers to the use of parasternal views whereas in human beings and small animals a wider range of views is possible because images can be obtained from cranial and/or caudal to the sternum. This does limit the ease with which some structures can be imaged in the horse and is particularly problematical for Doppler echocardiography, where sub-optimal images and quantitative data are obtained if the ultrasound beam cannot be aligned parallel to blood flow.

2D echocardiograms are obtained by sweeping an ultrasound beam in an arc to produce sector frames that are updated with time (Figs. 9.1–9.7). While these images provide the best spatial information, they are limited by frame rate. M-mode echocardiograms show the structure of the heart in a one-dimensional view where location is

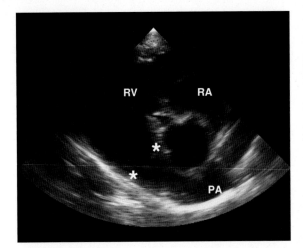

Figure 9.1 A right ventricular inflow–outflow echocardiogram obtained from the right fourth intercostal space with the transducer pointing towards the left third intercostal space in a normal 3-year-old Thoroughbred colt. * = landmarks to measure the pulmonary artery (PA). RA, right atrium; RV, right ventricle.

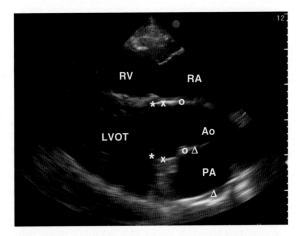

Figure 9.2 A right parasternal long-axis echocardiogram of the left ventricular outflow tract obtained from the right fourth intercostal space with the transducer pointing towards the left fourth intercostal space in a normal 3-year-old Thoroughbred colt. Landmarks to measure the aorta (Ao) at the valve (*), sinus of valsalva (x) and sinotubular junction (O) and pulmonary artery (PA, △) are shown. RA, right atrium; RV, right ventricle; LVOT, left ventricular outflow tract.

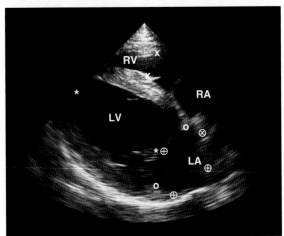

Figure 9.3 A right parasternal four-chamber long-axis echocardiogram obtained from the right fourth intercostal space with the transducer pointing towards the left fifth intercostal space in a normal 3-year-old Thoroughbred colt. Landmarks to measure the length of the left ventricle (LV, *), diameter of the right ventricle (RV, x), mitral annual diameter (O), left atrial (LA) length (⊕) and diameter (⊗) are shown. Note that subjectively the right atrium (RA) is smaller than the left atrium (LA) in this image plane.

Doppler echocardiography (ET)

Doppler echocardiography is a noninvasive means of interrogating intracardiac blood flow, or in the case of tissue velocity imaging (TVI, also known as Doppler tissue imaging), movement of cardiac structures. It is based on the Doppler principle: the frequency shift that occurs when sound of a known frequency is reflected by a moving structure. In echocardiography the moving structure can be the blood cells or, with TVI, various cardiac structures such as the chamber walls or valves. When an ultrasound beam of any given frequency is directed into the heart, it is reflected at a different frequency determined by the velocity and direction of the moving blood cells or cardiac structures. Objects that are moving towards the interrogating ultrasound beam produce an increase in frequency of reflected sound (a positive Doppler frequency shift), whereas those moving away from the interrogating sound beam produce a decrease in frequency (a negative Doppler frequency shift). Quantification of the frequency shift allows the velocity of that movement to be calculated from the following equations[2]:

$$f_d = f_r - f_t$$

$$f_d = \frac{2f_t \times v \times \cos\theta}{c}$$

$$v = \frac{f_d \times c}{2f_t(\cos\theta)}$$

displayed on the y-axis against time on the x-axis. Thus, the M-mode image shows motion of the cardiac structures and is not limited by frame rate. Most modern echocardiographic units allow the M-mode image planes to be guided from 2DE images.

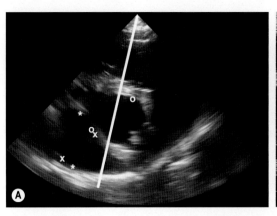 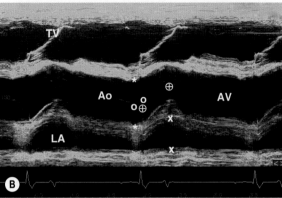

Figure 9.4 (A) A right parasternal short-axis echocardiogram of the left ventricular outflow tract obtained from the right fourth intercostal space with the transducer pointing dorsally in a normal 3-year-old Thoroughbred colt. Landmarks to measure the left atrial (LA) linear dimensions * and x, and aortic (Ao) diameter (O) are shown. The line indicates the cursor position to obtain an M-mode echocardiogram of the aorta. RA, right atrium; RV, right ventricle; Ao, aorta; LA, left atrium; PA, pulmonary artery. **(B)** An M-mode echocardiogram of the aorta obtained as indicated in **A**. The aortic valve (AV) has a box-like shape in systole. Landmarks to measure the Ao (*), LA (x), pre-ejection period (O) (the time from the Q wave to valve opening) and ejection period (the duration of valve opening, ⊕) are shown. RV, right ventricle; TV, tricuspid valve.

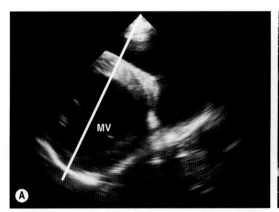 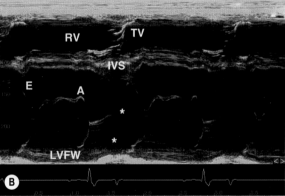

Figure 9.5 (A) A right parasternal short-axis echocardiogram obtained from the right fourth intercostal space with the transducer pointing horizontally in a normal 3-year-old Thoroughbred colt. The line indicates the cursor position to obtain an M-mode echocardiogram of the mitral valve (MV). **(B)** An M-mode echocardiogram of the mitral valve obtained as indicated in **A**. Note that the mitral valve opens maximally in early systole (E wave), in mid-diastole it is partially open and in late diastole it opens again following atrial contraction (A wave). The septal-E point separation is measured from the peak of the E wave to point of downward deflection of the septum (IVS). In this horse it is zero. The relaxation time index is the time from the maximal excursion of the left ventricular free wall (LVFW) and the opening of the mitral valve (MV)*. RV, right ventricle; TV, tricuspid valve.

The Doppler shift (f_d) is the difference between the received frequency (f_r) and the transmitted frequency (f_t). The velocity of the interrogated structure (v) is a function of f_d, f_t, the speed of sound in tissues (c) and the angle of interrogation (θ). Note: as θ increases the velocity estimate will become increasingly inaccurate; thus optimal data is obtained by aligning the interrogating ultrasound beam parallel to the blood flow under examination. (RCT) Most echocardiographic units provide good-quality Doppler signals at depths of no more than 18–24 cm, which can present difficulties in the horse. Unfortunately, in horses the acoustic windows are limited and optimum alignment to flow can be difficult to achieve.[3,4] Trans-oesophageal (TO) transducers can be placed directly over the heart to overcome some of these limitations.[5] However, although there are clear clinical advantages in a range of clinical settings in human patients, TO echocardiographic equipment has to be custom-built for equine patients, it

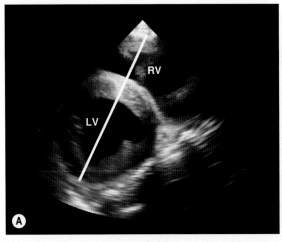
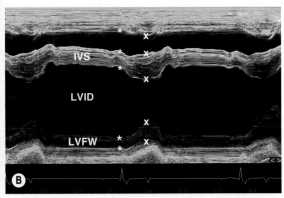

Figure 9.6 (A) A right parasternal short-axis chordal level echocardiogram obtained from the right fourth intercostal space with the transducer pointing ventrally in a normal 3-year-old Thoroughbred colt. Planimetry can be used to derive the LV lumen and wall areas from this image plane. The line indicates the cursor position to obtain an M-mode echocardiogram of the ventricles at chordal level. Measurements are made of the right ventricular lumen, ventricular septum (IVS), left ventricular internal diameter (LVID) and left ventricular free wall (LVFW). End-diastole (*) is taken as the onset of the QRS complex and peak systole (x) is the point of maximal deflection of the IVS.

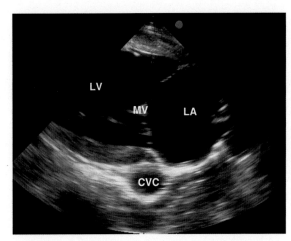

Figure 9.7 A left parasternal long-axis echocardiogram of the left atrium (LA) and ventricle (LV) obtained from the left fifth intercostal space with the transducer pointing towards the right fifth intercostal space in a normal 3-year-old Thoroughbred colt. Landmarks to measure the left atrial diameter (*) are shown. MV, mitral valve; CVC, caudal vena cava.

is expensive and it has only been used in anaesthetized horses, such that at the current time, its use has been restricted to research applications in horses.[6–15]

The simplest form of Doppler echocardiography is continuous wave (CW), a system where a continuous interrogating ultrasound beam is emitted from a piezoelectric crystal and a separate piezoelectric crystal receives the reflected sound. CW Doppler echocardiograms represent the velocity of blood cells moving in either direction along the entire path of the ultrasound beam displayed against time as a form of spectral display. CW is the most accurate in the detection of velocity as there is no limitation of aliasing; however, it provides limited spatial information[2,16] (Fig. 9.8). CW signals are more intense than those from PW (see below).

Pulsed-wave (PW) Doppler echocardiography overcomes the spatial limitations of CW by collecting Doppler data from an individual sampling site by emitting sound in pulses and measuring the frequency shift that occurs at an operator-determined location within the heart. PW is able to distinguish laminar flow, where all blood cells at one location are travelling at the same velocity, from turbulent flow, where multiple velocities will be detected at the same location. Turbulent flow is recognized on spectral PW because there is spectral broadening, i.e. a variety of velocities are depicted as a broad band rather than a tight envelope[17,18] (see Fig. 9.8).

When PW information is generated from a single sampling site and displayed as a graph of velocity against time, this is also a form of spectral display. Flow towards the transducer is displayed above the baseline of the time/velocity spectrum and flow away from the transducer is below the baseline. PW is used in conjunction with 2DE such that the operator can select a particular location within the heart for investigation. All forms of PW Doppler echocardiography are limited by the fact that they cannot accurately define high velocities. This is due to a phenomenon known as aliasing. In spectral PW, aliasing is represented by displaying the signal on the opposite side of the

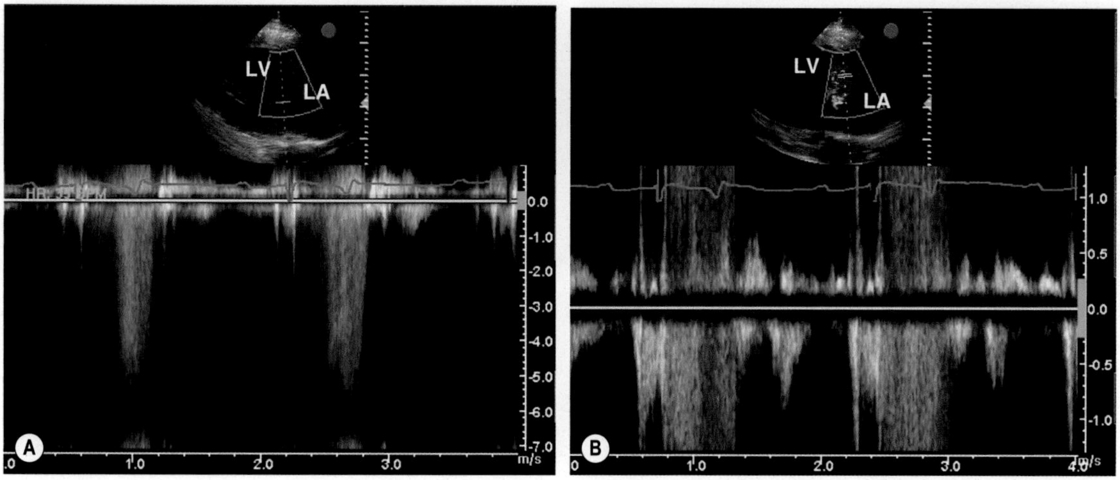

Figure 9.8 Continuous (**A**) and pulsed (**B**) wave spectral Doppler echocardiograms from a 5-year-old gelding with moderately severe mitral regurgitation. In continuous wave, the velocity is sampled along the entire length of the interrogating beam which has been placed across the left atrium (LA) near the mitral valve. This allows accurate measurement of velocity. In pulsed wave, a small sample volume can be placed within the regurgitant jet to map its location but velocity is not accurately recorded due to aliasing. Note that the jet is composed of a range of velocities displayed as a broad band. LV, left ventricle.

base line (i.e. forward flow is displayed at increasing velocities above the baseline until it exceeds the aliasing point and is represented below the baseline; see Fig. 9.8). The velocity at which aliasing occurs is determined by the Nyquist limit, which is dependent on the frequency of emission of the ultrasound pulses (the pulse repetition frequency) and the frequency of the emitted sound. Many echocardiographic units are equipped with a high pulse repetition frequency function that is effectively an intermediate between PW and CW, allowing higher velocities to be recorded accurately with some ability to localize the sampling site.[2,16]

Colour flow Doppler (CFD) echocardiography is a more sophisticated form of PW Doppler technology. Instead of a single sampling site, multiple sites within the heart are examined simultaneously. Flow is colour coded and superimposed on a two-dimensional image of the cardiac structures to produce a map of intracardiac flow (Fig. 9.9). Colour M-mode images provide the most accurate assessment of timing of flow events (Fig. 9.10). In all forms of CFD it is conventional to display flow towards the transducer encoded as red and flow away from the transducer encoded as blue. The intensity or shade of the colour varies to depict the velocity of blood flow. High-velocity turbulent jets appear as a mosaic pattern of high-intensity colour[17,18] (see Fig. 9.9). Some echocardiographic units add another colour, such as green, to display variance or turbulent flow (see Figs. 9.9 and 9.10). Where aliaising occurs, increasing velocities are indicated by moving through the colour sequence, thus rapid flow towards the transducer aliases from red, through orange and yellow to the blue shades, while rapid flow away from the trans-

ducer aliases from blue through turquoise and yellow to the red shades (see Fig. 9.9). In common with other ultrasonographic imaging modalities, CFD echocardiograms are updated many times per second to achieve a continuous, real-time image.[2,16–18] However, at the depths required in equine echocardiography, the addition of CFD can result in very slow frame rates. This limiting factor is highly machine dependent. (AR, RCT, VMD, VSD)

For conventional blood pool Doppler echocardiography, velocity filters are utilized to screen out low-velocity and high-amplitude signals that are likely to be due to the solid structures of the heart. In contrast, for TVI, velocity and amplitude filters are reversed and used to screen out high-velocity, low-amplitude signals that are likely to arise from the blood pool[19,20] (Fig. 9.11). Two TVI functions are available, each measuring different velocities: spectral TVI (Fig. 9.12) provides an estimate of the maximal velocity within a given region whereas colour TVI produces a trace of the mean velocity within the sampled region of myocardium.[21] TVI methods allow the velocity of individual areas of the myocardium to be determined.[22] These modalities provide a direct measure of intramural velocities during cardiac relaxation and contraction and have the potential to objectively quantify regional, in addition to global, mechanical function.[21,23]

ECHOCARDIOGRAPHIC EQUIPMENT

Imaging the heart requires a sector scanning transducer and in adult horses a 2.0–3.5-MHz transducer is ideal; in

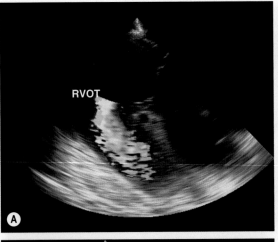

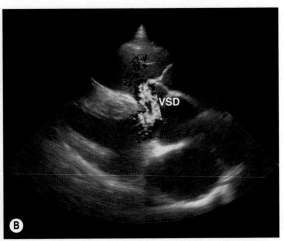

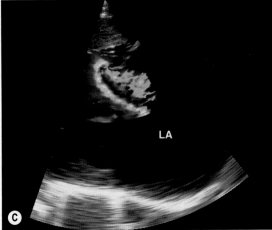

Figure 9.9 Colour-flow Doppler echocardiograms demonstrating aliasing and variance. (**A**) In this view of the right ventricular outflow tract (RVOT) rapid forward flow is away from the transducer (blue), but as it increases its velocity it has aliased to yellow. (**B**) In this view of a ventricular septal defect (VSD), flow is towards the transducer, but at the centre of the defect it has aliased to shades of blue that are darkest in the centre. (**C**). With mitral regurgitation, regurgitant flow approaching the ventricular aspect of the valve is blue then aliases to yellow as its velocity increases. As it regurgitates into the left atrium (LA), it becomes nonlaminar and a green area of variance is displayed.

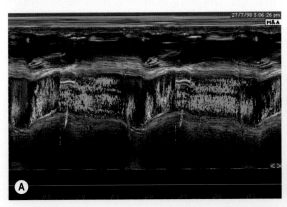

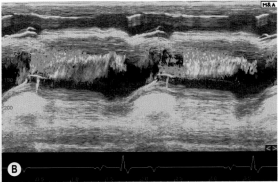

Figure 9.10 Colour Doppler M-mode echocardiograms of the aorta in which the blood flow is depicted in colour, allowing precise timing of events. Forward flow in systole is displayed in orange. Non-laminar flow represented by the green variance code in diastole represents aortic regurgitation which lasts throughout diastole with severe aortic regurgitation (**A**) and in mid to late diastole becomes less turbulent, changing green to yellow, and less rapid, changing from yellow to orange in a less severe example (**B**).

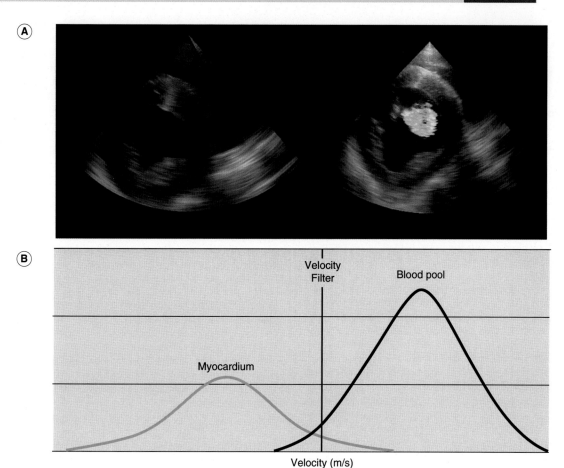

Figure 9.11 Right parasternal short-axis colour Doppler images of the right ventricle and interventricular septum (**A**) and the blood pool (**B**) from an 18-year-old horse with aortic regurgitation illustrating that velocity filters can be used to distinguish myocardial and blood pool movements.

foals 5.0–7.0 MHz may be more suitable. The relatively poor resolution of low-frequency transducers is more than compensated by their increased depth of penetration. The advent of harmonic imaging, with superior signal-to-noise, contrast-to-noise, spatial resolution and visualization of tissue at depth[2,24] may often improve the quality of images that can be obtained in large and overweight adult horses. A depth display of at least 30 cm facilitates imaging of the entire heart from the right side of the chest and equipment is now available that can image to depths of up to 36 cm. To be suitable for echocardiography, ultrasound machines should be equipped with an ECG display. A cine-loop facility, which allows previous frames to be analysed at the time of the examination, is also extremely useful and is included in most modern echocardiographic units.

THE ECHOCARDIOGRAPHIC EXAMINATION

Indications for echocardiography

Echocardiography is indicated in the following situations:

- When a murmur (other than a functional murmur) is heard (i.e. valvular or congenital heart disease is suspected).
- When dysrhythmias are detected.
- When heart sounds are muffled (e.g. due to pericardial or severe myocardial disease).
- When clinical signs of congestive heart failure are detected.

- In horses with pyrexia of unknown origin.
- In horses with unexplained reduced athletic performance once musculoskeletal and respiratory disease has been excluded.

Preparation of patient

Echocardiography is best performed in areas of subdued lighting and where the horse can be safely restrained. Hair should be clipped from the axilla, except in horses with a very fine hair coat. The skin should be cleaned of grease and dirt using surgical spirit or soap and water and acoustic coupling gel applied. Horses should not be sedated unless absolutely necessary because this will alter some cardiac dimensions and indices of function. If sedation is required to clip the horse it may be necessary to clip the horse under sedation and scan at least several hours later. Detomidine and romifidine primarily affect 2DE and M-mode measurements of the left ventricle (LV) and aorta (AO) in systole, reducing wall thickness and increasing the diameter of the ventricular lumen and aortic root.[25-27] One study has shown that detomidine can also increase the LV diameter in diastole.[21] Detomidine will also affect Doppler echocardiographic indices of systolic function.[26] Acepromazine appears to have less effect on echocardiographic variables[27,28] but has been shown to increase the diameters of the pulmonary artery (PA), AO and interventricular septum (IVS) and decrease the diameter of the left atrium (LA) in diastole.[27,28] If a horse has to be examined while sedated then structural information is still valid but the potential effects of sedation on the echocardiographic measurements should be taken into account.

Image planes

 ET)

In order to perform a thorough echocardiographic examination, standardized image planes should be obtained in a methodical manner before lesion-orientated views are studied. These image planes and the transducer positions used to obtain them have been described previously[29-31] and standardized views of 2D and M-mode image planes obtained from normal horses are shown in Figures 9.1–9.7 and cardiac anatomy is reviewed in Chapter 1. In brief, the right parasternal images are obtained by placing the transducer in the right fourth intercostal space (in most horses just under the triceps muscle), which is often facilitated by having the horse stand with its right fore in front of its left. The transducer should be tilted 5–10° from the vertical plane such that the ultrasound beam runs from a 1–2 o'clock position dorsally to a 7–8 o'clock position ventrally in long axis and from a 3–4 o'clock position cranially to a 9–10 o'clock position caudally in

short axis. In short-axis images at the heart base, a slight further clockwise rotation will often help produce clearer images of the aortic valve. In this way, the ultrasound beam will traverse the heart along its true long and short axes. Ideally, the images should be obtained in a consistent manner, for example, starting by orientating the transducer towards the left shoulder to view the right atrium (RA), ventricle (RV) and PA, sweeping caudally to the four-chamber view, then scanning the heart in short axis from the apex to the heart base and finally obtaining an M-mode series from the base to the apex. Left parasternal images are made with the horse standing square and the transducer located in the fifth intercostal space (in most horses just behind the border of the triceps muscle), orientated vertically or slightly rotated 5–10° in a clockwise direction to around 1 o'clock directed straight across the horse, or slightly caudally to image the LA and LV and then sweeping cranially while rotating the transducer in an anticlockwise direction to around 10–11 o'clock to visualize the left ventricular outflow tract (LVOT, Figs. 9.1–9.7). Standard images for Doppler imaging correspond to those used for 2DE[29-33] (Figs. 9.13–9.18). However, for imaging regurgitant jets, images must be selected so that the ultrasound beam can be aligned as closely as possible parallel to blood flow, and it is often necessary to supplement the standard images with lesion-orientated images optimized to align with regurgitant jets or intracardiac shunts.[34-38]

M-mode, 2DE and TVI assessment of cardiac dimensions and indices of cardiac function

One of the principal advantages of echocardiography is that it allows measurement of the size of cardiac structures and, with M-mode echocardiography, accurate timing of their motion. When these measurements are combined, valuable functional data can be obtained. Guidelines for measurements are available to ensure repeatability.[31,39,40] Strict adherence to these guidelines is mandatory if accurate measurements are to be made. It is extremely important that only perfect images are used for measurements. Measurements made from poor-quality images, and especially from images in the wrong anatomical plane, can be extremely misleading. Between three and five sets of measurements from different cardiac cycles should be made, with more if there is a dysrhythmia. Echocardiographic variables vary not only depending on the age and body weight of the horse but also between breeds and between different levels of fitness[41-48] (see Chapter 3). A range of measurements for adult Thoroughbred horses is presented in Table 9.1[39] and adult Standardbred horses in Table 9.2,[49] while a more limited range of measurements for mixed breed horses and ponies of a variety of sizes is listed in Table 9.3.[50] Regression equations allowing prediction

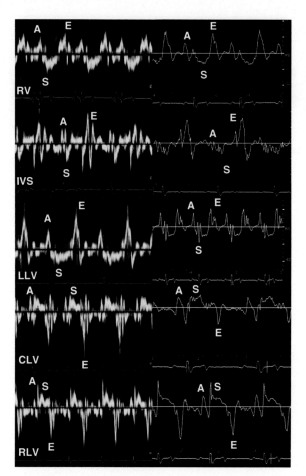

Figure 9.12 Spectral (left) and colour Doppler (right) tissue images showing regional differences in velocity of myocardial movement within the right ventricle (RV), interventricular septum (IVS), and the left (LLV), caudal (CLV) and right (RLV) regions of the left ventricle. The systolic (S), early (E) and late (A) diastolic waves are indicated. An ECG is superimposed for timing.

of cardiac sizes in Thoroughbred foals ranging from birth to 16 weeks of age are listed in Table 9.4.

The left ventricle

(AF, AR, IE, RCT, SFP, VMD)

The diameter of the LV is most repeatably and conveniently measured with M-mode[39] (see Fig. 9.6). M-mode also has the advantage of greater temporal resolution (see above). The appropriate M-mode trace is obtained from the 2DE right parasternal short-axis view at the level of the chordae tendineae (see Fig. 9.6). At this level neither the mitral valve nor the papillary muscles can be seen. When the LV appears as close to circular as possible (i.e. ensuring that the 2DE imaging plane is perpendicular to the long

axis of the ventricle), the M-mode cursor is placed across the major axis of the ventricle, between the chordae (see Fig. 9.6). If the cursor is placed too far dorsally, close to the membranous or nonmuscular portion of the IVS, it will appear to contract very little and/or portions of the mitral valve may be visible: both should prompt the echocardiographer to re-position the M-mode cursor. Once an appropriate image has been obtained, electronic calipers are used to measure by the leading-edge to leading-edge technique, from the IVS to the left ventricular free-wall (LVFW). Measurements are made at end-diastole, indicated by the onset of the QRS complex, and at peak systole, which is taken to be the point of maximum excursion of the septum. Note that the end-systolic point of the septal motion may not exactly co-incide with the maximum extent of LVFW motion but this apparent asynchrony in fact reflects movement of the entire heart within the thorax.

M-mode measurements of the LV internal diameter in diastole (LVIDd) and systole (LVIDs) are used to derive fractional shortening (FS%) and ejection fraction (EF%) using calculation packages available with most echo-cardiographic units[51]:

$$FS\% = \frac{(LVIDd - LVIDs) \times 100}{LVIDd}$$

$$EF\% = \frac{LVIDd^3 - LVIDs^3}{LVIDd^3}$$

An estimate of LV mass has also been validated by comparison with cadaver specimens:[52]

$$LV\ mass = 1.04 \times \left[(LVIDd + LVFWd + IVSd)^3 - LVIDd^3 \right] - 13.6$$

In Thoroughbreds, LV mass correlates with maximal oxygen uptake[53] and, combined with EF%, is correlated with racing performance in horses racing over long, but not short, distances[48] (see Chapter 3). With all derived indices, it is critical to remember that the information is only as good as the original images and should not be regarded as accurate if the measurements are not derived from optimal images.

The LV diameter and length can also be obtained from long- and short-axis 2DE images, respectively (Figs. 9.3 and 9.6) while planimetry can be used to derive the area of the LV lumen and walls. These methods of assessment of LV dimensions are less repeatable than guided M-mode techniques[39] and therefore are less relevant in assessing horses with cardiac disease. However, they can be used to derive estimates of the LV luminal volume in systole and diastole and from these, stroke volume and cardiac output (CO) can be estimated. One of these techniques, the Bullet method, has been compared with lithium dilution, partial carbon dioxide rebreathing and Doppler echocardiographic methods and been shown to be an accurate non-invasive estimate of CO in normal, anaesthetized foals.[54]

Table 9.1 Normal echocardiographic measurements in Thoroughbreds[39]

VARIABLE	MEAN	STANDARD DEVIATION	FIGURE OF IMAGE PLANE
M-mode echocardiography			
Interventricular septal thickness at end-diastole (cm)	2.85	0.278	9.6
Interventricular septal thickness at end-systole (cm)	4.21	0.463	9.6
Left ventricular internal diameter at end-diastole (cm)	11.92	0.76	9.6
Left ventricular internal diameter at end-systole (cm)	7.45	0.615	9.6
Left ventricular free wall thickness at end-diastole (cm)	2.32	0.382	9.6
Left ventricular free wall thickness at end-systole (cm)	3.85	0.414	9.6
Fractional shortening (%)	37.42	3.86	9.6
Interventricular septal thickness fraction (%)	48.27	15.4	9.6
Left ventricular free wall thickening fraction (%)	69.01	22.9	9.6
Left atrial appendage diameter at end-systole (cm)	6.2	0.737	9.4
Aortic diameter at end-diastole (cm)	7.95	0.534	9.4
Aortic diameter at end-systole (cm)	8.13	0.579	9.4
Two-dimensional echocardiography			
Left atrial diameter at end-diastole (cm)	12.82	0.782	9.7
Left atrial diameter at end-systole (cm)	12.87	0.782	9.7
Aortic diameter at valve at end-diastole (cm)	7.20	0.344	9.2
Aortic diameter at valve at end-systole (cm)	7.58	0.378	9.2
Aortic sinus diameter at end-diastole (cm)	8.72	0.504	9.2
Aortic sinus diameter at end-systole (cm)	9.02	0.495	9.2
Aortic sinotubular junction at end-diastole (cm)	7.45	0.388	9.2
Aortic sinotubular junction at end-systole (cm)	7.70	0.407	9.2
Pulmonary artery diameter at end-diastole (cm)	6.11	0.491	9.1
Left ventricular area at end-diastole (cm^2)	100.9	10.64	9.3
Left ventricular area at end-systole (cm^2)	40.84	6.90	9.3
Myocardial area at end-diastole (cm^2)	223.0	15.21	9.3
Myocardial area at end-systole (cm^2)	191.1	16.82	9.3
Fractional myocardial area change (%)	59.53	4.98	9.3

Using TVI, regional differences in systolic and early diastolic LV wall velocities have been demonstrated in normal horses (Fig. 9.12). Spectral TVI can be used more repeatably than colour Doppler TVI in the equine LV. The right and caudal regions of the LV at the chordal level move faster than other areas in all phases of the cardiac cycle and the systolic and early diastolic velocities are lowest in the IVS. There are no regional differences in the late diastolic velocities when it is likely that all regions of the LV walls will deflect at a similar rate as ventricular filling movement is due to atrial contraction in this phase.[19]

Table 9.2 Normal echocardiographic measurements in Standardbreds[49]

VARIABLE	MEAN	STANDARD DEVIATION	FIGURE OF IMAGE PLANE
M-Mode echocardiography			
Interventricular septal thickness at end-diastole (cm)	3.1	0.41	9.6
Interventricular septal thickness at end-systole (cm)	4.48	0.36	9.6
Left ventricular internal diameter at end-diastole (cm)	11.6	1.29	9.6
Left ventricular internal diameter at end-systole (cm)	7.42	1.05	9.6
Left ventricular free wall thickness at end-diastole (cm)	2.52	0.03	9.6
Left ventricular free wall thickness at end-systole (cm)	3.64	0.52	9.6
Fractional shortening (%)	36.2	3.9	9.6
Mitral E point:septal separation (cm)	0.59	0.21	9.5
Aortic diameter at end-diastole (cm)	7.79	0.46	9.4
Two-dimensional echocardiography			
Left atrial diameter at end-diastole (cm)	11.4	0.5	9.7
Mitral valve diameter at end-diastole (cm)	10.67	0.36	9.7
Aortic diameter at valve at end-diastole (cm)	7.24	0.29	9.2
Aortic sinus diameter at end-diastole (cm)	7.86	0.33	9.2
Aortic sinotubular junction at end-diastole (cm)	7.01	0.26	9.2
Pulmonary artery diameter at end-diastole (cm)	5.41	0.38	9.1

Table 9.3 M-mode echocardiographic measurements of cardiac dimensions in normal horses and ponies[50]

VARIABLE (MEAN ± S.D.)	SMALL PONIES 125–306 KG	LARGE PONIES 274–469 KG	HORSES 454–620 KG
Interventricular septal thickness at end-diastole (cm)	1.7 ± 0.3	2.4 ± 0.2	2.8 ± 0.2
Interventricular septal thickness at end-systole (cm)	2.3 ± 0.4	3.8 ± 0.5	4.6 ± 0.5
Left ventricular internal diameter at end-diastole (cm)	6.1 ± 1.0	8.9 ± 1.4	11.2 ± 0.8
Left ventricular internal diameter at end-systole (cm)	3.8 ± 0.4	5.9 ± 0.9	7.3 ± 0.8
Left ventricular free wall thickness at end-diastole (cm)	1.6 ± 0.4	2.2 ± 0.5	2.5 ± 0.3
Left ventricular free wall thickness at end-systole (cm)	2.2 ± 0.4	2.7 ± 0.8	3.8 ± 0.3
Aortic diameter at end-diastole (cm)	3.9 ± 0.5	5.9 ± 1.0	7.8 ± 0.6

Table 9.4 Regression equations that can be used to estimate echocardiographic variables from weight (kg) in healthy Thoroughbred foals from birth to 16 weeks of age[51]. Collins N, Palmer L, Marr CM. unpublished data.

VARIABLE	VARIABLE (Y) = SLOPE *WEIGHT (X) + INTERCEPT	STANDARD DEVIATION
M-mode echocardiography		
Interventricular septal thickness at end-diastole (cm)	$y = 0.0043x + 1.2239$	0.188
Interventricular septal thickness at end-systole (cm)	$y = 0.0073x + 1.7752$	0.223
Left ventricular internal diameter at end-diastole (cm)	$y = 0.0188x + 4.4265$	0.571
Left ventricular internal diameter at end-systole (cm)	$y = 0.0132x + 3.1092$	0.566
Left ventricular free wall thickness at end-diastole (cm)	$y = 0.0035x + 0.9868$	0.185
Left ventricular free wall thickness at end-systole (cm)	$y = 0.0052x + 1.543$	0.306
Aortic diameter at end-diastole (cm)	$y = 0.0134x + 2.3854$	0.346
Left atrial appendage diameter at end-systole (cm)	$y = 0.0097x + 1.9614$	0.411
Two-dimensional echocardiography		
Left atrial diameter at end-diastole (cm)	$y = 0.0238x + 4.1483$	0.436
Aortic diameter at valve at end-systole (cm)	$y = 0.01320x + 2.137$	0.213
Pulmonary artery diameter at end-systole (cm)	$y = 0.0091x + 2.4147$	0.270

The left atrium

 AF, IE, SFP, VMD, VSD)

Measurement of equine LA dimensions can be made using three separate methods. In the past in other species, the diameter of the LA and aorta were measured from a right parasternal M-mode image at the level of the heart base and using this technique the ratio of the aortic root to left atrial appendage should be less than 1 (see Fig. 9.4). However, there are significant problems with this method in horses and indeed other species. First, the dimension measured is actually the size of the left atrial appendage rather than the body of the LA and, since this is a roughly conical structure it is difficult to ensure that the diameter is measured consistently. Additionally, with many echocardiographic units, the far border of the LA will be out of range from a right parasternal view in larger horses, and particularly those with LA enlargement in whom the accurate measurement is most informative. The second method is to measure LA diameter from the left parasternal long-axis view. If care is taken to ensure that optimal angulation maximizes the diameter of the LA, the caudal vena cava appearing as a round structure deep to the LA (see Fig. 9.7), consistent measurements can be made.[39] In fact, this measurement is somewhat closer to the valve annulus than the middle of the atrium because there is the danger that the calipers will be placed in the pulmonary veins if they are positioned too far dorsally, and lung interference

sometimes prevents clear identification of the dorsal endocardial border. With this method, measurements can be made at both end-diastole and end-systole.[39] An alternative, more comprehensive, method of assessing LA size and function with 2DE involves obtaining LA linear dimensions, area and volume during maximal atrial filling, indexed to AO measurements, from right parasternal four-chamber long-axis (see Fig. 9.3) and right parasternal short-axis LV outflow tract (LVOT, see Fig. 9.4) images.[55] A range of functional indices can also be derived with this method. TVI can be applied in the same imaging planes to determine LA mechanical function.[55]

The aorta

 AR)

AO diameter can be measured using M-mode from a right parasternal short-axis LVOT image in order to compare it with LA size (see Fig 9.4) and, for consistent measurements, it is important to ensure that the M-mode cursor is placed across the widest part of the vessel, at the level of the aortic valve. Using 2DE from a right parasternal long-axis view of the LVOT (see Fig. 9.2), AO diameter can be measured at a number of different levels, including base (the level of the valve), sinus of Valsalva or the sino-tubular junction. Because measurements at different levels are significantly different, care should be taken to ensure consistency in caliper placement.

The right ventricle and right atrium

(AF, PH, VMD)

Measurement of the RV and RA can be difficult because of the lack of reliable landmarks and the trabeculation of the RV wall.[31] A subjective assessment of the RA can be made with 2DE and in the normal horse, the RA size should be less than the LA size in the right parasternal 4-chamber image[37] (Fig. 9.3) while the RV will be approximately one-third the size of the LV in the right parasternal image of the LVOT tract and AO.[37] With care, the RV can be measured in a repeatable manner from 2DE right parasternal long-axis four-chamber (see Fig 9.3) and short-axis chordal level (see Fig. 9.6) images.[56] In the long-axis image, the calipers are placed across the RV at the insertion of the tricuspid chordae with the IVS. The RV can also be measured at end-diastole and at end-systole from a ventricular M-mode image[56] (see Fig. 9.6).

The pulmonary artery

(PH, VMD)

The PA can be visualized in a variety of planes and is usually measured in two images: when measured at the level of the valve from the RV inflow–outflow view (see Fig. 9.1) it should be smaller than the AO, measured at the level of the valve from the right parasternal long-axis image of the LVOT tract (see Fig. 9.2). The right PA can also be measured, in short-axis, as it runs behind the AO in the right parasternal long-axis image of the LVOT (see Fig. 9.2) Absolute values for the PA in this image plane have not been published but in normal horses it will be noticeably smaller than the AO.

INTERPRETATION OF BLOOD POOL DOPPLER ECHOCARDIOGRAMS

Forward flow

Normal intracardiac forward flow should be laminar and of moderate velocity. This is recognized on spectral imaging as a tight envelope because all the blood cells are moving at approximately the same speed (see Fig. 9.8). When imaged from the right hemithorax, flow through the tricuspid valve is towards the transducer and, on CFD is coded in red (see Fig. 9.13). It occurs in two phases: an early peak (E peak) that relates to the predominant flow of rapid early diastolic filling and a peak in late diastole (A peak) which results from atrial contraction[3,4]. Alignment to flow is achieved using a right parasternal angled or long-axis image of the RV inflow tract from a dorsal location[3,4,31–33]. Similarly, when imaged from the left hemithorax, forward flow through the mitral valve is

towards the transducer (see Fig. 9.14) and occurs in two phases (see Fig. 9.15). Alignment to flow is achieved by using a 2D apical two-chambered long-axis view of the LV inflow tract[3,4,31–33] (see Figs. 9.14, 9.15).

Forward flow through the pulmonary valve can be imaged from either side of the thorax, but best alignment of the ultrasound beam parallel to the blood flow in the RV outflow tract (RVOT) and PA can usually be achieved using an angled long-axis image of the RV inflow and outflow from a dorsal location (see Fig. 9.16) or from a

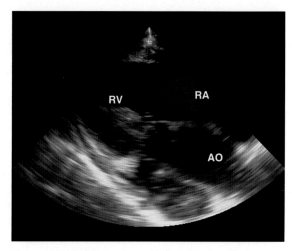

Figure 9.13 A right parasternal long-axis colour flow Doppler echocardiogram of the right ventricular inflow tract from a dorsal location showing normal forward flow (red, towards the transducer) through the tricuspid valve in early diastole. RV, right ventricle; RA, right atrium; Ao, aorta.

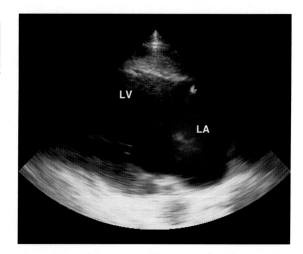

Figure 9.14 A left parasternal long-axis colour flow Doppler echocardiogram of the left ventricle (LV) and left atrium (LA) showing forward flow (red, towards the transducer) in early diastole.

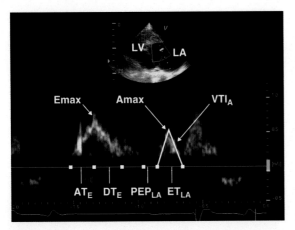

Figure 9.15 A left parasternal long-axis colour flow Doppler echocardiogram of the left ventricle (LV) and left atrium (LA) indicating the position of the sample volume to obtain a pulsed wave Doppler spectral trace of flow through the mitral valve. An ECG is displayed for timing of cardiac events. Emax = peak E velocity; AT_E = E wave acceleration time; DT_E = E wave deceleration time; Amax = peak A wave velocity; VTI_A = velocity time integral of the A wave; PEP_{LA}= LA pre-ejection period; ET_{LA} = LA ejection period.

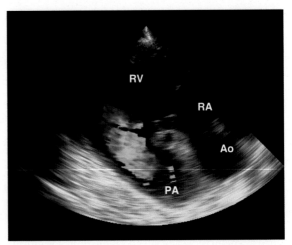

Figure 9.16 A right parasternal long-axis colour flow Doppler echocardiogram of the right ventricular outflow tract showing normal forward flow (blue, away from the transducer) in systole. RV, right ventricle; RA, right atrium; PA, pulmonary artery; Ao, aorta.

right parasternal apical image.[3,4,31-33] From the right hemithorax, forward flow in the RVOT and pulmonary artery are away from the transducer. Flow through the aortic valve is imaged from a left parasternal apical long axis image (see Fig. 9.17, 9.18), and again flow from this location is away from the transducer.[3,4,31-33]

Normal ranges for a variety of Doppler echocardiographic variables have been published previously[2,3] and are listed in Chapter 1 (see Tables 1.2 and 1.3). Doppler measurements from the outflow tracts that can be used to assess systolic function include systolic time intervals, peak acceleration, acceleration and ejection times and velocity time integral (VTI, the area under the curve of the Doppler envelope, see Fig. 9.18). Measurements which are typically recorded from spectral tracings of forward flow in the inflow tracts to assess diastolic function include peak E and A velocities, E:A ratio, VTI, and acceleration and deceleration times (see Fig. 9.15).

Cardiac output (CO) can be estimated by the equation:

$$CO = VTI \times vessel\ area \times heart\ rate$$

Studies comparing Doppler echocardiography with thermodilution, dye and lithium dilution have confirmed that it can be a reliable method of estimation of CO in adult horses.[8,15,57,58] The cross-sectional area of the AO is less likely to lead to an underestimation of CO than the cross-sectional area of the PA.[59] TO echocardiography provides a better estimate of CO than the transthoracic approach[15] reflecting the better alignment to flow that can be achieved with TO. Ideally, the angle of interrogation should be less than 20°[59] and in transthoracic images, improved alignment can be obtained by positioning the transducer towards the apex of the LV and angling dorsally towards the AO (see Fig. 9.17).

Aortic ejection time is reduced in states of high systemic resistance and with hypovolaemia; hypovolaemia will also reduce the peak outflow velocity.[59] Lower peak velocity and less steep peak acceleration suggest poor contractile function.[59] Horses with functional ejection murmurs also have lower peak aortic acceleration and longer acceleration time than those with no murmurs.[4] However, the potential for poor alignment to flow introduces considerable inaccuracies and variability in Doppler echocardiography and must be taken into consideration if these variable are being used.[40,60] Doppler assessments of haemodynamic status should be regarded as semiquantitative and are most likely to be useful for detecting changes while monitoring within individual patients as opposed to comparing individuals with reference ranges.[59]

Regurgitant flow and intracardiac shunts

Regurgitant flow and intracardiac shunts are of high velocity and are turbulent. Doppler echocardiography is ideally suited for their detection because it can characterize both of these features[17,18] (see Figs. 9.8 and 9.9). Regurgitant jets and intracardiac shunts can travel in a variety of directions and therefore rigid recommendations for detection of these jets cannot be given.[34-37] Examples of Doppler echocardiographic detection of abnormal flow in a variety of clinical problems are illustrated in a number of the

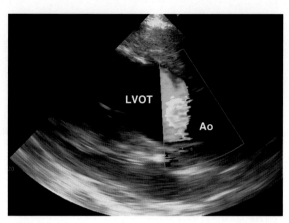

Figure 9.17 A left parasternal long-axis colour flow Doppler echocardiogram of the left ventricle outflow tract (LVOT) and aorta (Ao) showing normal forward flow (blue aliasing to yellow, away from the transducer) in systole.

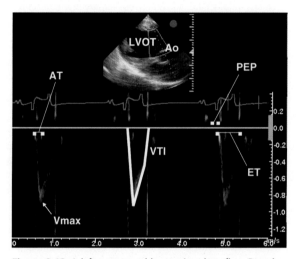

Figure 9.18 A left parasternal long-axis colour flow Doppler echocardiogram of the left ventricular outflow tract (LVOT) and aorta (Ao) indicating the position of the sample volume to obtain a pulsed-wave Doppler spectral trace of flow through the aortic valve in systole. An ECG is displayed for timing of cardiac events. Vmax = peak velocity; VTI = velocity time integral; PEP = pre-ejection period; ET = ejection time; AT = acceleration time.

digital case series (AF, AR, ET, RCT, RSD, SFP, VMD) The echographer should use the audio or visual signal to subtly modify the alignment of the ultrasound beam to obtain the maximal signal. Nevertheless, guidelines of typical locations are given below. As with any form of 2D imaging, when using Doppler echocardiography, it is essential to image the regurgitant jet or shunt in more than one image plane to obtain a full evaluation of the dimensions of the jet.

Tricuspid regurgitant (TR) jets are usually easily detected because the CFD beam can be aligned closely with their direction. Typically, they are found most easily in a long-axis image, optimized for the LVOT.[36] (AF, ET, VSD, VMD) Pulmonic regurgitation (PR) can be detected from both left and right sides of the thorax, but usually the jet is most closely aligned to the transducer in images from the right side. (AF, ET) Larger aortic regurgitant (AR) jets can also often be imaged from both sides of the thorax. (AR) Smaller AR jets are usually easier to see from the left thorax using, initially, a long-axis image and, if possible, a short-axis image of the LVOT.[35,36] (AF, ET, VSD) Jets of mitral regurgitation (MR) can be difficult to detect because Doppler is limited in its depth of penetration. Furthermore the large depth in horses means that the only images that can be obtained of the transmitral flow are made from the left parasternal location and even then the interrogating ultrasound beam is frequently very far from parallel to the jet, which can lead to underestimation of its velocity and area.[36] MR jets frequently skim along the surface of the valve or along the LA wall and may travel either towards or away from the transducer. (AF, AR, ET, IE, RCT, RSD, SFP, VMD, VSD)

Colour M-mode echocardiography is particularly valuable in precisely assessing timing (see Fig. 9.10). Flow mapping techniques have only a limited relationship to the degree of valvular regurgitation. Factors such as the instrument settings, the size and pressure of the chamber into which the regurgitant blood is flowing and, as frequently occurs in the horse, suboptimal imaging angles can influence the accuracy of the technique. Measurable characteristics of regurgitant jets include their duration and timing, maximal velocity, area, maximal width and width at the regurgitant orifice.[4,33,36,37,61,62] However, at the moment, there is limited information on the reliability and repeatability of Doppler estimates of the severity of regurgitation in horses but only changes in excess of 25% are likely to be indicative of genuine disease progression when serial measurements are compared.[60] A system of semiquantitation of the area of regurgitation has been proposed, and it is suggested that regurgitation should be classified as[36]:

- Insignificant – the regurgitant jet occupies a small area behind the valve. (ET)
- Mild – the jet occupies less than one-third of the chamber involved. (AF, AR, RSD, SFP, VSD)
- Moderate – the jet occupies less than two-thirds of the chamber involved. (AF, AR, VMD, VSD)
- Severe – regurgitant flow can be detected in greater than two-thirds of the chamber involved. (AF, AR, IE, RCT, VMD)

Contrast 2DE can be a useful alternative or supplement to Doppler echocardiography in demonstrating structural defects that are associated with a right to left, or bidirectional, shunt. In order to create a microbubble-laden

119

solution, 5–10 mL of the patient's blood is agitated with a similar volume of saline through a three-way tap. Alternatively simply small volumes of agitated saline or colloidal solutions such as dextrans can be used. The microbubble-laden solution is injected as a bolus via the jugular vein. The path of the microbubbles through the heart is visualized and if bubbles cross to the left structures, a right-to-left shunt is confirmed. (● *ACF, CCD, VSD*)

Estimation of pressure gradients

Doppler echocardiography can be used to estimate pressure gradients between cardiac chambers and vessels and across intracardiac shunts based on the modified Bernoulli equation[38,58,33]:

$$\text{Pressure gradient} = 4 \times \text{maximal velocity}^2$$

This technique is useful in the estimation of pressure increases within the right ventricle in horses with ventricular septal defects (VSD)[38] (● *VSD* see Chapter 15). The "normal" pressure gradient between the LV and RV is around 80–90 mmHg, so velocities of 4.5 m/second or greater suggest normal RV pressures. Where right ventricular pressure in horses with a VSD has increased due to pulmonary hypertension the shunt velocities will fall to around 3.5–4 m/second, assuming good alignment with flow.[1] Similarly, the acceleration and deceleration characteristics of regurgitant jets are indicative of the associated pressure changes. In severe aortic insufficiency, there may be large differences in pressure between the aorta and left ventricle in early diastole leading to high maximal velocities of the regurgitation, and the pressure in the left ventricle rises rapidly in late diastole causing an abrupt deceleration of the regurgitant jet.[35,63] (● *AR*)

Physiological regurgitation
(AF, ET, SFP)

In human beings and small animals, regurgitant jets which are located in a small area, close behind the valve leaflets, can be detected in a large number of normal individuals with no cardiac murmurs or signs of cardiovascular disease, and this valvular regurgitation is considered to be physiological.[64–66] Similarly, in horses it has been recognized that physiological regurgitation is common. In one study of young Standardbred and Thoroughbred racehorses, physiological AR was present in 80%, TR in 46% and MR in 26% of cases[33]. In another study of clinically normal Thoroughbreds, regurgitant jets were detected at the tricuspid valve in 77.5%, the mitral valve in 67.5% and the aortic valve in 47.5% of the horses.[32] It is important that physiological valvular regurgitation be identified to avoid misinterpretation of echocardiographic findings. Physiological regurgitation can be distinguished from pathological regurgitant regurgitation because it is usually transient, frequently associated with valve closure and jets

are very small. The valves usually appear to be structurally normal on 2DE, although there may be mild prolapse.[33] Physiological TR and MR is common in racing breeds with no impact on racing performance[33,67–69] and is more prevalent and severe in Thoroughbreds engaged in Steeplechasing compared to those in flat racing.[67]

IDENTIFICATION OF DISEASE-INDUCED CHANGES IN CARDIAC ANATOMY AND FUNCTION

Dimensions of the cardiac chambers and great vessels

MR can result in dilatation of the LV and LA,[70] while AR may also result in dilatation of the LV.[71] (● *AF, IE, RCT*) Volume overload of the RV and RA may occur with TR, pulmonary hypertension and some congenital heart defects. (● *CCD, VMD*) Gross enlargement of these chambers therefore indicates that these conditions are severe. The AO diameter increases slightly during systole, and can be reduced in animals with poor CO. A dilated AO is found in some horses with AR,[71] aneurysms[72,73] or in those with VSDs in which the root has prolapsed into the defect.[38] The PA can be dilated in horses with pulmonary hypertension, usually secondary to left-sided congestive heart failure. (● *AF, IE, VMD*) Because this can be a precursor to rupture in horses with severe cardiac disease, these cases need to be identified and the owner advised not to ride the horse.[70] Pulmonary hypertension also arises in a variety of disease states that involve hypoxia and/or pulmonary vasoconstriction, for example, severe interstitial pneumonia, systemic inflammatory response syndrome and severe recurrent airway obstruction. Studies comparing direct PA pressures with echocardiographic estimates in adult horses with cardiac disease[74] and with recurrent airway obstruction,[75] and in experimentally induced, short-term hypoxia in foals[76] have been shown that measurement of echocardiography is potentially a useful noninvasive tool for monitoring PA pressure. (● *PH, VMD*)

The ability to evaluate the severity of cardiac disease by its impact on chamber and vessel size is one of the most valuable features of echocardiography in horses. Serial echocardiographic measurements made over time allow the clinician to document progression of cardiac disease in many cases. Day-to-day and inter-observer variation in echocardiographic measurements has been reported in a variety of studies of normal horses. In general 2DE and M-mode variables are less variable than Doppler echocardiographic measurements and differences from 4–14% and 11.4–21.8%, respectively, are needed to document significant changes between serial measurements in normal horses.[40,55,56,60,77] Unpublished studies on horses with moderate or severe aortic regurgitation in one of the authors' clinics suggest similar variability can be expected in horses with cardiac disease. The M-mode LVIDd is the least variable parameter, with experienced examiners achieving intra-observer variation of around 5% and inter-observer variation is around 7%. Doppler echocardiographic variables are much less repeatable and only serial differences in dimensions of regurgitant jets of greater than around 25% should be considered likely to be due to progression of disease, as opposed to simply intra- or inter-observer variation.

Structure and position of the cardiac chambers

The structure of the myocardium is seldom identified as abnormal on echocardiography and small areas of ischaemia or myocarditis are unlikely to be identified. With extensive fibrosis, echogenic lesions may be found but similar "changes" may be seen with slight changes in gain settings and are therefore not necessarily clinically significant. (💿 VSD) Large areas of myocardial inflammation[78] and neoplastic infiltrates can cause echogenic, anechoic or heterogeneous areas within the myocardium and/or valves. (💿 CN, VMD)

Gross abnormalities of the structure and position of the cardiac chambers are mostly likely due to congenital heart disease. The most common congenital abnormality is the VSD. This is usually located at the junction of the IVS and the AO, just beneath the right coronary cusp of the aortic valve and the septal (💿 VSD) valve[38,79] (Fig. 9.9). Occasionally, VSD enter the RV just beneath the pulmonary valve, and others occur in the muscular portion of the septum (see Chapter 15). These variants are much less common and are more commonly associated with significant volume overload. Atrial septal defects (ASD) are uncommon and appear as an incongruity in the atrial septum, best seen in a long-axis view.[80] However, it is possible to create a similar appearance artefactually. A genuine ASD has very echogenic ends to the septum either side of the defect.

Complex congenital cardiac disease can lead to a range of malformations of the cardiac chamber and great arteries. In congenital heart disease, each structure should be identified by its specific anatomical features and its relationship to the surrounding structures assessed.[79] (💿 CCD) For a method of examination of cases of complex congenital cardiac disease, the reader is referred to a detailed protocol for sequential segmental analysis involving[81]:

1. Determination of the atrial arrangement: the RA has a triangular broad-based appendage, a terminal crest and extensive pectinate muscles whereas the LA appendage is tubular and narrow with no terminal crest. (💿 VSD)

2. Determination of the ventricular arrangement: the ventricles can be defined as morphologically right if there is a coarse trabeculated structure, valve leaflet attaching to the septum and moderator band; morphologically left if characterized by fine trabeculations and smooth upper septum; or morphologically interdeterminate if there is a solitary ventricle with no septum. Ventricles can also be hypoplastic but complete or hypoplastic and incomplete.

3. Characterization of atrioventricular connections.

4. Assessment of the morphology of the atrioventricular valves.

5. Assessment of the ventriculo-arterial connections: the great vessels are distinguished by the vessels that arise from them, i.e. the coronary arteries and brachiocephalic trunk originate from the AO while the right and left PA arise from the main PA.

6. Assessment of the morphology of the semi-lunar valves.

7. Identification of associated malformation affecting the septum, outflow tracts, great vessels and systemic and pulmonary venous connections.

Shape of the cardiac chambers

The shape of the ventricles can be altered by the presence of volume and/or pressure overload. Volume overload from MR, AR or congenital disease give the LV a globular appearance, with the apex appearing rounded rather than oval. (💿 AR, VMD) Volume or pressure overload of the RV results in the loss of its usual crescent shape in short axis, largely due to displacement of the IVS, which may be flattened or even bowed into the LV and, in long axis, the development of a double-apex appearance. The LA also adopts a rounded, globular appearance if its pressure and/or volume rises due to MR or congenital disease. (💿 AF, RSD, SFP, VMD, VSD)

Motion of the chamber walls

The extent to which the ventricular walls move is governed by preload, afterload and contractility. FS% can be a useful indicator of changes in these factors.[16] Unfortunately, it is not always possible to distinguish which factor is altered but, when evaluated in conjunction with clinical and other echocardiographic findings, the measurement can be very useful. A reduction in FS% due to poor myocardial contractility can be found in cases of myocarditis, myocardial fibrosis or cardiomyopathy. Measurement of FS% immediately before and after exercise has been used to try to identify subtle myocardial disease causing poor athletic performance that is apparent only after exercise[82,83] but decreases in FS% after exercise may also reflect changes in preload associated with redistribution of blood flow after strenuous exercise[84] (see Chapters 3 and 11). FS% can be expected to decrease with AF due to decreased preload. (AF) Sedative drugs also cause a decrease in FS%[25] while an increase in FS% may be found when preload is increased as a result of volume overload and when after-load is significantly reduced. Consequently, FS% can be expected to increase with severe MR and AR, at least until the point that myocardial failure ensues. Thus, where normal FS% is found in the presence of severe MR or AR, concurrent ventricular failure should be suspected. A sig-nificant increase in LVIDs may also be indicative of myo-cardial failure. (VMD)

The motion of the IVS can be affected by changes in ventricular filling or emptying and by the pressure gradi-ent between the LV and RV. In severe MR, the systolic motion of the IVS may be exaggerated because of the low afterload that results from the incompetence of the mitral valve and the concurrent increased filling volume. In AR, the diastolic motion of the IVS is also often exaggerated because of increased ventricular filling and reduced after-load. Whereas, if RV pressure or volume overload is severe, paradoxical motion of the septum may be seen,[85] with the IVS moving towards the LV free-wall during diastole. In some animals, both LV and RV volume and/or overload are present and the IVS may give the impression of "flap-ping" as it is influenced by both sides. (AR, PH, VMD)

Valvular thickening

Valvular incompetence most commonly results from degenerative disease within the leaflets but can also be due to infective endocarditis, congenital dysplasia or non-septic valvulitis (see Chapters 16 and 17). Degenerative valvular disease may result in diffuse or localized thicken-ing in the atrioventricular valves. Nodular or band-like

thickening often affect the aortic valve, most commonly on the right and left coronary cusps, and may or may not result in AR. Thickening of the atrioventricular valves due to mild or moderate degenerative disease is often subtle and in a substantial number of cases of degenera-tive MR, thickening of the valves is not detected echo-cardiographically. Conversely, it is possible to create the appearance of thickening by inappropriate use of the gain controls. Care must therefore be taken in interpreting diffuse thickening. An echogenic appearance to the tip of the left coronary cusp in a right parasternal long-axis view is a common echocardiographic artifact and should not be mistaken for a nodule. Aortic nodules are more com-monly situated a little way from the free border of the cusp and are often most easily seen in a short-axis view (Fig. 9.19). Echocardiography is helpful in establishing a diagnosis in animals with infective endocarditis (see Chapter 17). Identification of large vegetative lesions is diagnostic of infective endocarditis but moderately sized nodular lesions could be due to either degenerative or infective pathology and the clinical and laboratory find-ings may also help to differentiate the pathogenesis (see Chapter 17). (AR, IE, VMD)

Valvular motion

Motion of the valves can be affected by valvular disease, myocardial disease and by arrhythmias. Many cases of MR, TR and AR are associated with prolapse of the valves and in most of these instances the regurgitation is fairly mild and nonprogressive.[33] Localized prolapse occurs when the valve buckles into the atrium or ventricle and the change in the shape of the valve can result in incompetence. (AF, SFP) Prolapse may also be detected in animals in

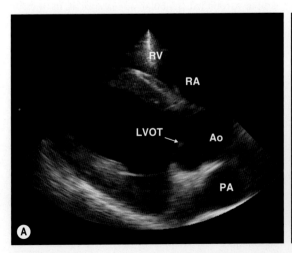
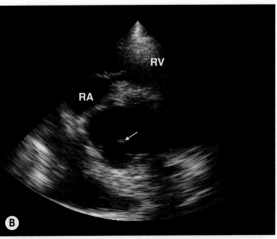

Figure 9.19 Right parasternal long-axis (**A**) and short-axis (**B**) echocardiograms of the left ventricular outflow tract from an 8-year-old Cleveland Bay gelding. A nodule is present on the left coronary cusp (arrow). RA, right atrium; RV, right ventricle; LVOT, left ventricular outflow tract; Ao, aorta; PA, pulmonary artery.

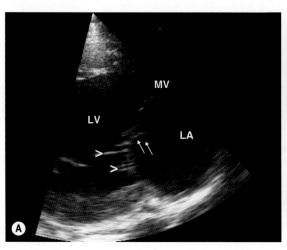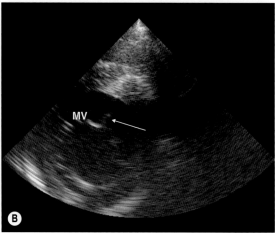

Figure 9.20 Left parasternal long-axis (**A**) and short-axis (**B**) echocardiograms of the left atrium (LA) and left ventricle (LV) from an 8-year-old Cleveland Bay gelding with a ruptured chorda tendinea of the mitral valve (MV). The ruptured chorda tendinea is visible within the left atrium (arrows). Some of the intact chordae tendineae (arrowheads) are also visible.

which the competence of the valve is maintained. Valvular prolapse is less likely to progress to result in clinical progression than degenerative valvular disease, therefore, it is important to distinguish prolapse from thickening. More exaggerated valve motion is seen if chordae tendineae rupture.[70] This results in a "flail" leaflet, in which the tip of the valve is seen within the atrium. The right commissural cusp of the mitral valve is most commonly affected, and this may be seen most clearly from a left parasternal long-axis view (Fig. 9.20). (RCT)

M-mode echocardiography, with its excellent temporal resolution, can demonstrate valve motion extremely well. The atrioventricular valves have a typical M-shaped pattern of motion associated with early diastolic filling (E wave) and atrial contraction (A wave) (see Fig. 9.5) The ratio of the E wave and A wave gives some indication of the relative contribution to ventricular filling.[16] For example, the A peak of AV valve motion will be absent in atrial fibrillation, and may be replaced by small undulations[86] (AF) and with atrioventricular block there may be extra A waves during diastole. (AR) Abnormal filling of the ventricles may result in a change in the E wave to A wave ratio[16]; however, examples of the use of valve motion to assess abnormal diastolic function in horses are poorly documented. High-frequency vibration of the aortic valve and/or anterior mitral leaflet in diastole is diagnostic of AR.[71] (AR)

The motion of the semilunar valves can be used, in association with the ECG, to measure the time taken for different systolic events known as systolic time intervals (see Fig. 9.4) Useful information about ventricular function can be derived from these measurements: prolongation of the pre-ejection period and decreases in ejection time suggested reduced global ventricular function which may be due to one or more of decreased myocardial

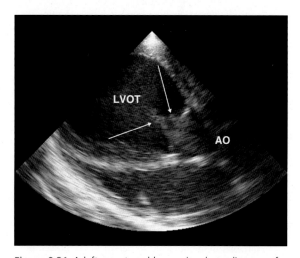

Figure 9.21 A left parasternal long-axis echocardiogram of the left ventricular outflow tract (LVOT) and aorta (Ao) from a horse with congestive heart failure. The sluggish blood flow has become so echogenic that a jet of aortic regurgitation is visible (arrows).

function, decreased preload or increased afterload[25,87] (see Chapter 1). (AF, CN, PC, VMD)

Spontaneous contrast

In most species, moving blood is anechoic; however, in normal horses, blood within the heart may appear echogenic depending on the gain settings of the echocardiographic unit. It can be particularly prominent when blood is slow moving such as in sedated animals, and it can be very striking in animals with congestive heart failure (Fig. 9.21). In the past, an association between spontaneous contrast and poor athletic performance, in particular in horses with a history of exercise-induced pulmonary haemorrhage (EIPH), was suggested.[88] However, spontaneous contrast is often found in healthy horses, particularly after deep inspiration or sudden excitement during an echocardiographic examination and any link with EIPH remains unproven. (AF, PC, VT)

REFERENCES

1. Bonagura JD, Blissitt KJ. Echocardiography. Equine Vet J Suppl 1995;19:5–17.

2. Armstrong W. Echocardiography. In: Zipes D, Libby P, Bonow RO, Braunwald EB, editors. Braunwald's Heart Disease: A Textbook of Cardiovascular Medicine, 7th ed. Philadelphia: WB Saunders; 2005. p. 187–270.

3. Reef VB, Lalezari K, De Boo J, et al. Pulsed-wave Doppler evaluation of intracardiac blood flow in 30 clinically normal Standardbred horses. Am J Vet Res 1989;50(1):75–83.

4. Blissitt KJ, Bonagura JD. Pulsed wave Doppler echocardiography in normal horses. Equine Vet J Suppl 1995;19:38–46.

5. Young LE, Blissitt KJ, Clutton RE, et al. Feasibility of transoesophageal echocardiography for evaluation of left ventricular performance in anaesthetised horses. Equine Vet J Suppl 1995;19:63–70.

6. Young L, Long KJ, Darke PGG, et al. Effects of detomidine, dopamine and dobutamine on selected Doppler echocardiographic variables in the horse. Br J Anaesth 1993;69:222P.

7. Young L. Measurement of left ventricular function in anaesthetised horses using transoesophageal echocardiography. PhD thesis, University of Edinburgh, 1995:1–282.

8. Young LE, Blissitt KJ, Bartram DH, et al. Measurement of cardiac output by transoesophageal Doppler echocardiography in anaesthetized horses: comparison with thermodilution. Br J Anaesth 1996;77(6):773–780.

9. Young LE, Blissitt KJ, Clutton RE, et al. Temporal effects of an infusion of dopexamine hydrochloride in horses anesthetized with halothane. Am J Vet Res 1997;58(5):516–523.

10. Young LE, Blissitt KJ, Clutton RE, et al. Temporal effects of an infusion of dobutamine hydrochloride in horses anesthetized with halothane. Am J Vet Res 1998;59(8):1027–1032.

11. Young LE, Blissitt KJ, Clutton RE, et al. Haemodynamic effects of a sixty minute infusion of dopamine hydrochloride in horses anaesthetised with halothane. Equine Vet J 1998;30(4):310–316.

12. Raisis AL, Young LE, Blissitt KJ, et al. A comparison of the haemodynamic effects of isoflurane and halothane anaesthesia in horses. Equine Vet J 2000;32(4):318–326.

13. Blissitt KJ, Raisis AL, Adams VJ, et al. The effects of halothane and isoflurane on cardiovascular function in dorsally recumbent horses undergoing surgery. Vet Anaesth Analg 2008;35(3):208–219.

14. Raisis AL, Blissitt KJ, Henley W, et al. The effects of halothane and isoflurane on cardiovascular function in laterally recumbent horses. Br J Anaesth 2005;95(3):317–325.

15. Linton RA, Young LE, Marlin DJ, et al. Cardiac output measured by lithium dilution, thermodilution, and transesophageal Doppler echocardiography in anesthetized horses. Am J Vet Res 2000;61(7):731–737.

16. Feigenbaum H. Echocardiography. In: Braunwald E, editor. Heart Disease; A Textbook of Cardiovascular Medicine, 3rd ed. Philadelphia: WB Saunders; 1998. p. 83–139.

17. Mark D, Robertson DB, Adams D, Kisslo J. Doppler evaluation of valvular regurgitation. In: Kisslo J, Adams D, Mark DB, editors. Basic Doppler Echocardiography. New York: Churchill Livingstone; 1986. p. 91–92.

18. Cooper J, Fan PH, Nanda NC. How to perform a color Doppler examination. In: Nanda N, editor. Textbook of Color Doppler Echocardiography. Philadelphia: Lea & Febiger; 1989. p. 116–140.

19. Sepulveda MF, Perkins JD, Bowen IM, et al. Demonstration of regional differences in equine ventricular myocardial velocity in normal 2-year-old Thoroughbreds with Doppler tissue imaging. Equine Vet J 2005;37(3):222–226.

20. Estrada A, Chetboul V. Tissue Doppler evaluation of ventricular synchrony. J Vet Cardiol 2006;8:129–137.

21. Katz W, Gulati VK, Mahler CM, Gorcsan J. Quantitative evaluation of the segmental left ventricular response to dobutamine stress by tissue Doppler echocardiography. Am J Cardiol 1997;79:1036–1042.

22. Garcia M, Rodriguez L, Ares M, Griffin BP, Klein AL, Stewart WJ, et al. Myocardial wall velocity assessment by pulsed Doppler tissue imaging; characteristic findings in normal subjects. Am Heart J 1996;132:648–656.

23. Sutherland C, Lange A, Palka P, et al. Does Doppler myocardial imaging give new insights or simply old information revisited? Heart 1996;76:197–199.

24. Tranquart F, Grenier N, Eder V, Pourcelot L. Clinical use of ultrasound tissue harmonic imaging. Ultrasound Med Biol 1999;25:889–894.

25. Patteson MW, Gibbs C, Wotton PR, et al. Effects of sedation with detomidine hydrochloride on echocardiographic measurements of cardiac dimensions and indices of cardiac function in horses. Equine Vet J Suppl 1995;(19):33–37.

26. Gehlen H, Kroker K, Deegen E, et al. [Influence of detomidine on echocardiographic function parameters and cardiac hemodynamics in horses with and without heart murmur]. Schweiz Arch Tierheilkd 2004;146(3): 119–126.

27. Buhl R, Ersboll AK, Larsen NH, et al. The effects of detomidine, romifidine or acepromazine on echocardiographic measurements and cardiac function in normal horses. Vet Anaesth Analg 2007; 34(1):1–8.

28. Menzies-Gow NJ. Effects of sedation with acepromazine on echocardiographic measurements in eight healthy thoroughbred horses. Vet Rec 2008;163(1): 21–25.

29. Long KJ, Bonagura JD, Darke PG. Standardised imaging technique for guided M-mode and Doppler echocardiography in the horse. Equine Vet J 1992;24(3):226–235.

30. Reef V. Echocardiographic examination in the horse: the basics. Compend Contin Educ Pract Vet 1990;12:1312–1319.

31. Long K, Bonagura JD, Darke PGG. Standardised imaging technique for guided M mode and Doppler echocardiography in the horse. Equine Vet J 1992;24:226–235.

32. Blissitt KJ, Bonagura JD. Colour flow Doppler echocardiography in normal horses. Equine Vet J Suppl 1995;(19):47–55.

33. Marr CM, Reef VB. Physiological valvular regurgitation in clinically normal young racehorses: prevalence and two-dimensional colour flow Doppler echocardiographic characteristics. Equine Vet J Suppl 1995;(19): 56–62.

34. Long KJ. Doppler echocardiography in the horse. Equine Vet Educ 1990;2:15–17.

35. Marr CM. Equine echocardiography: sound advice at the heart of the matter. Br Vet J 1994;150(6): 527–545.

36. Reef VB. Advances in echocardiography. Vet Clin North Am Equine Pract 1991;7(2): 435–450.

37. Reef VB. Heart murmurs in horses: determining their significance with echocardiography. Equine Vet J Suppl 1995;(19):71–80.

38. Reef VB. Evaluation of ventricular septal defects in horses using two-dimensional and Doppler echocardiography. Equine Vet J Suppl 1995;(19):86–95.

39. Patteson MW, Gibbs C, Wotton PR, et al. Echocardiographic measurements of cardiac dimensions and indices of cardiac function in normal adult thoroughbred horses. Equine Vet J Suppl 1995;(19):18–27.

40. Young LE, Scott GR. Measurement of cardiac function by transthoracic echocardiography: day to day variability and repeatability in normal Thoroughbred horses. Equine Vet J 1998;30(2):117–122.

41. Lescure F, Tamzali Y. Valeurs de reference en echocardiographie TM chez le cheval de sport. Rev Vet Med 1984;135:405–418.

42. Bakos Z, Voros K, Jarvinen T, et al. Two-dimensional and M-mode echocardiographic measurements of cardiac dimensions in healthy standardbred trotters. Acta Vet Hung 2002;50(3):273–282.

43. Gehlen H, Haubold A, Stadler P. [Reference values for echocardiographic parameters of trained and untrained Icelandic horses]. Dtsch Tierärztl Wochenschr 2007;114(10): 374–377.

44. Buhl R, Ersboll AK, Eriksen L, et al. Changes over time in echocardiographic measurements in young Standardbred racehorses undergoing training and racing and association with racing performance. J Am Vet Med Assoc 2005;226(11):1881–1887.

45. Kriz NG, Hodgson DR, Rose RJ. Changes in cardiac dimensions and indices of cardiac function during deconditioning in horses. Am J Vet Res 2000;61(12):1553–1560.

46. Gehlen H, Marnette S, Rohn K, et al. [Precision-controlled echocardiographic left ventricular function parameters by repeated measurement on three consecutive days in trained and untrained warmblood horses]. Dtsch Tierärztl Wochenschr 2005;112(2):48–54.

47. Young LE. Cardiac responses to training in 2-year-old thoroughbreds: an echocardiographic study. Equine Vet J Suppl 1999;30:195–198.

48. Young LE, Rogers K, Wood JL. Left ventricular size and systolic function in Thoroughbred racehorses and their relationships to race performance. J Appl Physiol 2005;99(4):1278–1285.

49. Zucca E, Ferrucci F, Croci C, et al. Echocardiographic measurements of cardiac dimensions in normal Standardbred racehorses. J Vet Cardiol 2008;10(1):45–51.

50. Slater JD, Herrtage ME. Echocardiographic measurements of cardiac dimensions in normal ponies and horses. Equine Vet J Suppl 1995;(19):28–32.

51. Armstrong WF. Echocardiography. In: Zipes DP, Libby P, Bonow RO, Braunwald E. Braunwald's Heart Disease: a textbook of cardiovascular medicine. 7th ed. 2005. p. 187–260.

52. O'Callaghan MW. Comparison of echocardiographic and autopsy measurements of cardiac dimensions in the horse. Equine Vet J 1985;17(5):361–368.

53. Young LE, Marlin DJ, Deaton C, et al. Heart size estimated by echocardiography correlates with maximal oxygen uptake. Equine Vet J Suppl 2002;(34):467–471.

54. Giguere S, Bucki E, Adin DB, et al. Cardiac output measurement by partial carbon dioxide rebreathing, 2-dimensional echocardiography, and lithium-dilution method in anesthetized neonatal foals. J Vet Intern Med 2005;19(5):737–743.

55. Schwarzwald CC, Schober KE, Bonagura JD. Methods and reliability of echocardiographic assessment of left atrial size and mechanical function in horses. Am J Vet Res 2007;68(7):735–747.

56. Helwegen MM, Young LE, Rogers K, et al. Measurements of right ventricular internal dimensions and their relationships to severity of tricuspid valve regurgitation in national hunt thoroughbreds. Equine Vet J Suppl 2006;(36):171–177.

57. Mizuno Y, Aida H, Hara H, et al. Comparison of methods of cardiac output measurements determined by dye dilution, pulsed Doppler echocardiography and thermodilution in horses. J Vet Med Sci 1994;56(1):1–5.

58. Blissitt KJ, Young LE, Jones RS, et al. Measurement of cardiac output in standing horses by Doppler echocardiography and thermodilution. Equine Vet J 1997;29(1):18–25.

59. Corley KT, Donaldson LL, Durando MM, et al. Cardiac output technologies with special reference to the horse. J Vet Intern Med 2003;17(3):262–272.

60. Buhl R, Ersboll AK, Eriksen L, et al. Sources and magnitude of variation of echocardiographic measurements in normal standardbred horses. Vet Radiol Ultrasound 2004;45(6):505–512.

61. Blissitt KJ, Bonagura JD. Colour flow Doppler echocardiography in horses with cardiac murmurs. Equine Vet J Suppl 1995;(19): 82–85.

62. Lightfoot G, Jose-Cunilleras E, Rogers K, et al. An echocardiographic and auscultation study of right heart responses to training in young national hunt thoroughbred horses. Equine Vet J Suppl 2006;(36):153–158.

63. Stadler P, Hoch M, Fraunhaul B, Deegen E. Echocardiography in horses with and without heart murmurs in aortic regurgitation. Pferdeheilkunde 1995;11:373–383.

64. Adin D, McCloy K. Physiologic valve regurgitation in normal cats. J Vet Cardiol 2005;7:9–13.

65. Nakayama T, Wakao Y, Takiguchi S. Prevalence of valvular regurgitation in normal beagle dogs detected by color Doppler echocardiography. J Vet Med Sci 1994;56:973–975.

66. Simpson M, Valdes-Cruz LM, Recusani F. Color flow Doppler mapping studies of "physiologic" pulmonary and tricuspid regurgitation: evidence for true regurgitation as opposed to a valve closing volume. J Am Soc Echocardiogr 1991;4:589–597.

67. Young LE, Rogers K, Wood JL. Heart murmurs and valvular regurgitation in thoroughbred racehorses: epidemiology and associations with athletic performance. J Vet Intern Med 2008;22(2):418–426.

68. Young LE, Wood JL. Effect of age and training on murmurs of atrioventricular valvular regurgitation in young thoroughbreds. Equine Vet J 2000;32(3):195–199.

69. Buhl R, Ersboll AK, Eriksen L, et al. Use of color Doppler echocardiography to assess the development of valvular regurgitation in Standardbred trotters. J Am Vet Med Assoc 2005;227(10):1630–1635.

70. Reef VB, Bain FT, Spencer PA. Severe mitral regurgitation in horses: clinical, echocardiographic and pathological findings. Equine Vet J 1998;30(1):18–27.

71. Reef VB, Spencer P. Echocardiographic evaluation of equine aortic insufficiency. Am J Vet Res 1987;48(6):904–909.

72. Reef VB, Klumpp S, Maxson AD, et al. Echocardiographic detection of an intact aneurysm in a horse. J Am Vet Med Assoc 1990;197(6): 752–755.

73. Roby KA, Reef VB, Shaw DP, et al. Rupture of an aortic sinus aneurysm in a 15-year-old broodmare. J Am Vet Med Assoc 1986;189(3):305–308.

74. Durando M, Slack J, Reef VB, Seco-Diaz O, Smith G, Birks EK. Echocardiographic estimation of pulmonary arterial pressures in horses with cardiac disease. J Vet Intern Med 2006;20:742.

75. Slack J, Durando MM, Ainsworth DM, Reef VB, Jesty SA, Smith G, et al. Non-invasive estimation of pulmonary arterial pressure in horses with recurrent airway obstruction. J Vet Intern Med 2006;20:757.

76. Durando M, Collins N, Slack J, Marr CM, Ousey J, Palmer L, et al. Echocardiographic estimation of pulmonary arterial pressures in hypoxemic foals. J Vet Emerg Crit Care 2008;18:422.

77. Kriz NG, Rose RJ. Repeatability of standard transthoracic echocardiographic measurements in horses. Aust Vet J 2002;80(6): 362–370.

78. Traub-Dargatz JL, Schlipf JW Jr, Boon J, et al. Ventricular tachycardia and myocardial dysfunction in a horse. J Am Vet Med Assoc 1994;205(11): 1569–1573.

79. Reef V. Echocardiographic findings in horses with congenital heart disease. Compend Contin Educ Pract Vet 1991;13:109–117.

80. Taylor FG, Wotton PR, Hillyer MH, et al. Atrial septal defect and atrial fibrillation in a foal. Vet Rec 1991;128(4):80–81.

81. Schwarzwald C. Sequential segmental analysis: a systematic approach to the diagnosis of congenital cardiac defects. Equine Vet Educ 2008;20:305–309.

82. Martin BB Jr., Reef VB, Parente EJ, et al. Causes of poor performance of horses during training, racing, or showing: 348 cases (1992–1996). J Am Vet Med Assoc 2000;216(4): 554–558.

83. Reef VB. Stress echocardiography and its role in performance assessment. Vet Clin North Am Equine Pract 2001;17(1):179–189, viii.

84. Marr CM, Bright JM, Marlin DJ, et al. Pre- and post exercise echocardiography in horses performing treadmill exercise in cool and hot/humid conditions. Equine Vet J Suppl 1999;30: 131–136.

85. DeMadron E, Bonagura, JD, O'Grady, MR. Normal and paradoxical ventricular septal motion in the dog. Am J Vet Res 1985;46:2546–2552.

86. Wingfield WE, Miller CW, Voss JL, et al. Echocardiography in assessing mitral valve motion in 3 horses with atrial fibrillation. Equine Vet J 1980;12(4):181–184.

87. Atkins C, Snyder, PE. Systolic time intervals and their derivatives for evaluation of cardiac function. J Vet Intern Med 1992;6:55–63.

88. Mahony C, Rantanen NW, DeMichael JA, et al. Spontaneous echocardiographic contrast in the thoroughbred: high prevalence in racehorses and a characteristic abnormality in bleeders. Equine Vet J 1992;24(2):129–133.

Chapter | **10** |

Ambulatory electrocardiography and heart rate variability

I Mark Bowen

INTRODUCTION

Electrocardiography is used for the diagnosis of cardiac rhythm disturbances that may have been identified during a physical examination. However, some arrhythmias are not present at the time of electrocardiography, despite being obvious during physical examination, or may be suggested by a clinical history of intermittent reduction in cardiac output and not identified clinically. There are several reasons why the arrhythmia may not be detected at the time of recording a patient-side ECG and may be related to changes in autonomic tone such that they only occur during exercise or during rest. In these situations ambulatory electrocardiography can be very useful in order to document cardiac rate and rhythm at the times when clinical signs have been reported, such that a dysrhythmia may be reproduced. In addition, ambulatory electrocardiography can be useful in the critical care setting where cardiac rhythm disturbances may occur as a result of electrolyte and fluid status or even following drug administration such as quinidine sulfate for the treatment of atrial fibrillation (AF).

Traditionally ambulatory ECG devices were defined as being either continuous ambulatory monitors that recorded the ECG signal for subsequent analysis or radio-telemetric devices that transmitted the ECG signal to a terminal where they could be viewed in real time. These boundaries have now been blurred and devices are able to both store and transmit ECG data to be viewed in real-time and interrogated more thoroughly at a later stage. Despite this, the traditional definitions are still valid in terms of how the ECG signal will be used, although since they are all ambulatory monitors, the clinical uses will be defined as resting or exercising ambulatory electrocardiography.

Continuous ambulatory (Holter) electrocardiography traditionally refers to an ECG device that records the ECG signal for subsequent analysis. There is no requirement for the ECG to be monitored during the recording, with the possible exception of ensuring an adequate signal is present. The ECG signal can be recorded using a variety of technologies ranging from analogue audiotapes, mini-discs, or solid state memory devices. The duration of the recording can be variable, traditional tape-based analogue systems used to provide a 24-hour recording period while modern solid state devices can record for up to a week. The longer periods of recording are more likely to be representative of any intermittent dysrhythmia but require more time to process and since the automated algorithms used are designed for use in human patients they are not always accurate when analysing equine ECGs. This form of device is most appropriate for stable/paddock rest or low intensity/endurance exercise where it is not possible to follow the path of the horse or stay within range of a radio signal.

© 2010 Elsevier Ltd.
DOI: 10.1016/B978-0-7020-2817-5.00015-8

Radiotelemetric ECG devices transmit an ECG signal to a distant terminal where it can be visualized without immediate detailed analysis. This brings with it a requirement for trained observers to be present to identify abnormalities and react to these as they occur. Recently, internet and mobile phone ready devices have been established allowing remote monitoring by trained personnel. The obvious advantage of this system is that it allows the observer to intervene should any dysrhythmia occur, and therefore is ideal for exercise and in a critical care setting.

ELECTRODE PLACEMENT FOR AMBULATORY ELECTROCARDIOGRAPHY

In order to obtain a diagnostic ambulatory ECG it is usual to use a chest-lead system so that electrodes can be placed underneath a girth or surcingle that will ensure appropriate contact between the electrode and the skin, will reduce movement artifact and will provide a point for attachment of the device. In order to optimize the ECG for automated processing the lead placement is usually such that the positive electrode (right arm) is placed at the top of the thorax on the left-hand side at the level of the vertebral bodies while the negative electrode (left arm) is placed on the sternum. If multiple leads are being used the neutral (left leg) is placed on the right-hand side of the thoracic wall. The earth (right leg) electrode can be placed anywhere around the girth area. It is usual to clip the horse where the electrodes will be placed and to use self-sticking electrodes that contain contact gel. It may be necessary to apply surgical spirit to maintain electrical contact especially in hot climates. The girth should be applied tightly to prevent movement of the electrodes. This arrangement of electrodes should record an ECG with a negative QRS, positive P and T waves (Fig. 10.1).

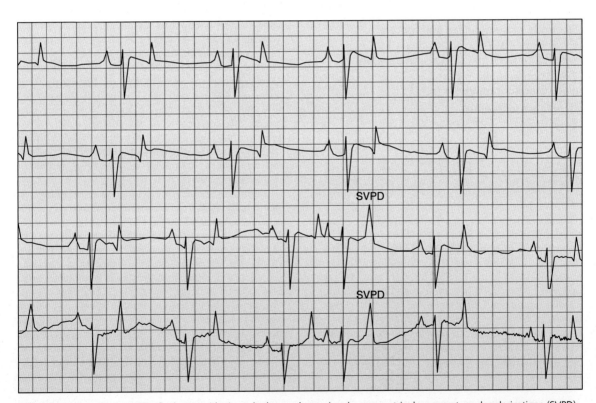

Figure 10.1 Continuous ECG of a horse with sinus rhythm and occasional supraventricular premature depolarizations (SVPD) obtained via a 24-hour continuous Holter recorder. Notice both SVPD have normal appearing premature QRS complexes that are preceded by a P wave and normal P–R interval. The sinus rhythm returns to normal following SVPD. Isolated ectopy is not uncommon in resting ambulatory recordings at a frequency of around one per hour. Modified base-apex ECG, 25 mm/second paper speed.

RESTING AMBULATORY ELECTROCARDIOGRAPHY

Resting ambulatory electrocardiography can be useful in order to establish true resting heart rate and rhythm as well as to document the frequency of any intermittent dysrhythmia. Resting ambulatory electrocardiography is indicated in animals that are presented for investigation of poor performance and/or collapse where the purpose of the recording is to identify intermittent dysrhythmias that may themselves be clinically significant or that suggest underlying myocardial disease. Resting electrocardiography is also indicated in the clinical care setting.

When interpreting resting ambulatory ECGs some dysrhythmias are often found that are of no clinical significance; the prevalence of second degree atrioventricular block (AVB)[1] is much higher during ambulatory recordings at rest than during patient-side ECG recording as a result of reduced sympathetic stimulation when the animal is returned to a more natural environment. This is a normal physiological dysrhythmia and should be of no significance if it resolves during light exercise. Occasional ventricular (VPD) and supraventricular premature depolarizations (SVPD) can also be seen on resting ambulatory recordings and provided that they occur less than 1 per hour and are not present at exercise are not considered abnormal (Figs. 10.1 and 10.2).

AF most frequently presents as a persistent dysrhythmia, but can also present as a paroxysmal form where the dysrhythmia spontaneously resolves. Although resting ambulatory electrocardiography is unlikely to identify this, if not present on a patient-side ECG, horses may have frequent isolated SVPD between episodes. If these are present and the horse has a history of a dysrhythmia following exercise, often associated with a sudden loss of performance,[2] then this may support a tentative diagnosis of paroxysmal atrial fibrillation. If isolated SVPD are frequent without a history that supports a diagnosis of

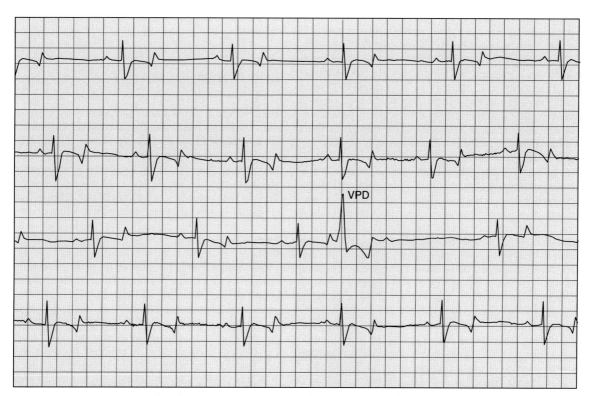

Figure 10.2 Continuous ECG of a horse with sinus rhythm and occasional ventricular premature depolarizations (VPD) obtained via a 24-hour continuous Holter recorder. Notice the ventricular premature depolarization with its QRS complex that is widened and bizarre in appearance when compared to the other normally conducted QRS complexes. The T wave of the ventricular premature depolarization is oriented in the opposite direction of the QRS complex. The next normal sinus beat occurs but is not conducted through to the ventricle, resulting in a compensatory pause. Modified base-apex ECG, 25 mm/second paper speed.

paroxysmal atrial fibrillation the horse should undergo a full cardiovascular assessment. Although SVPD are unlikely to destabilize and compromise cardiac function they may be evidence of underlying atrial myocardial disease. (⬭ *AF, SFP, VMD*)

Frequent VPD (see Fig. 10.2) that are present on an ambulatory resting ECG may be suggestive of underlying myocardial disease or may occur in horses with aortic valve disease and should prompt a thorough investigation in an attempt to document underlying pathology and determine whether treatment is likely to be effective (see Chapter 13). In a study of 38 horses with ventricular dysrhythmias, 14 had frequent VPD and were managed by pasture rest and the administration of corticosteroids based on a presumptive diagnosis of myocarditis. There was an improvement of dysrhythmia frequency in nine horses, in five of which the dysrhythmia was completely abolished suggesting that these dysrhythmias represent underlying myocardial pathology (Bowen IM, Marr CM, unpublished observations). Frequent or complex VPD are reported to be associated with sudden cardiac death in humans[3] and horses[4] and it is believed that they persist or deteriorate in horses that are kept in exercise. Therefore, rest is an important aspect of management of these animals and glucocorticoids are sometimes recommended in the belief that the period of rest required would be shorter. Where horses have frequent isolated ventricular premature complexes their prevalence should be evaluated during exercise. Although isolated single VPD have little effect on cardiac output, they may become more frequent with exercise or result in ventricular tachycardia, which could result in collapse during exercise or even sudden death should ventricular tachycardia develop into ventricular fibrillation. (⬭ *AF, AR, RCT*)

Ventricular tachycardia is most likely to be seen in the critical care setting with the use of ambulatory or telemetric electrocardiography (see Chapter 21). There is a particular association between horses with gastrointestinal tract disease and ventricular dysrhythmias, and electrocardiography should be considered when heart rates are higher than would be expected for the degree of pain and hypovolaemia.[5] These dysrhythmias may represent changes in electrolyte, acid-base or fluid status or endotoxaemia and therefore an assessment of the underlying cause is important. Cardiac troponin I concentrations may be increased in horses undergoing exploratory laparotomy for the correction of strangulating small intestinal lesions. This suggests a degree of cardiac myocyte damage, which in one study was shown to be related to hypovolaemia rather than endotoxaemia.[6] Therefore, volume expansion should be considered in these animals. Criteria for diagnosis and specific management of ventricular dysrhythmias are detailed in Chapter 13. The aim of diagnosis, management and monitoring of these animals is to identify those at risk from progression to ventricular fibrillation which is rarely amenable to intervention.

EXERCISING AMBULATORY ELECTROCARDIOGRAPHY

Exercising electrocardiography can be used to assess the significance of dysrhythmias detected at rest and to identify dysrhythmias that were otherwise undetected and that only occur during exercise. The advantage of ambulatory electrocardiography in this setting is that the animal can be examined in the same conditions that provoke clinical signs. Exercising ambulatory electrocardiography is indicated for investigation of horses that are presented for investigation of poor performance and collapse and should form part of the evaluation of a horse with aortic valve regurgitation. In addition to providing information about cardiac rhythm cardiac rate can be obtained and can be compared to speed of the horse at the time using either a high-speed treadmill or GPS-based velocity devices. Further details regarding exercise testing and interpretation of exercising electrocardiography can be found in Chapter 11.

HEART RATE VARIABILITY

Heart rate variability describes and quantifies the beat-to-beat variability in heart rate that occurs due to neurohormonal control of heart rate. Currently the technique is not in routine clinical use for the diagnosis or monitoring of cardiovascular disease in the horse; however many large-scale studies have shown it to be a useful method of predicting prognosis in various cardiac disease states in human beings. Therefore an understanding of these methods may prove useful in further improving the veterinarian's ability to stratify risk in horses with cardiac disease.

Heart rate is not static, even in the resting horse, and changes in beat-to-beat intervals occur in the normal healthy animal. As such, the classical view of the heart possessing a metronome-like character only applies to the decentralized heart. In vivo the heart is under the influence of both the autonomic nervous system and the neuroendocrine system in order to maintain normal arterial blood pressure and result in cyclical changes in heart rate (R–R intervals). Techniques of assessing heart rate variability therefore quantify neurohormonal control and do so independently of heart rate providing an indicator of cardiovascular well being. The greater the heart rate variability, the healthier the heart. For example, both respiratory sinus arrhythmia and second degree atrioventricular block are considered normal physiological dysrhythmias[1,7] and are a result of autonomic control of the heart.

Determination of heart rate variability

Heart rate variability can be determined from a recorded ECG by extraction of normal R–R intervals (termed N–N intervals; normal–normal) either manually or automatically. These data can then be used to create a tachogram of R–R data (Fig. 10.3) and used for subsequent analysis. The duration of recording and environment in which the recording is made is important to consider. Most heart rate variability indices are obtained from continuous ambulatory recordings where the influence of external stimuli such as handling and transport can be excluded while providing large amounts of data that can be analysed. Accurate detection of normal intervals is essential and therefore the quality of ECG recording is vital in calculating accurate heart rate variability indices. The author's recommendations for obtaining ECG recordings for heart rate variability analysis are shown in Table 10.1.

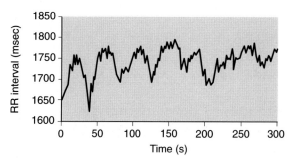

Figure 10.3 Tachogram of normal R–R (N–N) intervals from a horse showing cyclic fluctuations in heart rate.

Table 10.1 Clinical recommendations for the use of heart rate variability in the horse

- Horses should be maintained in a familiar environment
- Recordings should be made during minimal disruption, and for at least 4 hours (preferably at night)
- Ensure good quality recordings with R wave amplitudes at least twice that of T waves
- Exclude dysrhythmias, including physiological second degree atrioventricular block using electronic filters (65–175%)
- Time domain analysis: hourly calculations using SDNN, TI, RMSSD and sNN100
- Vaso-vagal tonus index calculated from 20 complexes
- Frequency domain: perform hourly calculations using 1024 N–N intervals using high frequency >0.07 Hz and low frequency 0.05–0.07 Hz

For most applications automated processing of the ECG is essential to provide N–N data since manual processing would be too labour intensive. This can be done using computer-based algorithms that determine shape, size and timing of the ECG waveforms in order to identify normal intervals. Since the extraction of N–N data usually relies upon algorithms designed for use in human cardiology it is important to optimize the ECG recording to provide large QRS complexes and small T waves with minimal movement artifact. As previously discussed it is often helpful to place electrodes for ambulatory recordings under a girth or surcingle to ensure adequate contact is maintained.

Having obtained an ECG and identified normal intervals the tachogram can be further filtered to remove mis-detected prematurity or movement artifact using timing-based filters that remove intervals if they differ excessively from the previous interval durations. This is important as heart rate variability is used to assess fluctuations brought about by autonomic control, not due to abnormal conduction within the myocardium (dysrhythmia). Since physiological changes in heart rate are not sudden, acute changes are likely to represent artifact, premature complexes, prolonged pauses and second-degree atrioventricular block. However, filtering all episodes of second-degree AV block from equine ECG recordings may remove important information about autonomic control of the equine heart since second-degree AV block is brought about by similar control mechanisms that induce respiratory sinus arrhythmia in other species; vagal outflow results in blocked conduction through the AV node, rather than slowing discharge from the sinoatrial node. Removing this from heart rate variability calculations removes a large amount of information, but to include it would result in a greater amount of heterogeneity of heart rate variability in normal animals. In addition, it would prevent the use of time-based filters which often overcome the shortcomings of shape-based algorithms based on human ECG recordings. Consequently the author recommends that time-based filters are set to remove intervals that are less than 65% or more than 175% of preceding intervals (see Table 10.1).

Time domain analysis of heart rate variability

Time domain analyses of heart rate variability are simple robust methods that use statistical or geometric techniques to quantify changes in heart rate. There are many different types of time domain analyses and these provide a global view of autonomic control of the heart. They can be applied to long-duration recordings as well as short but are relatively resistant to the effects of artifact or mis-detected complexes so are most likely to be clinically useful in the horse. Other time domain analyses are used in human medicine but those in equine use include the following.

Standard deviation of normal intervals (SDNN)

SDNN is the simplest method of assessing variability of normal intervals and gives an overall assessment of autonomic function. It is important that results are compared from the same duration of recordings and since 24 hours of artifact and stimulation free recording are difficult to obtain in horses, 4-hour recording may be an appropriate compromise.[8] SDNN has been widely used in a range of physiological studies in both equine and human studies. There is no information about the repeatability of SDNN calculation from horses obtained on consecutive days.

Vasovagal tonus index (VVTI)

VVTI is a simple method of assessing autonomic control based on the natural logarithm of standard deviation of normal intervals (VVTI = $\ln_{(SDNN)}{}^2$). VVTI has been described as a method for assessing heart rate variability over short periods using just 20 consecutive beats. In dogs, VVTI has been shown to be reduced in animals suffering from congestive heart failure. Preliminary studies in eight horses showed relatively good repeatability of results from consecutive days using this technique.[9] Since VVTI uses only short-term recordings these data are an indicator of vagal control of heart rate and therefore may be appropriate in the resting horse, which is primarily under vagal influence without the need for ambulatory monitoring.

Other statistical methods

The root mean square of successive intervals (RMSSD) and number of intervals greater then 50 ms (sNN50) are estimates of high-frequency fluctuations that have been used in human cardiology. Due to the lower heart rate in horses than in humans the sNN100 is recommended by the author, and results in similar normal range (approximately 200 per hour) to the sNN50 in humans. However, since this index is affected by heart rate it is only applicable to the resting horse.

Geometric methods

Geometric methods convert N–N intervals into geometric shapes which provide a further method of filtering aberrant data by forcing a geometric filter over this data. The simplest method is the triangular index (TI; Fig. 10.4) which plots a histogram of N–N data. The index is then calculated as the number of N–N intervals divided by the peak of the histogram. Because outliers are excluded from the data set by this method it overcomes many of the

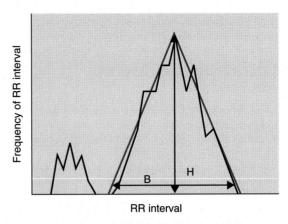

Figure 10.4 Geometric filter for heart rate variability analysis, showing the method of calculation of triangular index. Mechanical filter derived by fitting shape to triangular distribution. Light-shaded area shows area used for calculations. Outliers are excluded. B, base of triangle; H, height of triangle.

problems in terms of artifact detection and interval-based filtering. However, this technique requires more N–N intervals to construct a useful histogram and in human cardiology is not recommended for recordings less than 30 minutes. Therefore, in equine use they would require an ECG recording of at least 60 minutes to provide useful clinical data.

Frequency domain analysis (power spectral analysis) of heart rate variability

Frequency domain analysis of heart rate variability uses spectral analysis techniques to attempt to separate the effects of different components of the neuroendocrine system on fluctuations of heart rate. The renin–angiotensin–aldosterone system affects heart rate over a long period of time (seconds to minutes), the sympathetic nervous system over a short period of time (seconds) and the parasympathetic nervous system on a beat-to-beat basis (seconds). Frequency domain analysis is highly susceptible to the effects of artifact on its results and therefore is usually only calculated over 5–10-minute intervals per hour in humans. Spectral analysis shows the effect (power) of each influence over a range of frequencies. Very low frequency (30 seconds to 5 minutes) and ultra low frequency fluctuations (more than 5 minutes 30 seconds) in heart rate are brought about by posture and the renin–angiotensin–aldosterone system, respectively. Low frequency fluctuations (6 seconds) are brought about by the sympathetic nervous system and high frequency fluctuations (2–6 seconds) are brought about by the parasympathetic nervous system (Fig. 10.5). Frequency domains

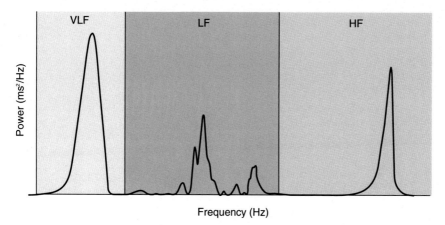

Figure 10.5 Frequency domain analysis of heart rate variability showing typical power spectral recording. Normal R–R (N–N) data is extracted from ECG recording, and power of frequency influences calculated in each domain. Trace shows high frequency (HF), influenced on a beat-to-beat basis by parasympathetic tone, low frequency (LF), influenced by sympathetic function and very low frequency, influenced by hormonal control (VLF). Frequency ranges are shown in Table 10.3.

Table 10.2 Frequency domains defined for use in power spectral analysis in human beings and in the horse

	FREQUENCY RANGE FOR DOMAIN (HZ)			
	MAN[30]	**HORSE**[12]	**HORSE**[13]	**CONTROL MECHANISM**[1]
Ultra low frequency	<0.003	ND	ND	RAAS
Very low frequency	0.003–0.04	ND	0.001–0.005	
Low frequency	0.04–0.15	0.01–0.07	0.005–0.07	Sympathetic Parasympathetic
High frequency	0.15–0.40	0.07–0.6	0.07–0.5	Parasympathetic RAAS, renin-angiotensin-aldosterone system

ND, not defined.
From Malik[30]; Kuwahara et al[12]; Bowen and Marr[13].

have been described in the horse using both respiratory plesmography[10] and pharmacological dissection[11] (Table 10.2) and show many similarities. The author recommends using 1024 N–N intervals (see Table 10.1) rather than an arbitrary 5-minute time frame for use in frequency domain analysis. This should provide sufficient data in order to quantify the effects of both the high frequency and low frequency fluctuations in heart rate.

Clinical applications of heart rate variability

Heart rate variability has been investigated in a variety of clinical scenarios and disease states and has been shown to provide prognostic information in cardiac and vascular diseases (Table 10.3). In almost all cases heart rate variability is used as a research tool although the evidence to suggest its use in clinical medicine is growing. There is little published work investigating the use of heart rate variability in disease in the horse, although it has received some interest in exercise physiology and potentially for performance testing.

Ventricular dysrhythmias

Prediction of ventricular tachydysrhythmias is of considerable importance in human medicine and in some cases can be fatal. Heart rate variability has been shown to decrease, with a particular fall in high frequency variability

Table 10.3 Some examples of clinical application for heart rate variability analysis in humans

Post myocardial infarction	Hypertension, congestive heart failure
Heart transplantation	Mitral regurgitation and valve prolapse
Sudden death	Ventricular and supraventricular arrhythmias
Long QT syndrome	Hypertrophic and dilated cardiomyopathy
Syncope	Diabetes mellitus, Chagas syndrome, systemic sclerosis
Alcoholism	Systemic lupus erythematosus
Aerobic fitness	Fitness training
Effect of antiarrhythmic, ACE inhibitors and other cardioactive drugs	
After Camm and Fei.[29]	

Table 10.4 Time domain variables for heart rate variability analysis for 14 normal horses and 12 horses with ventricular arrhythmias (mean ± SD)

	NORMAL HORSES	HORSES WITH VENTRICULAR ARRHYTHMIA	CRITICAL LIMIT
SDNN (ms)	158 (±70)	90 (±53)*	75
Triangular index	37 (±±7)	24 (±9)*	25

SDNN, standard deviation of normal intervals; critical limit, value below which suggestive of autonomic dysfunction.
*Significantly different (p < 0.05).

and an increase in low frequency (increased sympathetic and decreased parasympathetic function) in a variety of studies[12,13] and has been proposed to be a method for identifying patients at increased risk who may benefit from early intervention. Changes in heart rate variability occur independently of the frequency of ectopy on an ambulatory ECG and therefore are an independent risk factor for the development of significant tachydysrhythmias.

In horses there is less evidence to suggest that heart rate variability could be used as a predictor for horses that are likely to suffer from ventricular tachydysrhythmias that may subsequently lead to collapse. However, in one small study of t12 horses that had ventricular dysrhythmias SDNN and TI were both lower than in age-matched controls (p < 0.05; Table 10.4), although there was some overlap between these groups which may represent differences in severity of the condition in the horses with dysrhythmias. The critical limits that the author considers abnormal in a clinical population are shown in Table 10.4. These data suggest that further investigation of the use of heart rate variability in this group of animals may lead to a better understanding of the pathophysiology of ventricular dysrhythmias and may, in the future, help clinicians to have a better understanding of which cases are likely to develop either life-threatening dysrhythmias or collapse during exercise.

Congestive heart failure

Congestive heart failure is a syndrome resulting from neurohormonal activation which can be documented using heart rate variability analysis in human patients, and subsequently can be improved with pharmacological manipulation with beta-blockers, ACE inhibitors and spironolactone.[14] Heart rate variability failed to offer prognostic information for Doberman Pinschers with cardiomyopathy,[15] being different only in severely diseased animals, although VVTI was significantly reduced in a separate study of dogs with congestive heart failure.[16] There are no reports of heart rate variability being used in horses with congestive heart failure. It would seem unlikely that the technique would offer any significant advantage over existing diagnostic methodologies and in view of the general poor response to therapy for congestive heart failure in this species.

Valvular heart disease

Time domain indices of heart rate variability has been investigated as a prognostic tool for both aortic and mitral valve disease in human patients and has been shown to predict mortality or subsequent deterioration such that valve replacement is required.[17,18] VVTI has also been shown to correlate with the severity of left atrial enlargement in Cavalier King Charles Spaniels with mitral valve disease. In horses VVTI has been shown to be reduced (7.90 ± 0.9; n = 17) compared to a group of horses without cardiac disease (9.10 ± 0.9; n = 21)[9] although there was no difference between those with mild aortic regurgitation (normal left ventricular diameter, n = 8) compared to those with severe aortic regurgitation (increased left ventricular diameter, n = 9). These changes in heart rate variability are presumed to represent changes in autonomic function as with other forms of congestive heart failure. This study was undertaken retrospectively and did not address which animals subsequently developed significant complications and therefore the value of VVTI as a method of predicting risk cannot be assessed. However, if heart rate variability could offer this prognostic information this would be a relatively simple technique since it uses only 20 consecutive beats.

Atrial fibrillation

In general, heart rate variability should not be calculated from animals with dysrhythmias since this will represent myocardial activity rather than changes in autonomic function. However, heart rate variability has been determined in horses with AF and demonstrates an underlying periodicity in horses brought about by parasympathetic modulation of heart rate that modulates the ventricular response.[19,20] This demonstrates an ability to document physiological states but offers little clinical information in horses undergoing treatment for this condition.

Dysautonomias

Cardiac dysautonomia in human patients with diabetes mellitus has been documented using time domain indices of heart rate variability and correlates with the severity of neuropathy.[21] Horses with equine grass sickness also have evidence of cardiac dysautonomia by changes in time domain indices of heart rate variability.[22] This may explain, in part, the excessively high heart rates in horses with equine grass sickness that usually cannot be explained by the degree of hypovolaemia or pain. This finding is supported by chromolytic changes seen in the parasympa-

thetic terminal ganglia of affected horses. Although this finding does not constitute a clinical pre-mortem diagnostic test it provides further evidence that heart rate variability provides valid clinical information in the horse.

Effects of exercise and stress on heart rate variability

Training and detrain have both been shown to affect heart rate variability in humans, in particular in relation to increased low frequency fluctuations from frequency domain analysis.[23] Similar changes are found in horses, especially in relation to low frequency fluctuations suggesting limited effects of training on the parasympathetic function of the horse.[24] During exercise heart rate variability decreases until heart rates reach approximately 130 bpm, after which time non-neural mechanisms result in an increase in high frequency fluctuations. These are likely to be influenced by external factors such as locomotion forces. As a result heart rate variability only provides information about autonomic control of the heart during moderate intensity of exercise.[25,26] There are no data to suggest that exercise performance can be predicted by heart rate variability scores.

Since heart rate variability reflects cardiac autonomic tone it is unsurprising that stress and pain both affect these indices. Transport has been shown to result in a reduction in heart rate variability[27] suggesting that it could be a noninvasive method of determining stress. In horses with laminitis there was no correlation between heart rate variability indices and plasma cortisol concentrations, although pain was associated with a decrease in high frequency and increased low frequency fluctuations.[28] These effects were offset by administration of analgesic agents. Although it may be difficult to use heart rate variability as a method for assessing the impact of management factors on welfare of single animals, changes brought about by interventions may become apparent using these techniques.

CONCLUSIONS

Ambulatory electrocardiography provides considerable information relating to both the frequency of intermittent dysrhythmias and to identify critical dysrhythmias associated with clinical signs. In addition ambulatory recordings can be used for the quantification of heart rate variability in the horse. Although this technique has, as yet, no clinical indication, further investigations in this field may build on several small preliminary studies and provide additional prognostic information for the determination of heart rate variability in the horse. There are many factors that influence the reliability of heart rate variability analysis, and repeatability and reliability of the different measures needs to be established and standardized criteria used to ensure results can be transferred and interpreted between laboratories. Until these can be agreed, the author recommends a range of criteria shown in Table 10.1.

REFERENCES

1. Vibe-Petersen G, Nielsen K. Electrocardiography in the horse (a report of findings in 138 horses). Nord Vet Med 1980;32(3–4):105–121.

2. Holmes JR, Henigan M, Williams RB, et al. Paroxysmal atrial fibrillation in racehorses. Equine Vet J 1986;18(1):37–42.

3. Abdalla IS, Prineas RJ, Neaton JD, et al. Relation between ventricular premature complexes and sudden cardiac death in apparently healthy men. Am J Cardiol 1987;60(13): 1036–1042.

4. Kiryu K, Machida N, Kashida Y, et al. Pathologic and electrocardiographic findings in sudden cardiac death in racehorses. J Vet Med Sci 1999;61(8):921–928.

5. Bowen IM. Post operative complications: cardiac arrhythmias. In: Mair T, Divers T, Ducharme N, editors. Manual of Equine Gastroenterology. London: WB Saunders; 2001, p. 232–237.

6. Hallowell GD, Bowen IM. Cardiac Troponin-I in equine surgical colic patients: myocardial damage due to endotoxaemia or hypoperfusion? Paper presented at the 9th International Equine Colic Symposium, Liverpool, UK, 2008.

7. Reimer JM. Cardiac arrhythmias. In: Robinson NE, editor. Current Therapy in Equine Medicine 3. Philadelphia: WB Saunders; 1992, p. 383–393.

8. Bowen IM, Marr CM. Analysis of heart rate variability in horses with ventricular arrhythmias. Paper presented at 37th British Equine Veterinary Association Congress, Birmingham, UK, 1998.

9. Hammond L. Activation of the Autonomic Nervous System in Horses with Aortic Valve Disease. London: Royal Veterinary College; 2006, p. 32.

10. Kuwahara M, Hashimoto S, Ishii K, et al. Assessment of autonomic nervous function by power spectral analysis of heart rate variability in the horse. J Auton Nerv Syst 1996;60(1–2):43–48.

11. Bowen IM, Marr CM. Assessment of glycopyrrolate and propanolol on frequency domain analysis of heart rate variability in the horse. J Vet Intern Med 1998. 12(3):255.

12. Lanza GA, Cianflone D, Rebuzzi AG, et al. Prognostic value of ventricular arrhythmias and heart rate variability in patients with unstable angina. Heart 2006;92(8): 1055–1063.

13. Reed MJ, Robertson CE, Addison PS. Heart rate variability measurements and the prediction of ventricular arrhythmias. QJM 2005;98(2):87–95.

14. Routledge HC, Chowdhary S, Townend JN. Heart rate variability: a therapeutic target? J Clin Pharm Ther 2002;27(2):85–92.

15. Calvert CA, Wall M. Effect of severity of myocardial failure on heart rate variability in Doberman pinschers with and without echocardiographic evidence of dilated cardiomyopathy. J Am Vet Med Assoc 2001;219(8):1084–1088.

16. Doxey S, Boswood A. Differences between breeds of dog in a measure of heart rate variability. Vet Rec 2004;154(23):713–717.

17. Freed LA, Stein KM, Borer JS, et al. Relation of ultra-low frequency heart rate variability to the clinical course of chronic aortic regurgitation. Am J Cardiol 1997;79(11):1482–1487.

18. Stein KM, Borer JS, Hochreiter C, et al. Prognostic value and physiological correlates of heart rate variability in chronic severe mitral regurgitation. Circulation 1993;88(1):127–135.

19. Gelzer AR, Moise NS, Vaidya D, et al. Temporal organization of atrial activity and irregular ventricular rhythm during spontaneous atrial fibrillation: an in vivo study in the horse. J Cardiovasc Electrophysiol 2000;11(7):773–784.

20. Kuwahara M, Hiraga A, Nishimura T, et al. Power spectral analysis of heart rate variability in a horse with atrial fibrillation. J Vet Med Sci 1998;60(1):111–114.

21. Balcioglu S, Arslan U, Turkoglu S, et al. Heart rate variability and heart rate turbulence in patients with type 2 diabetes mellitus with versus without cardiac autonomic neuropathy. Am J Cardiol 2007; 100(5):890–893.

22. Perkins JD, Bowen IM, Else RW, et al. Functional and histopathological evidence of cardiac parasympathetic dysautonomia in equine grass sickness. Vet Rec 2000;146(9): 246–250.

23. Gamelin FX, Berthoin S, Sayah H, et al. Effect of training and detraining on heart rate variability in healthy young men. Int J Sports Med 2007;28(7):564–570.

24. Kuwahara M, Hiraga A, Kai M, et al. Influence of training on autonomic nervous function in horses: evaluation by power spectral analysis of heart rate variability. Equine Vet J Suppl 1999;30:178–180.

25. Physick-Sheard PW, Marlin DJ, Thornhill R, et al. Frequency domain analysis of heart rate variability in horses at rest and during exercise. Equine Vet J 2000;32(3):253–262.

26. Cottin F, Medigue C, Lopes P, et al. Effect of exercise intensity and repetition on heart rate variability during training in elite trotting

horse. Int J Sports Med 2005; 26(10):859–867.

27. Ohmura H, Hiraga A, Aida H, et al. Changes in heart rate and heart rate variability in Thoroughbreds during prolonged road transportation. Am J Vet Res 2006;67(3):455–462.

28. Rietmann TR, Stauffacher M, Bernasconi P, et al. The association between heart rate, heart rate variability, endocrine and behavioural pain measures in horses suffering from laminitis. J Vet Med A Physiol Pathol Clin Med 2004;51(5):218–225.

29. Camm AJ, Fei L. Clinical significance of heart rate variability. In: Moss AJ, Stern S, editors. Noninvasive Electrocardiography: Clinical Aspects of Holter Monitoring. London: WB Saunders; 1996, p. 225–247.

30. Malik M. Heart rate variability: time domain. In: Moss AJ, Stem S, editors. Noninvasive Electrocardiography: Clinical Aspects of Holter Monitoring. London: WB Saunders; 1996, p. 161–173.

Chapter | 11 |

Exercise and stress testing

Mary Durando

INTRODUCTION

Horses are most commonly used as athletes, whether for professional purposes or for pleasure riding. Because of this, veterinary expertise is often sought if horses are unable to complete the desired work level or are no longer performing at the previous level of ability. Because evaluations of poor performance athletes have become more common, the importance of functional evaluation during exercise has been increasingly recognized in recent years. Musculoskeletal and respiratory problems are the most common reasons horses may be unable to perform adequately, but in many cases a cardiovascular cause is suspected. These horses may appear healthy on physical examination, and be capable of performing lower workloads or living a non-athletic life, but are unable to compete successfully in more strenuous activities because of cardiac disease. Return to previous function is generally the goal of diagnosing and treating cardiac problems in horses with performance limitations. This differs from human and small animal medicine, where the goal of management of cardiac disease is often primarily to increase longevity and to improve quality of life, rather than restore or improve performance.

When asked to evaluate a horse for poor athletic performance, it is not uncommon for the veterinary clinician to encounter cardiac murmurs or dysrhythmias on physical examination, and for the horses presented for poor performance to also have concurrent mild cardiac disease. The clinician must determine if an observed cardiac abnormality is causing the decrement in atheletic performance, or if another body system is more likely to be responsible. Because murmurs and dysrhythmias that may be either physiological or not clinically important are extremely prevalent in horses, this can be challenging and in these cases, an exercise test can be useful to determine whether the horse's performance is actually limited by an observed cardiac problem.

Although resting examinations are critical and will allow recognition of many clinical problems that affect performance, exercise tests have become more important in recent years, and in particular they may help the clinician to assess dynamic problems. Exercise results in tremendous changes in the cardiovascular system of the horse, such as increases in heart rate, myocardial contractility, venous return, blood pressure and blood supply to working muscles. These adaptations are responsible for their superior athletic ability. Horses have a remarkable cardiovascular reserve: cardiac output can increase by 8–10 times over resting values in the more elite athletes, and heart rate can increase sevenfold over resting heart rates. Because of their large cardiovascular reserve, subtle abnormalities may not be obvious at rest. It is often not until stressed closer to physical limits with exercise that abnormalities become apparent. In addition, they may have exercise-induced problems such as dysrhythmias, which are not present at rest. Therefore, exercise testing is

DOI: 10.1016/B978-0-7020-2817-5.00016-X

used in an attempt to reproduce the working conditions causing clinical signs.

Several advances in techniques in recent years have helped improve clinicians' abilities to diagnose cardiac abnormalities. While cardiovascular diseases have been recognized as a potential cause of poor athletic performance for years, documentation has been difficult because of technical limitations of examinations and other reasons mentioned above. The development of the high-speed treadmill has been one of the critical factors facilitating diagnosis of dynamic abnormalities in several body systems. It has allowed physiologists to study normal exercise function and clinicians to recognize abnormal function, in a controlled setting. Some of the techniques currently available in clinical situations include exercising electrocardiography and pre- and post-exercise echocardiography. Other more invasive techniques that may become more widely used in the future would include exercising cardiac output and evaluation of exercising systemic and pulmonary arterial blood pressures. In addition, recent attention has turned to pharmacological cardiac stress testing and the possibility of using this as a substitute for exercise stress testing in some situations, as is done in human medicine.

ELECTROCARDIOGRAPHY

Exercising electrocardiographic methods

Electrocardiography (ECG) is the gold standard for definitively diagnosing rhythm disorders,[1,2] and permits monitoring of the horse's heart rate and rhythm during exercise. Continuous monitoring of the ECG can be accomplished with telemetry, with electrodes positioned in a modified base-apex configuration and attached to a transmitter that sends signals to a receiver.[3,4] Electrodes can either be placed on the neck base and flank or positioned, under a surcingle, at the level of the sixth or seventh intercostal space (Fig. 11.1). The signal is then displayed on an oscilloscope, which can be digitized or printed to permanently record the ECG. These types of systems can be used in conjunction with various exercise tests that best mimic or exceed the usual level of exercise of the horse. This can include simply lungeing the horse, riding the horse on the flat or over jumps, or exercising it at high speed on a racetrack, training gallop or on a high-speed treadmill.

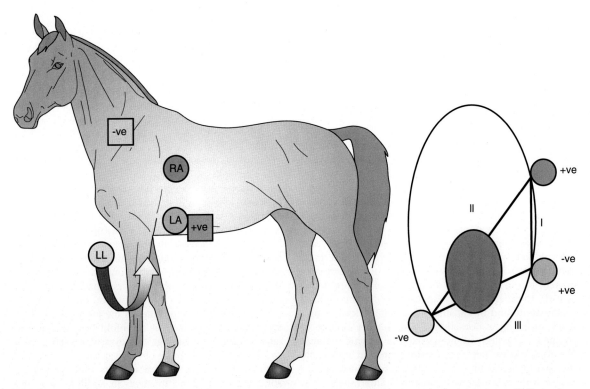

Figure 11.1 Options for electrode placement during exercising ECG. The inset illustrates a transverse section and shows the relationship of the electrodes around the heart. RA, right arm; LA, left arm; LL, left leg.

Although less desirable than telemetry, continuous 24-hour ambulatory ECG monitoring (see Chapter 10) can also be used to monitor heart rate and rhythm during exercise. The main disadvantage with Holter monitors is that they do not display the ECG in real time. However, in some situations, when the exercise area is beyond the range of a telemetry unit, they may be more appropriate to use. For example, if it is not practical to reproduce exercising conditions using a treadmill, arena or racetrack, such as may occur with dysrhythmias suspected during endurance exercise, a Holter monitor can be placed during a long distance ride. This allows the potential to re-create similar environmental conditions and stresses. Holter montitors can also be used to identify the presence of dysrhythmias in a 24-hour period that warrants assessment for dysrhythmias during exercise.

Heart rate

Monitoring the heart rate at different exercise intensities and as the horse recovers from exercise has been utilized to determine fitness and the presence of possible cardiac disease. A range of heart rates for various exercise intensities has been described, with an expected heart rate of 80–120 beats per minute (bpm) at the trot (nonracing), 120–150 bpm at the canter, 150–180 bpm at a hand gallop and >200 (200–240) bpm at maximum exercise intensity[4] (Fig. 11.2). If the heart rate deviates from these ranges, cardiac disease or lack of fitness may be a cause; however, it is important to remember that noncardiac factors may play a role in determining heart rate, including pain, respiratory disease, dehydration, or environmental conditions such as high heat or humidity. These other causes must first be ruled out before attributing heart rate deviations to cardiac disease. These ranges are also useful to determine if the horse is capable of performing its expected workload. If a horse can attain the desired level of work before reaching its maximal heart rate, it should theoretically be able to maintain that intensity, barring other problems. If it reaches a maximal heart rate at low speeds or exertion, it is unlikely it will be able to perform more vigorously. (AF, VSD)

Heart rate decrease following exercise has also been used as a guide to fitness or cardiovascular problems. Generally, after very high-intensity exercise the horse's heart rate decreases to below 100 bpm within 5 minutes, and returns to normal within 45 minutes. The same caveats for interpretation of delayed return of heart rate to normal values are true with heart rate recovery. This can be influenced by many other factors including pain, respiratory disease, dehydration, heat and humidity.

Variations in ECG configuration

Although changes in the configuration of the ECG, in particular, the T wave have been used to predict perform-

ance or organic heart disease, caution must be used in the interpretation of some deviations. Some of the components may have a different appearance from that expected, depending on changes in autonomic nervous system tone, with the most notable changes occurring in the T wave. During strenuous exercise the ECG becomes more difficult to critically evaluate because of high heart rates and motion artifacts. There are several changes that occur in the ECG during exercise. The T wave will often change polarity during exercise, from biphasic or negative to positive, with an increase in amplitude, if a modified base-apex lead system is used. The T wave may remain positive for some time after exercise has ended and the heart rate decreases, before returning to a resting configuration. The amplitude of the QRS may increase and be variable during exercise, and depending on the positioning of the electrodes, there may be motion-related artifacts. The P–R and Q–T intervals will shorten as the heart rate increases, however there will be little change in the QRS duration. The P wave will often become difficult to discern with increasing heart rates, as it can become buried in the preceding T wave. However, the R–R interval should always remain absolutely regular, and the polarity of the QRS should remain the same.

Dysrhythmias associated with exercise

Monitoring for the presence of dysrhythmias is the most important benefit of performing an exercising ECG. Continuous monitoring of the heart rhythm during exercise is vital to the diagnosis of dysrhythmias that may impact performance, or potentially even result in collapse or death. (AF) Paroxysmal atrial fibrillation (PAF) is an important cause of poor performance;[5–7] however, it can be difficult to document because horses often convert to sinus rhythm before it is possible to complete a detailed electrocardiographic examination.[6,8] Therefore, it may be difficult to confirm PAF in those horses in which an irregularly irregular rhythm is auscultated after fading or stopping in a race, unless an ECG is obtained at that time. However, the presence of frequent supraventricular premature depolarizations (SVPD) in a 24-hour period might support a tentative diagnosis of PAF in these situations. If numerous ventricular premature depolarizations (VPD) are observed in a 24-hour period, shortly after an exercise-associated dysrhythmia is auscultated, this may suggest that the dysrhythmia could have been ventricular in origin. (AF)

Horses have a high prevalence of dysrhythmias at rest that are vagally mediated and disappear with exercise. They may also have occasional premature depolarizations at rest; however, if they are infrequent, isolated and disappear with exercise they are unlikely to be of consequence (see Figs. 10.1 and 10.2). Conversely, horses may have a

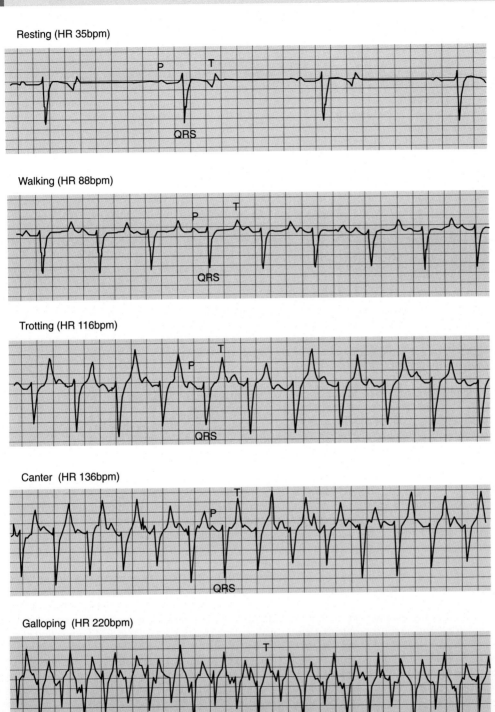

Resting (HR 35bpm)

Walking (HR 88bpm)

Trotting (HR 116bpm)

Canter (HR 136bpm)

Galloping (HR 220bpm)

Figure 11.2 Continuous base-apex ECG of a horse exercising at various speeds on a high-speed treadmill. This shows the normal heart rate response to exercise and the appearance of the ECG. The resting ECG shows a bifid P wave and a bidirectional T wave. As the heart rate and sympathetic tone increase, the T wave becomes positive and increases in amplitude. Also, as the heart rate increases maximally, the P waves become more difficult to distinguish from the preceding T wave. However, the R–R interval remains regular, and the configuration of the R waves remain similar.

Table 11.1 Prevalence of cardiac arrhythmias as detected using ambulatory recordings around exercise in normal race horses (n = 99) and in racehorses presented for assessment of poor performance (n = 88)

	PREVALENCE IN NORMAL RACE HORSES (%)[9]			PREVALENCE IN HORSES PRESENTED WITH POOR PERFORMANCE (%)[11]
Relationship to exercise	Before	During	After	At least one exercise period
Physiological bradyarrhythmias	55	0	30	NR
Supraventricular premature depolarizations	10 (1–37)	0	7 (1–2)	36 (1–9)
Ventricular premature depolarizations	12 (1–33)	3 (1–2)	8 (1–19)	43 (1–30)

Numbers in brackets represent range of abnormal depolarizations seen in different horses.

NR, not recorded.

normal sinus rhythm at rest; however, this does not preclude them from developing dysrhythmias during peak exercise. That may impact performance. Cardiac dysrhythmias may be present before, during and after exercise in horses with no underlying cardiac disease and their interpretation can be difficult. A recent study examined the occurrence of dysrhythmias during warm-up, exercise and in the immediate post-exercise period in clinically healthy horses performing up to expectations[9]. In this study, isolated SVPD and VPD prior to exercise were a relatively common occurrence in these clinically normal horses. The etiology of these premature beats was unknown, although may relate to psychological factors. As many as 33 SVPD and 37 VPD were reported during that time period[9]. (Table 11.1).

Cardiac dysrhythmias were found to be the most common cardiac abnormality diagnosed in horses presented for poor performance by one group.[10] This study showed that almost 30% of horses presented for poor performance had dysrhythmias detected during exercise or in the immediate post-exercise period. Although many of these were determined to be clinically insignificant because they occurred in the immediate post-exercise period, about 10% had exercising dysrhythmias deemed significant, and a likely contributing factor to poor performance. Dysrhythmias were determined to be clinically significant if more than two premature depolarizations occurred during peak exercise. These ranged from SVPD or VPD to episodes of ventricular tachycardia during peak exercise (Fig. 11.3). The study evaluating the occurrence of dysrhythmias in normal horses supported these guidelines, as only 3 out of 101 horses had premature depolarizations during maximal exercise, and none of them had more than two isolated premature depolarizations during maximal exercise.[9] Ventricular and supraventricular ectopy was common in a group of horses that were presented for

investigation of poor performance (see Table 11.1).[11] In this study[11], 55 of 88 horses had at least one premature beat, either before, during or after the exercise test, with 22 horses meeting the criteria for clinical significance determined by Martin et al[10]. However only 2 horses had clinically significant dysrhythmias during exercise, with the majority occurring in the immediate post-exercise period. (AF)

Premature depolarizations occurring during peak exercise or cardiovascular demand and at maximal heart rates can dramatically reduce cardiac output because of a decrease in ventricular filling and stroke volume. This can result in slowing of the horse during a race, fatigue and poor finishing ability. Depending on the severity of the dysrhythmia, collapse or even sudden death may result. Sudden death may occur if an unstable ventricular arrhythmia results in ventricular fibrillation.[12] The cause of these dysrhythmias is not always determined; however, they have been linked to hypoxemia, ischemia, electrolyte disorders, metabolic disorders or pre-existing cardiac disease such as myocarditis. Ventricular ectopy has also been observed at exercise in horses with aortic valve disease. Although these are generally isolated their occurrence during exercise suggests concurrent underlying myocardial disease.

When an exercise-associated dysrhythmia is documented, it is very important to perform a complete evaluation of other body systems in these horses to try to determine an etiology, or to document multifactorial problems. Dynamic upper airway evaluation with endoscopy and analysis of arterial blood gases and electrolyte status during exercise should be done to determine an etiology or assess the presence of other problems. In addition, echocardiography, a 24-hour ambulatory (Holter) ECG and evaluation of cardiac troponin I (cTnI) concentrations should be performed to try to pinpoint a primary

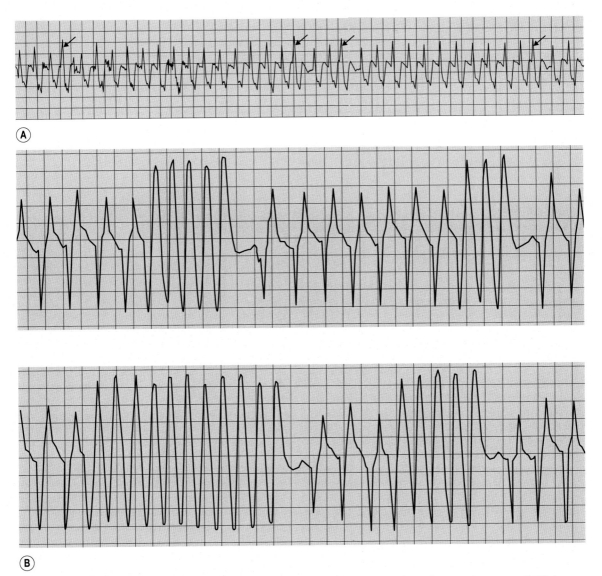

Figure 11.3 (**A**) Frequent ventricular premature depolarizations (four) occurring at peak exercise at a heart rate of 220 bpm. The ventricular premature depolarizations are occurring earlier than normal and are followed by a compensatory pause, but appear similar in orientation to the normally conducted sinus beats and are probably originating from an area in the ventricle near the specialized conduction system. Base-apex ECG, 25 mm/second paper speed. (**B**) Runs of ventricular tachycardia near peak exercise in a stallion with a history of poor performance. Notice the paroxysms of ventricular tachycardia with widened QRS and T wave complexes and a nearly sine wave pattern to the wide QRS tachycardia. This rapid wide ventricular tachycardia with a rate of nearly 300 bpm could potentially degenerate into a fatal ventricular arrhythmia. The underlying sinus rate is approximately 180 bpm. Modified base-apex lead, 25 mm/second paper speed.

cardiac disorder. These horses should not be kept in training while dysrhythmias are present, as they are unlikely to disappear without adequate rest, and the horse is unlikely to perform well while dysrhythmias are present. Because ventricular dysrhythmias may deteriorate during exercise, horses with isolated ventricular premature depolarizations at maximal exercise, not induced by respiratory tract disorders, are generally considered unsafe to ride. Although these may resolve with rest, if persistent then retirement from ridden exercise may be recommended. Most episodes of ventricular and supraventricular ectopy are not life threatening and have minimal impact on perform-

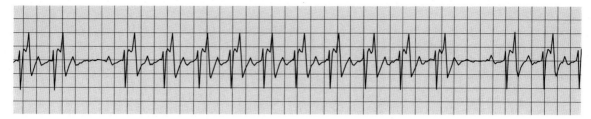

Figure 11.4 Second-degree AV block following high-intensity exercise at a heart rate of 120 bpm. Notice the two periods of second-degree AV block with a P wave, not followed by a QRS complex. All QRS complexes present are preceded by a P wave at a normal P–R interval. The P–P interval is fairly regular, as is the R–R interval, except for the periods of second-degree AV block. Modified base-apex lead, 25 mm/second paper speed.

ance. However, the goal of interpretation of these findings is to identify those animals at risk of developing more significant dysrhythmias that may lead to collapse or even sudden cardiac death.[12] (AR)

Dysrhythmias after exercise

Normal horses frequently develop dysrhythmias in the postexercise period.[9] Many of these dysrhythmias are considered to be normal, and most likely to be caused by rapidly changing autonomic nervous system control.[13] At this time, sympathetic input is decreasing rapidly, and vagal tone is becoming more prominent. This can lead to dysrhythmias such as second-degree atrioventricular block and sinus arrhythmias, pauses or block at relatively high heart rates (Fig. 11.4). These will typically disappear as the heart rate slows further. (SFP) SVPD and VPD may also occur immediately following exercise (see Table 11.1, Fig. 11.5). These are not likely to cause a problem, and are considered normal, if they are fairly infrequent and isolated.[9,14] Up to 20 isolated SVPD or VPD were observed in the first 2 minutes after pulling up from strenous exercise in one group of apparently healthy young Thoroughbreds.[9] Conversely, very frequent or multiform VPD or runs of ventricular tachycardia immediately after exercise are not considered to be normal (Fig. 11.6); nevertheless, their significance can be very difficult to determine if they do not occur during peak exercise. However, they could lead to prolonged recovery after work, weakness or ataxia. It is also possible that the exercise test did not adequately mimic racing conditions, and that these dysrhythmias may be more severe under natural circumstances. Thus, as in horses with dysrhythmias during peak exercise, horses with numerous premature depolarizations following exercise should also be subject to detailed cardiological investigations including echocardiography, cTnI concentrations and a 24-hour ambulatory (Holter) ECG to try to document or eliminate a cardiac problem. Complete evaluations of other body systems such as upper airway endoscopy and arterial blood gases during exercise is also warranted to assess the potential contribution of noncardiac disease.

ECHOCARDIOGRAPHY

The value of echocardiography to assess cardiac chamber size and valvular and myocardial function at rest is undisputed.[15,16] Horses with significant abnormalities at rest generally do not make successful athletes. While dysrhythmias are probably the most common cardiac cause of poor performance, myocarditis, congenital abnormalities and some valvular diseases can affect performance. Horses may not have obvious structural or functional deficits at rest, but still have exercise-induced abnormalities. As with upper airway function, gas exchange and heart rhythm, normal cardiac structure and function at rest may not exclude abnormalities induced by strenuous exercise, under maximal demands. Horses that appear normal at rest may have exercise-induced wall motion abnormalities that are seen only after high-intensity exercise, and a standardized, rigorous treadmill test including postexercise echocardiography is needed for their recognition.

Exercise stress echocardiography (SE)

Cardiac stress testing has been employed in people for many years to help recognize abnormalities that are not seen at rest, but that are induced by increased cardiovascular demands.[17–21] In human beings, exercise stress echocardiography utilizing treadmills or stationary bicycles is most common. It is primarily used to diagnose coronary artery disease and ischaemic events; however, it has also been used to determine exercise capabilities and assess valvular and left ventricular function during exercise in patients with various other cardiac diseases, such as valvular diseases and cardiomyopathy.[22–26] Left ventricular inward wall motion and endocardial thickening in standardized views are evaluated at rest, and then compared with the same views obtained during the exercise or immediate post-exercise examination. The computer program digitizes these images and displays them adjacent to one another, in a continuous loop format, at matching heart

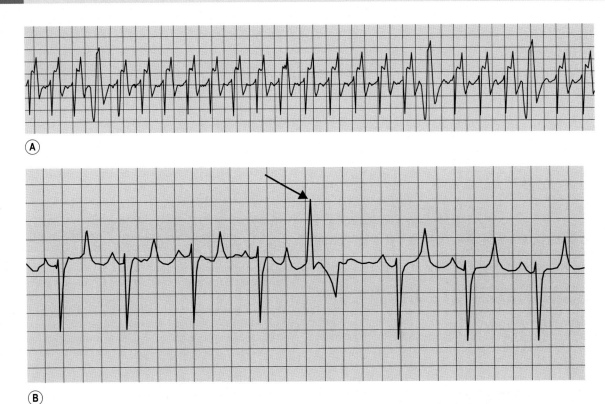

Figure 11.5 (A) Occasional ventricular premature depolarizations in the immediate post-exercise period at a heart rate of 160 bpm. Notice the three premature depolarizations that appear somewhat widened and bizarre when compared to the normal sinus beats and which are followed by a compensatory pause. The underlying sinus rhythm is otherwise regular. Modified base-apex lead, 25 mm/second paper speed. **(B)** One single ventricular premature depolarization in the post-exercise period at a heart rate of 80 bpm (arrow). Notice the slightly premature depolarization that is opposite in direction to the normal sinus beats, and that is followed by a slight, compensatory pause. Modified base-apex lead, 25 mm/second paper speed.

rates. Segments are graded for inward wall motion and thickening. If this is decreased post-exercise, the specific segments are described as hypokinetic, akinetic or dyskinetic, and given a score. Stress echocardiography has been found to have high sensitivity and specificity for the diagnosis of coronary artery disease.

Postexercise stress echocardiography has been adapted from human medicine for use in horses performing a standardized exercise test on a high-speed treadmill, to recognize exercise-induced myocardial dysfunction.[27] For stress echocardiography in horses, four standardized views of the left ventricle are obtained, maximizing visualization of the ventricular myocardium. These are obtained pre- and immediately post-exercise, and displayed side-by-side at matching heart rates, as in human medicine, for comparison of wall motion and thickening. Because echocardiography cannot currently be performed during exercise in horses, examinations are limited to the immediate post-exercise time. Myocardial contractility should increase with exercise (or increased sympathetic stimulation), causing an increase in fractional shortening, and an

increase in free wall and interventricular septal thickness during systole. This increased contractility will persist into the immediate post-exercise period, while the heart rate is still very elevated.[13] Studies in horses exercising at speeds eliciting maximal oxygen consumption on a high-speed treadmill have shown that invasive estimates of contractility calculated within the first 30 seconds are representative of exercising values, but by 2 minutes have decreased significantly compared with exercising values.[28,29] Therefore, it is critical to perform the echocardiogram as soon after treadmill exercise as possible, preferably within 1 minute. As the heart rate decreases below 100 bpm, fractional shortening and wall motion indices will decrease, and return to baseline values. If thickening of the ventricular free wall or septum during systole is decreased immediately post-exercise compared with pre-exercise, while the heart rate remains greater than 100 bpm, it is highly suggestive of exercise-induced myocardial dysfunction. Some of these horses may have exercising ventricular premature depolarizations, but more commonly no other cardiac abnormalities are seen. A complete workup, including

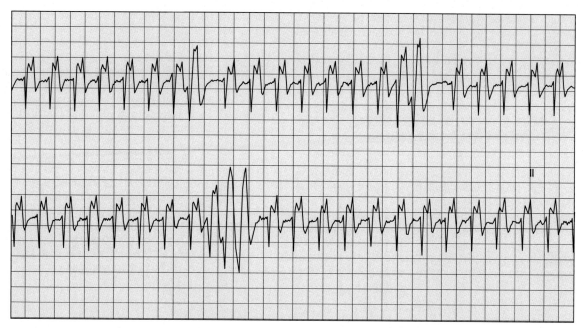

Figure 11.6 Frequent ventricular premature depolarizations in the immediate post-exercise period in a horse with a sinus tachycardia and a rate of 160 bpm. Notice the ventricular premature depolarizations that appear widened and bizarre and are occurring earlier than normal and are followed by a compensatory pause. Modified base-apex lead, 25 mm/second paper speed.

exercising upper respiratory tract endoscopy, exercising arterial blood gas determinations and measurement of cTnI should be performed, to try to separate a primary cardiac problem from a secondary one. The aetiology of exercise-induced ventricular dysfunction is unknown, but possible causes may be related to hypoxaemia, ischaemia or primary myocardial disease.

Pharmacological stress echocardiography

Other forms of cardiac stress testing have been used in people who are physically incapable of exercising adequately. Pharmaceutical agents such as dobutamine, dobutamine and a parasympatholytic agent, or adenosine have been employed to mimic exercise.[30-34] Studies have shown that the results using these drugs are similar in sensitivity and specificity to exercise in diagnosing coronary artery disease. Recently, pharmacological stress echocardiography has been evaluated in horses.[35-37] High-dose dobutamine alone is not recommended as a pharmacological stressor, due to safety problems in healthy horses; however, the combination of a parasympatholytic agent with a lower dose of dobutamine has also been evaluated, and deserves further study. Advantages to pharmacological stress testing are a potentially prolonged time to perform more detailed echocardiographic examinations, and somewhat easier working conditions than pos-

sible during immediate post-exercise echocardiography. In addition, not all hospitals have access to a high-speed treadmill, and some horses cannot or will not perform an adequate exercise test, due to musculoskeletal problems or lack of mental aptitude, making this a possible substitute. Disadvantages would include the inability to monitor and test other body systems, such as the musculoskeletal and respiratory systems. These are more commonly the cause of poor performance, and so abnormalities in these systems should always be ruled out. Many performance problems are multifactorial, so that even if a cardiac cause is confirmed, it is important to investigate other body systems. In addition, rhythm disturbances are the most commonly recognized cardiac cause of poor performance. The pharmacological agents used for these protocols have the potential to cause dysrhythmias. Therefore, if dysrhythmias are observed during a pharmacological stress test, they could be drug-related, rather than exercise-induced. Their presence would need to be confirmed with an exercise test. Conversely, it is not known if these agents would mimic the effects of exercise in those horses that develop exercise-induced dysrhythmias.

Evaluation of pharmacological stress testing is still in the early stages in horses. At this time, it is not clear if pharmacological stress testing mimics exercise closely enough to be useful, or if it is capable of unmasking exercise-induced problems, as it does in people. Its use has only been reported in healthy horses, so its effects in horses with cardiac disease are unknown. However, if it is found to induce changes similar to exercise, it would potentially allow longer and more detailed studies of myocardial and valvular dysfunction under conditions mimicking exercise, or effects of higher heart rates on shunts such as ventricular septal defect.

CARDIAC OUTPUT AND DIRECT PRESSURE MEASUREMENTS

Future additions to exercise stress testing to monitor cardiac function include slightly more invasive approaches. Measurement of cardiac output, which is perhaps the best indicator of global cardiac function, is currently only performed in research settings. The main reason for this is the invasive nature of instrumentation for determination of cardiac output using the Fick method of calculating cardiac output. However, adaptation of lithium dilution cardiac output (LIDCO) measurements to horses during exercise may be possible, and is considerably less invasive than the Fick method. For this method, the primary requirements are a jugular venous catheter and a peripheral artery catheter, which many horses instrumented for treadmill tests already have in place. LIDCO has recently been validated during exercise, although it may be less accurate than the Fick method, and has limitations such as the number of repetitive measurements that can be performed, it has promise to be useful to obtain an estimate of cardiac output in horses during exercise.[38]

Measurements of arterial and pulmonary arterial pressures in horses during exercise can also be performed; however, this does require sophisticated equipment that may not be available, and, in the case of pulmonary arterial pressure measurement, is considered more invasive. However, these indices can sometimes give important information regarding cardiovascular function under the stress of exercise, in the face of normal values at rest.

REFERENCES

1. Fregin GF. The equine electrocardiogram with standardized body and limb positions. Cornell Vet 1982;72(3): 304–324.

2. Fregin GF. Electrocardiography. Vet Clin North Am: Equine Pract 1985;1(2):419–432.

3. Holmes JR, Alps BJ, Darke PGG. A method of radiotelemetry in equine electrocardiography. Vet 1966;79:90–94.

4. Senta T, Smetzer DL, Smith CR. Effects of exercise on certain electrocardiographic parameters and cardiac arrhythmias in the horse: a radiotelemetric study. Cornell Vet 1970;60(4):552–569.

5. Ohmura H, Hiraga A, Takahashi T, et al. Risk factors for atrial fibrillation during racing in slow-finishing horses. J Am Vet Med Assoc 2003;223(1):84–88.

6. Holmes JR. Cardiac arrhythmias on the racecourse. In: Gillespie J, Robinson N, editors. Equine Exercise Physiology 2. Davis, CA: ICEEP Publications; 1987, p. 781–785.

7. Amada A, Kurita H. Five cases of paroxysmal atrial fibrillation in the racehorse. Exp Rep Equine Health Lab 1975;12:89–100.

8. Holmes JR. Paroxysmal atrial fibrillation in racehorses. Equine Vet J 1986;18(1):37–42.

9. Ryan N, Marr CM, McGladdery AJ. Survey of cardiac arrhythmias during submaximal and maximal exercise in Thoroughbred racehorses. Equine Vet J 2005;37(3):265–268.

10. Kiryu K, Machida N, Kashida Y, et al. Pathologic and electrocardiographic findings in sudden cardiac death in racehorses. J Vet Med Sci 1999;61(8):921–928.

11. Martin BB Jr, Reef VB, Parente EJ, et al. Causes of poor performance of horses during training, racing, or showing: 348 cases (1992–1996). J Am Vet Med Assoc 2000;216(4): 554–558.

12. Jose-Cunilleras E, Young LE, Newton JR, et al. Cardiac arrhythmias during and after treadmill exercise in poorly performing thoroughbred racehorses. Equine Vet J Suppl 2006;36:163–170.

13. Reef VB, Maxson AD, Lewis M. Echocardiographic and ECG changes in horses following exercise. Paper presented at Proceedings of the 12th Anual Convention of the American College of Veterinary Internal Medicine, San Francisco, CA, 1994:256–258.

14. Senta T, Smetzer DL, Smith CR. Effects of exercise on certain electrocardiographic parameters and cardiac arrhythmias in the horse.:a radiotelemetric study. Cornell Vet 1970;60(4):552–569.

15. Reef VB, Whittier M, Allam LG. Echocardiography. (Special issue: Ultrasonography). Clin Tech Equine Pract 2004;3(3):274–283.

16. Reef VB. Heart murmurs in horses: determining their significance with echocardiography. Equine Vet J Suppl 1995;19:71–80.

17. Ryan T, Feigenbaum H. Exercise echocardiography. Am J Cardiol 1992;69(20):82H–89H.

18. Armstrong WF. Treadmill exercise echocardiography: methodology and clinical role. Eur Heart J 1997;18(Suppl D):D2–D8.

19. Marwick TH. Application of stress echocardiography to the evaluation of non-coronary heart disease. Eur J Echocardiogr 2000;1(3): 171–179.

20. Armstrong WF. Stress echocardiography: introduction, history, and methods. Progr Cardiovasc Dis 1997;39(6): 499–522.

21. Marwick T. Current status of stress echocardiography in the diagnosis of coronary artery disease. Cleveland Clin J Med 1995;62(4): 227–234.

22. Wu W-C, Aziz GF, Sadaniantz A. The use of stress echocardiography in the assessment of mitral valvular disease. Echocardiography 2004;21(5):451–458.

23. Pierard LA, Hoffer EP. Role of stress echocardiography in heart failure. Am J Cardiol 1998;81(12A):111G–114G.

24. Wu W-C, Bhavsar JH, Aziz GF, et al. An overview of stress echocardiography in the study of patients with dilated or hypertrophic cardiomyopathy. Echocardiography 2004;21(5): 467–475.

25. Wu W-C, Ireland LA, Sadaniantz A. Evaluation of aortic valve disorders using stress echocardiography. Echocardiography 2004;21(5): 459–466.

26. Decena BF 3rd, Tischler MD. Stress echocardiography in valvular heart disease. Cardiol Clin 1999;17(3): 555–572.

27. Reef VB. Stress echocardiography and its role in performance assessment. Vet Clin North Am: Equine Pract 2001;17(1):179–189.

28. Durando MM, Reef VB, Birks EK. Correlation of echocardiographic stress tests with left ventricular pressure dynamics. J Vet Intern Med 2001;19:851.

29. Durando MM, Reef VB, Birks EK. Right ventricular pressure dynamics during exercise: relationship to stress echocardiography. Equine Vet J Suppl 2002;34:472–477.

30. Ostojic M, Picano E, Beleslin B, et al. Dipyridamole-dobutamine echocardiography: a novel test for the detection of milder forms of coronary artery disease. J Am College Cardiol 1994;23(5): 1115–1122.

31. Beleslin BD, Ostojic M, Stepanovic J, et al. Stress echocardiography in the detection of myocardial ischemia: head-to-head comparison of exercise, dobutamine, and dipyridamole tests. Circulation 1994;90(3):1168–1176.

32. Sharp SM, Sawada SG, Segar DS, et al. Dobutamine stress echocardiography: detection of coronary artery disease in patients with dilated cardiomyopathy. J Am College Cardiol 1994;24(4):934–939.

33. Geleijnse ML, Vigna C, Kasprzak JD, et al. Usefulness and limitations of dobutamine-atropine stress echocardiography for the diagnosis of coronary artery disease in patients with left bundle branch block: a multicentre study. Eur Heart J 2000;21(20):1666–1673.

34. Kosmala W, Spring A. [Comparison of usefulness of dobutamine-atropine and dobutamine-adenosine stress echocardiography in detection of coronary artery disease]. Polski Merkuriusz Lekarski 2004;16(94):313–315.

35. Frye MA, Bright JM, Dargatz DA, et al. A comparison of dobutamine infusion to exercise as a cardiac stress test in healthy horses. J Vet Intern Med 2003;17:58–64.

36. Sandersen CF, Detilleux J, Delguste C, et al. Atropine reduces dobutamine-induced side effects in ponies undergoing a pharmacological stress protocol. Equine Vet J 2005;37(2):128–132.

37. Durando MM, Slack J, Reef VB, Birks EK. Right ventricular pressure dynamics and stress echocardiography in pharmacological and exercise stress testing. Equine Vet J Suppl 2006;36:183–192.

38. Durando MM, Corley KTT, Boston RC, Birks EK. Cardiac output determination by use of lithium dilution during exercise in horses. Am J Vet Research 2008;69:1054–1060.

Chapter | 12 |

Biochemical markers of cardiovascular disease

Celia M Marr

INTRODUCTION

Biochemical markers of cardiovascular disease are important tools in assessing human heart disease. Assays based on natriuretic peptides and biochemical mediators of activation of the sympathetic nervous and renin–angiotensin–aldosterone system can be used for diagnosis, prognosis and treatment monitoring in a range of heart diseases. Measurement of cardiac troponins is the gold-standard for identification of myocardial disease in human beings. While it is extremely tempting to reach for an "off-the-shelf" assay kits developed for use in human beings and apply these to equine patients, this is often not appropriate for a number of reasons. Firstly, immunoassays developed in one species do not necessarily cross-react with the equivalent molecule in another species and it is important that any biochemical assay is either developed specifically for equine use, or if developed for another species, it should have been validated for horses before it is applied in clinical practice. Secondly, the prevalence of the target disorder within the species of interest must be considered. Diagnostic tests are often described in terms of their sensitivity (the proportion of true positives) and specificity (the proportion of true negatives). These can be regarded as inherent characteristics of the test; however, from a clinical perspective, it is much more relevant to know a test's predictive value or how likely it is that the test will give a correct diagnosis of whether the tested animal is diseased or disease free.[1] The predictive value is not only influenced by the accuracy of the test but also by the prevalence of disease within a given population and predictive values decrease as prevalence decreases. This issue is particularly relevant to biomarkers of cardiovascular disease in horses because disease states that are common in human beings such as heart failure and myocardial necrosis are extremely uncommon in horses. Consequently, biomarkers that are extremely important in human beings are not necessarily so useful in horses. A test may be extremely sensitive and specific in detecting a specific form of cardiovascular pathology, but this is not very helpful when the problem faced by the equine clinician is in finding the horse that actually has the pathology in question. Finally, in-depth knowledge of the neuroendocrine changes that accompany heart disease in horses is lacking compared to the wealth of data available in human beings. Nevertheless, research on equine cardiovascular biomarkers is underway and this is an interesting and exciting area of development in equine cardiology.

CATECHOLAMINES

Activation of the sympathetic (adrenergic) nervous system is a hallmark of heart failure[2] (see Chapters 2 and 5). The β_1- and β_2-adrenoreceptors are important regulators of cardiac function and their characteristics change in human and canine cardiac disease. Atypical β-adrenoreceptors (β_3 and β_4) are also found in the cardiovascular system of

DOI: 10.1016/B978-0-7020-2817-5.00017-1

some species. Myocardial tissues from failing human ventricles demonstrate a reduction in β-adrenoreceptor density and contractile response to β-adrenergic agonists. These changes are mediated by increased concentrations of noradrenaline (norepinephrine) in the vicinity of the receptors.[2] There is wide variation in the distribution of cardiac β-adrenoreceptor types among species: in the equine heart the predominant adrenoreceptor is the β_1 subtype and there is also evidence for atypical adrenoreceptors within the heart although these have not been fully characterized.[3] In contrast to human beings, in horses, the density of β-adrenoreceptors did not change in heart failure but, in some cases, heart failure increases the expression of β_2-adrenoreceptors.[3]

One method of documenting the increase of sympathetic outflow is by measurement of plasma catecholamine concentrations and these have been used as prognostic indicators in human congestive cardiac failure.[4,5] Plasma concentrations of noradrenaline are increased in human heart failure and the clinical outcome is related to plasma noradrenaline concentrations.[5] In contrast, plasma concentrations of noradrenaline did not differ among healthy horses and those with aortic insufficiency with and without clinical signs of cardiovascular compromise at rest whereas adrenaline (epinephrine) concentrations were significantly different among healthy horses and those with aortic regurgitation (Fig. 12.1).[6] Although this finding is of interest as it provides evidence on the pathophysiology of equine heart disease, measurement of plasma catecholamines is limited in its usefulness in the clinical setting because there are circadian variations in plasma concentrations and samples must be kept on ice and processed very quickly. Furthermore, the sensitivity and specificity of plasma catecholamines in distinguishing horses with mild and severe and nonprogressive and progressive aortic regurgitation are low.[6]

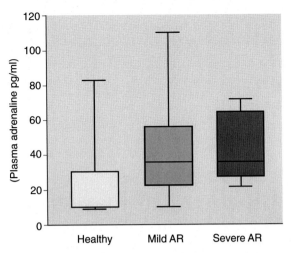

Figure 12.1 Plasma concentrations of adrenaline in healthy horses and those with aortic regurgitation (AR; n = 40) that had no clinical signs at rest (mild AR; n = 59) and those that did (severe AR; n = 9). Plasma adrenaline concentrations are significantly lower in healthy horses compared to those with mild (p < 0.01) and severe (p < 0.05) AR. The box extends from the 25th–75th percentile with a line at the median; the whiskers show the range in the data. Reproduced with permission from Horn JNR (2002, Sympathetic nervous control of cardiac function and its role in equine heart disease, PhD thesis, University of London.)

RENIN–ANGIOTENSIN–ALDOSTERONE SYSTEM

The renin–angiotensin–aldosterone system (RAAS) is activated in low cardiac output states and serves to maintain arterial blood pressure by retaining sodium and water (see Chapters 2 and 5). Angiotensin II is a potent peripheral vasoconstrictor and together with increased adrenergic activity contributes to excessively increased systemic vascular resistance in heart failure. Angiotensin II also enhances release of noradrenaline. Sodium retention, mediated by aldosterone, contributes to oedema formation. Tissue angiotensin and aldosterone also have a key role in cardiovascular remodelling and fibrosis and this leads to reduced vascular compliance and ventricular diastolic dysfunction.[2] Plasma renin activity and plasma aldosterone concentration increase and correlate with

severity in canine dilated cardiomyopathy.[7] There is also early activation of the RAAS in some dogs with mitral valvular insufficiency[8] whereas other studies have shown that plasma aldosterone and angiotensin II decrease as cardiac decompensation ensues.[9] Studies in horses with valvular insufficiency have shown that plasma aldosterone concentrations rise as the severity of valvular disease increases with significant differences detected between healthy horses and those with left ventricular and atrial dilation.[10] In contrast, another equine study showed no activation of the RAAS in horses with aortic insufficiency (n = 25) compared to healthy horses (I. M. Bowen, C. M. Marr, J. Elliott, unpublished data).

NATRIURETIC PEPTIDES

There are three natriuretic peptides: atrial natriuretic peptide (ANP), brain natriuretic peptide (BNP) and C-type natriuretic peptide (CNP). ANP is stored mainly in the right atrium and is released in response to increased atrial pressure (see Chapter 2). ANP causes vasodilation and sodium excretion and thus counteracts the effects of the adrenergic system, RAAS and arginine vasopressin. BNP is stored mainly in the ventricles and is released in response to increased ventricular pressure. BNP has similar effects to ANP. CNP is located in the vasculature and its physiological role remains to be clearly defined.[2] Plasma concentrations of ANP, BNP and their pro-hormones are increased in human heart failure. Because plasma BNP release is less affected by atrial filling pressures, it provides a better indication of myocardial disease than ANP and is regarded as a quantitative marker for heart failure.[11] BNP is a cost-effective screening tool for left ventricular systolic dysfunction[12] and plasma BNP concentrations independently predicted nonsurvival in a large prospective study on left ventricular dysfunction conducted over 4 years in people who were asymptomatic upon entry to the study.[13] BNP is also increased in dogs with congestive heart failure,[14] mitral valve disease,[15] aortic stenosis[16] and subclinical dilated cardiomyopathy.[17] As is the case in human heart disease, BNP has better predictive value than ANP in dogs[17] although ANP has thus far received most attention in veterinary medicine and it has been shown in a large number of studies to increase in canine heart disease.[9,14,18,19]

In horses, plasma ANP concentration rises during exercise[20-23] and is higher in old exercising horses compared to young horses.[24] Plasma ANP concentrations are increased with hypovolaemia and fall in response to fluid resuscitation in both foals and mature horses.[25] To date, there is only one study on the effects of equine heart disease on plasma ANP in which it was not possible to demonstrate any difference between healthy horses and those with heart disease[26] and further work in this area of equine cardiology is needed. ANP is well conserved across species and thus assays developed for use in other species can be used in the horse.[27] Unfortunately, BNP, the more useful test in human patients, is not well conserved across species and commercial assays developed for human use do not identify equine BNP.[28]

CARDIAC TROPONIN, CREATINE KINASE AND LACTATE DEHYDROGENASE (AF, PC, VT)

In the past the cardiac isoenzymes of creatine kinase (CK-MB) and lactate dehydrogenase (HBDH, isoenzymes 1 and 2) were used as biomarkers of myocardial disease.[29] However, these assays have now been superseded in human cardiology in favour of cardiac troponins. Troponin is a complex of three proteins to which calcium binds to regulate muscle contraction. It has three subunits: troponin C (TnC) binds to calcium ions to produce a conformational change in troponin I (TnI), troponin T (TnT) binds to tropomyosin and troponin I binds to actin to hold the troponin–tropomyosin complex in place. Cardiac troponins are released into the circulation with myocardial injury[30] and cardiac TnI (cTnI) remains in the circulation for longer than other sub-units and thus is the most clinically applicable assay.[31,32] Cardiac troponin I is highly conserved across species and assay cross-reactivity has been demonstrated in the horse and, thus, commercially available assays can be used in equine cardiology.[31,32] At rest, both horses at pasture and those in race-training have low concentrations of cTnI[33] but mild increases can be expected in response to endurance racing,[34] treadmill exercise[35] and racing.[36] The clinical significance of this is uncertain but it must be borne in mind when interpreting cTnI results from clinical patients. Increases in cTnI have been reported in horses with idiopathic myocardial disease[37] and myocardial injury due to a ruptured aortic regurgitation jet lesion,[38] myocardial necrosis[39] and piroplasmosis,[40] demonstrating the usefulness of this biomarker in equine myocardial disease. Plasma cTnI concentrations were significantly higher in septic foals compared to healthy neonates but did not correlate with survival.[41] The test must be interpreted with caution as myocardial disease is not the only cause of increased cTnI and increases can also be expected in renal disease, pulmonary embolism[42] and in endotoxaemia.[43] Also, because myocardial injury is relatively uncommon in horses, it is important to consider the impact of disease prevalence on predictive values when positive results, particularly modest increases, are obtained with cTnI assays.[1]

REFERENCES

1. Petrie A, Watson P. Statistics for Veterinary and Animal Science. Oxford: Blackwell Publishing; 1999.
2. Colucci W, Braunwald E. Pathophysiology of heart failure. In: Zipes DP, Libby P, Bonow RO, Braunwald E, editor. Braunwald's Heart Disease: A textbook of Cardiovascular Medicine. Philadelphia: Elsevier Saunders; 2005, p. 509–538.
3. Horn J, Bailey S, Berhane Y, et al. Density and binding characteristics of beta-adrenoceptors in the normal and failing equine myocardium. Equine Vet J 2002;34(4):411–416.

4. Cohn JN, Levine TB, Olivari MT, et al. Plasma norepinephrine as a guide to prognosis in patients with chronic congestive heart failure. N Engl J Med 1984;311(13): 819–823.

5. Esler M, Kaye D, Lambert G, et al. Adrenergic nervous system in heart failure. Am J Cardiol 1997;80(11A):7L–14L.

6. Horn J. Sympathetic Nervous Control of Cardiac Function and its Role in Equine Heart Disease. PhD thesis, Royal Veterinary College, University of London, 2002.

7. Koch J, Pedersen HD, Jensen AL, et al. Activation of the renin-angiotensin system in dogs with asymptomatic and symptomatic dilated cardiomyopathy. Res Vet Sci 1995;59(2):172–175.

8. Pedersen HD, Koch J, Poulsen K, et al. Activation of the renin-angiotensin system in dogs with asymptomatic and mildly symptomatic mitral valvular insufficiency. J Vet Intern Med 1995;9(5):328–331.

9. Haggstrom J, Hansson K, Kvart C, et al. Effects of naturally acquired decompensated mitral valve regurgitation on the renin-angiotensin-aldosterone system and atrial natriuretic peptide concentration in dogs. Am J Vet Res 1997;58(1):77–82.

10. Gehlen H, Sundermann T, Rohn K, et al. Aldosterone plasma concentration in horses with heart valve insufficiencies. Res Vet Sci 2008;85(2):340–344.

11. Maurellet JD, Liu PT. B-type natriuretic peptide in the management of heart failure. Hong Kong Med J 2008;14(3):216–219.

12. Nielsen OW, McDonagh TA, Robb SD, et al. Retrospective analysis of the cost-effectiveness of using plasma brain natriuretic peptide in screening for left ventricular systolic dysfunction in the general population. J Am Coll Cardiol 2003;41(1):113–120.

13. McDonagh TA, Cunningham AD, Morrison CE, et al. Left ventricular dysfunction, natriuretic peptides, and mortality in an urban population. Heart 2001;86(1): 21–26.

14. Asano K, Masuda K, Okumura M, et al. Plasma atrial and brain natriuretic peptide levels in dogs with congestive heart failure. J Vet Med Sci 1999;61(5):523–529.

15. Tarnow I, Olsen LH, Kvart C, et al. Predictive value of natriuretic peptides in dogs with mitral valve disease. Vet J 2009;180(2): 195–201.

16. Hori Y, Tsubaki M, Katou A, et al. Evaluation of NT-pro BNP and CT-ANP as markers of concentric hypertrophy in dogs with a model of compensated aortic stenosis. J Vet Intern Med 2008;22(5): 1118–1123.

17. Oyama MA, Sisson DD, Solter PF. Prospective screening for occult cardiomyopathy in dogs by measurement of plasma atrial natriuretic peptide, B-type natriuretic peptide, and cardiac troponin-I concentrations. Am J Vet Res 2007;68(1):42–47.

18. Haggstrom J, Hansson K, Karlberg BE, et al. Plasma concentration of atrial natriuretic peptide in relation to severity of mitral regurgitation in Cavalier King Charles Spaniels. Am J Vet Res 1994;55(5):698–703.

19. Haggstrom J, Hansson K, Kvart C, et al. Relationship between different natriuretic peptides and severity of naturally acquired mitral regurgitation in dogs with chronic myxomatous valve disease. J Vet Cardiol 2000;2(1):7–16.

20. Kokkonen UM, Hackzell M, Rasanen LA. Plasma atrial natriuretic peptide in standardbred and Finnhorse trotters during and after exercise. Acta Physiol Scand 1995;154(1):51–58.

21. Kokkonen UM, Hyyppa S, Poso AR. Plasma atrial natriuretic peptide during and after repeated exercise under heat exposure. Equine Vet J Suppl 1999;30: 184–189.

22. Kokkonen UM, Poso AR, Hyyppa S, et al. Exercise-induced changes in atrial peptides in relation to neuroendocrine responses and fluid balance in the horse. J Vet Med A Physiol Pathol Clin Med 2002;49(3):144–150.

23. Nyman S, Kokkonen UM, Dahlborn K. Changes in plasma atrial natriuretic peptide concentration in exercising horses in relation to hydration status and exercise intensity. Am J Vet Res 1998;59(4):489–494.

24. McKeever KH, Malinowski K. Endocrine response to exercise in young and old horses. Equine Vet J Suppl 1999;30:561–566.

25. Hollis AR, Boston RC, Corley KT. Plasma aldosterone, vasopressin and atrial natriuretic peptide in hypovolaemia: a preliminary comparative study of neonatal and mature horses. Equine Vet J 2008;40(1):64–69.

26. Gehlen H, Sundermann T, Rohn K, et al. Plasma atrial natriuretic peptide concentration in warmblood horses with heart valve regurgitations. J Vet Cardiol 2007;9(2):99–101.

27. Richter R, Magert H, Mifune H, et al. Equine cardiodilatin/atrial natriuretic peptide: primary structure and immunohistochemical localization in auricular cardiocytes. Acta Anat (Basel) 1998;162(4): 185–193.

28. Mifune H, Richter R, Forssmann WG. Detection of immunoreactive atrial and brain natriuretic peptides in the equine atrium. Anat Embryol (Berl) 1995;192(2): 117–121.

29. Reef VB, Bain FT, Spencer PA. Severe mitral regurgitation in horses: clinical, echocardiographic and pathological findings. Equine Vet J 1998;30(1):18–27.

30. Peacock WFT, De Marco T, Fonarow GC, et al. Cardiac troponin and outcome in acute heart failure. N Engl J Med 2008;358(20): 2117–2126.

31. O'Brien PJ, Dameron GW, Beck ML, et al. Differential reactivity of cardiac and skeletal muscle from various species in two generations of cardiac troponin-T immunoassays. Res Vet Sci 1998;65(2):135–137.

32. O'Brien PJ, Landt Y, Ladenson JH. Differential reactivity of cardiac and skeletal muscle from various species in a cardiac troponin I immunoassay. Clin Chem 1997;43(12): 2333–2338.

33. Phillips W, Giguere S, Franklin RP, et al. Cardiac troponin I in

pastured and race-training Thoroughbred horses. J Vet Intern Med 2003;17(4):597–599.

34. Holbrook TC, Birks EK, Sleeper MM, et al. Endurance exercise is associated with increased plasma cardiac troponin I in horses. Equine Vet J Suppl 2006;36:27–31.

35. Durando M, Reef VB, Kine K, Birks EK. Acute effects of short duration maximal exercise on cardiac troponin I in healthy horses. Equine Comp Exerc Physiol 2006;4:217–223.

36. Nostell K, Haggstrom J. Resting concentrations of cardiac troponin I in fit horses and effect of racing. J Vet Cardiol 2008;10(2):105–109.

37. Johnson A, Jesty SA, Gelzer ARM, Divers TJ, Kraus MS. ECG of the

month. J Am Vet Med Assoc 2007;231:706–708.

38. Cornelisse CJ, Schott HC 2nd, Olivier NB, et al. Concentration of cardiac troponin I in a horse with a ruptured aortic regurgitation jet lesion and ventricular tachycardia. J Am Vet Med Assoc 2000;217(2): 231–235.

39. Schwarzwald CC, Hardy J, Buccellato M. High cardiac troponin I serum concentration in a horse with multiform ventricular tachycardia and myocardial necrosis. J Vet Intern Med 2003;17(3):364–368.

40. Diana A, Guglielmini C, Candini D, et al. Cardiac arrhythmias associated with piroplasmosis in the horse:

a case report. Vet J 2007;174(1): 193–195.

41. Slack JA, McGuirk SM, Erb HN, et al. Biochemical markers of cardiac injury in normal, surviving septic, or nonsurviving septic neonatal foals. J Vet Intern Med 2005;19(4):577–580.

42. Rosenbaum LS, Januzzi JL. Moving troponin testing into the 21st century: will greater sensitivity be met with greater sensibility? Cardiovasc Hematol Disord Drug Targets 2008;8(2):118–126.

43. Peek SF, Apple FS, Murakami MA, et al. Cardiac isoenzymes in healthy Holstein calves and calves with experimentally induced endotoxemia. Can J Vet Res 2008;72(4):356–361.

Section | 3 |

Clinical problems

Chapter | **13** |

Dysrhythmias: assessment and medical management

Virginia B Reef and Celia M Marr

INTRODUCTION

Cardiac dysrhythmias occur frequently in horses and can be associated with a wide range of cardiac and noncardiac diseases. They can be associated with valvular disease,[1] congenital defects, pericardial disease and primary myocardial pathology,[2] for example, myocarditis,[3] myocardial fibrosis,[4] myocardial ischaemia,[5] cardiomyopathy,[6] ionophore toxicosis,[7-9] myocardial trauma or myocardial neoplasia.[10] However, more commonly, horses develop dysrhythmias in association with hypoxia, metabolic acidosis and electrolyte disturbances,[11,12] alterations in local or circulating catecholamine concentrations and autonomic tone,[13] septicaemia,[14] endotoxaemia,[15,16] or various drugs including some that are used to treat dysrhythmias such as quinidine and digoxin,[17,18] and the reader is referred to Chapter 6 for a detailed description of arrhythmogenesis.

An important diagnostic goal in horses with dysrhythmias is to identify any contributing cardiac or noncardiac disease. Initial therapy should also be aimed at the underlying causes and cardiac dysrhythmias relatively rarely require specific antidysrhythmic therapy.

IDENTIFICATION AND ASSESSMENT OF DYSRHYTHMIAS

To determine if a cardiac dysrhythmia is present, the horse's heart rate should be obtained (normal, slow or fast) and the rhythm characterized (regular, regularly irregular or irregularly irregular). The normal adult horse has a heart rate of 28–44 bpm at rest with a regular (sinus) rhythm. The normal heart rate in foals is as high as 80 bpm (average in the equine neonate is 70 bpm). The heart sounds should be identified and their timing and intensity described. It is particularly pertinent to attempt to distinguish all four heart sounds in horses with dysrhythmias as their presence or absence may alert the clinician to the specific dysrhythmias described below. The arterial pulses should be palpated simultaneously with auscultation of the heart to determine if the arterial pulses are synchronous with every heart beat. The arterial pulse quality should be assessed in the facial or transverse facial artery and in the extremities for variation in the intensity of the pulses or pulse deficits. The jugular vein, saphenous vein and other peripheral veins should be evaluated for distention and pulsations. Auscultation of both lung fields should be performed at rest and, if possible, with the horse breathing into a rebreathing bag.

An ECG must be performed to definitively diagnose any dysrhythmia (see Chapter 6). The normal components of the surface ECG are:

- *P wave:* generated by atrial depolarization
- *PR segment:* representing the duration of atrioventricular (AV) conduction
- *QRS complex:* produced by ventricular depolarization

© 2010 Elsevier Ltd.
DOI: 10.1016/B978-0-7020-2817-5.00018-3

- *ST segment*: representing the duration of the ventricular refractory period
- *T wave*: produced by ventricular repolarization

Thus, the surface ECG provides a "road map" of electrical events within the heart and allows the origin of any abnormalities to be identified. A variety of options for lead placement are available (Table 13.1). However, a base-apex lead is often the only lead needed to accurately diagnose the rhythm disturbance present, because this lead produces large, easy to read complexes and is usually well tolerated by the horse (see Chapter 6). It is conventional to display the base-apex lead with negative QRS complexes; however, some clinicians, particularly in the UK, prefer to invert the leads to produce positive QRS complexes. Either is appropriate and the choice is dictated by personal preference. The base-apex lead is the most con-

venient monitoring lead for critically ill patients, for example, during antidysrhythmic therapy or while performing a pericardiocentesis or other invasive procedure. Occasionally it may be difficult to determine if a rhythm disturbance is of ventricular or supraventricular origin from just one ECG lead, particularly with supraventricular dysrhythmias. In these horses at least two different leads are needed to determine the origin of the abnormal depolarization (see Table 13.1).

Echocardiography is used to identify valvular disease, pericarditis congenital defects and myocardial pathology although a normal echocardiogram does rule out the presence of myocardial disease (see Chapter 9). Assays of serum cardiac troponin I and other biomarkers (see Chapter 12) may also provide evidence of myocardial disease while haematology, blood biochemistry, serum electrolyte and blood gas analysis, and other laboratory

Table 13.1 Electrode placement for complete 12-lead electrocardiogram

Lead 1: LA–RA	Left foreleg (left arm) electrode placed just below the point of the elbow on the back of the left forearm – right foreleg (right arm) electrode placed just below the point of the elbow on the back of the right forearm
Lead II: LL–LA	Left hindleg (left leg) electrode placed on the loose skin at the left stifle in the region of the patella – left foreleg (left arm) electrode placed just below the point of the elbow on the back of the left forearm
Lead III: LL–RA	Left hindleg (left leg) electrode placed on the loose skin at the left stifle in the region of the patella – right foreleg (right arm) electrode placed just below the point of the elbow on the back of the right forearm
aVr: RA–CT	Right foreleg (right arm) electrode placed just below the point of the elbow on the back of the right forearm – the electrical centre of the heart or central terminal × 3/2
aVl: LA–CT	Left foreleg (left arm) electrode placed just below the point of the elbow on the back of the left forearm – the electrical centre of the heart or central terminal × 3/2
aVf: LL-CT	Left hindleg (left leg) electrode placed on the loose skin at the left stifle in the region of the patella – the electrical centre of the heart or central terminal × 3/2
CV6LL: VI–CT	VI electrode placed in the 6th intercostal space on the left side of the thorax along a line parallel to the level of the point of the elbow – the electrical centre of the heart (central terminal)
CV6LU: V2–CT	V2 electrode placed in the 6th intercostal space on the left side of the thorax along a line parallel to the level of the point of the shoulder – the electrical centre of the heart (central terminal)
V10: V3–CT	V3 electrode placed over the dorsal thoracic spine of T7 at the withers – electrical centre of the heart. The dorsal spine of T7 is located on a line encircling the chest in the 6th intercostal space (central terminal)
CV6RL: V4–CT	V4 electrode placed in the 6th intercostal space on the right side of the thorax along a line parallel to the level of the point of the elbow – the electrical centre of the heart (central terminal)
CV6RL: V5–CT	V5 electrode placed in the 6th intercostal space on the right side of the thorax along a line parallel to the level of the point of the shoulder – the electrical centre of the heart (central terminal)
Base-apex: LA–RA	Left foreleg (left arm) electrode placed in the 6th intercostal space on the left side of the thorax along a line parallel to the level of the point of the elbow – right foreleg (right arm) electrode placed on the top of the right scapular spine

assessments such as blood culture, virus isolation and serology are also helpful in identifying possible contributing factors in horses presenting with dysrhythmias.

CLASSIFICATION OF DYSRHYTHMIAS

There are several different classifications of rhythm disturbances. From a clinical perspective, it is useful to categorize cardiac dysrhythmias by their site of origin (supraventricular or ventricular) and by their rate (bradydysrhythmias or tachydysrhythmias)[19-21] as these factors determine their clinical significance and most appropriate management. In horses, most bradydysrhythmias are physiological and associated with high vagal (parasympathetic) tone while most tachydysrhythmias are abnormal. Profound bradydysrhythmias and rapid tachydysrhythmias, particularly those of ventricular origin, are the rhythm disturbances most likely to need immediate treatment to control the ventricular rate and relieve the clinical signs of cardiovascular collapse.

Bradydysrhythmias

Bradydysrhythmias are commonly detected in healthy horses and are associated with high parasympathetic tone. Second-degree atrioventricular (AV) block is the most common bradydysrhythmia detected in resting horses. Sinus arrhythmia, sinus bradycardia, sinoatrial (SA) block and SA arrest also occur in normal horses with high vagal tone.[20,22] These normal dysrhythmias are present at rest and should disappear with a decrease in parasympathetic tone and/or an increase in sympathetic tone such as occurs with excitement or exercise.

Second-degree AV block
(🔵 AF, AR, RSD, SFP)

Second-degree AV block is the most common vagally mediated dysrhythmia detected in normal horses. In this dysrhythmia, conduction is blocked intermittently at the level of the AV node whereas first-degree AV block is defined as delayed conduction at the AV node that is not blocked. Second-degree AV block is detected in over 40% of healthy horses during 24-hour continuous electrocardiographic monitoring. Horses with second-degree AV block have a slow to normal heart rate (usually 20–40 bpm). The first (S1) and second (S2) heart sounds are regularly spaced and a fourth (S4) heart sound precedes each S1 and is present in the diastolic pause during the period of second-degree AV block. In most normal horses only one period of second-degree AV block occurs before the next conducted impulse but occasionally two blocks occur in sequence which should still be regarded as a normal physiological variant, providing that the dysrhythmia disappears with exercise or excitement.

The ECG reveals a slow to normal heart rate with a regular R–R interval and a normal QRS complex. Each QRS complex is preceded by a P wave with a normal to near normal PR interval but there are occasional P waves not followed by a QRS complex. The P–P interval is regular or may vary slightly. The frequency of blocked beats is usually, but not always, fairly regular and can range upwards from one in every three beats in healthy horses. In the majority of normal horses there is only one blocked P wave before P waves that are followed by a conducted QRS complex but occasionally there are two. This normal dysrhythmia should be replaced by sinus tachycardia with excitement, exercise or the administration of a vagolytic drug.

Advanced second-degree AV block

Advanced second-degree AV block, rare in horses, is a pathological form of conduction block at the AV node and can be caused by electrolyte imbalances, digitalis toxicity and AV nodal disease (inflammatory or degenerative).[2,20] Horses with advanced second-degree AV block usually have severe exercise intolerance and may collapse. A complete cardiovascular examination, biochemistry screen and complete blood count should be performed on all horses presenting with advanced second-degree AV block to attempt to determine the underlying cause of the dysrhythmia. Affected horses have a slow heart rate (usually 8–24 bpm). On auscultation S1 and S2 is regularly spaced with an audible S4 preceding each S1. S4 is heard in the diastolic pauses with one, or more, S4 for each period of second-degree AV block.

The ECG reveals a slow heart rate with a regular R–R interval between episodes of AV block and normally configured QRS complexes. The QRS complexes are each preceded by a P wave at a normal to near normal P–R interval, evidence of AV conduction. The P–R interval may be slightly prolonged as first-degree AV block may also be present. The P–P interval is regular and the atrial rate is rapid with numerous (two or more) P waves not followed by QRS complexes (Fig. 13.1). Appropriate treatment should be instituted as soon as possible, based upon the probable aetiology of the dysrhythmia to hopefully prevent the progression of the conduction block to complete AV block (see treatment of complete heart block below).

Complete (third-degree) AV block

Complete heart block is rare in horses and is usually associated with inflammatory or degenerative changes in the AV node,[23] although it may occur with electrolyte imbalances or other metabolic abnormalities such as is seen with foals with uroperitoneum, particularly when anaesthetized.[24,25] Complete heart block has also been

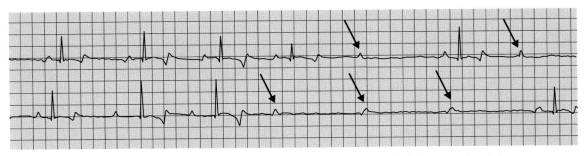

Figure 13.1 Lead II ECG obtained from a horse. Advanced second-degree AV block. Blocked P waves (arrows) occur frequently, singly and in runs. Recorded at paper speed of 25 mm/second, sensitivity of 5 mm = 1 mV.

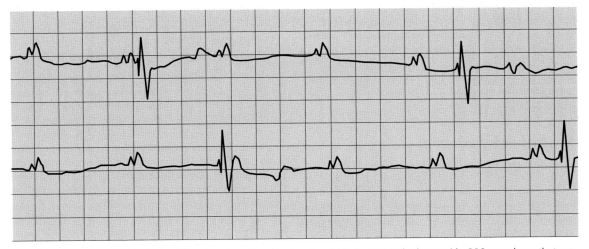

Figure 13.2 Base-apex ECG obtained from a horse with complete heart block. Notice the large wide QRS complexes that are not associated with the preceding P waves. There is complete AV dissociation with a rapid regular atrial rate of 70/minute and a slow regular ventricular rate of 20 bpm. The P–P interval is regular and the R–R interval is regular. Recorded at paper speed of 25 mm, sensitivity of 10 mm = 1 mV.

observed as a congenital defect[26] and associated with mediastinal lymphoma[27] and rattlesnake envenomation.[28] Horses with third-degree AV block will typically have severe exercise intolerance and frequent syncope. The resting heart rate (ventricular rate) is very slow (usually ≤20 bpm) but regular with a more rapid, independent atrial rate. The heart rate does not increase appropriately with a decrease in vagal tone or an increase in sympathetic tone. The S1 and S2 are usually loud and regularly spaced with more rapid independent S4 (usually ≤60/minute), which are also regularly spaced. Occasional "bruit de cannon" sounds, caused by the summation of S4 with another heart sound (S1, S2 or S3) are detected. An irregular rhythm may be detected in some horses with concurrent paroxysms of ventricular tachycardia.

The ECG usually reveals regular P waves that are not followed by QRS complexes (i.e. there is no evidence of AV conduction) and QRS complexes that are widened and bizarre in their appearance because they are originating from an idionodal or idioventricular pacemaker (Fig. 13.2). If the QRS complexes are regularly spaced, they should all look alike because they are originating from the same idionodal or idioventricular pacemaker. These are known as escape complexes because they represent the ventricles' attempt to escape in the absence of AV conduction. If there is other ventricular ectopy present, there will be more than one QRS configuration and the R–R interval may vary (Fig. 13.3). The P–R intervals will be of varying lengths with no consistent relationship between the P waves and the QRS complexes (see Figs. 13.2, 13.3). The atrial rate is usually very rapid with a regular P–P interval and there are many more P waves than QRS complexes.

Treatment of complete heart block in horses should be initiated as soon as the diagnosis is made. If the underlying cause of the complete heart block cannot be corrected or removed, the definitive treatment for third-degree AV block is a pacemaker (see Chapter 14). Corticosteroids, for example, dexamethasone at 0.05–0.2 mg/kg IV, are usually

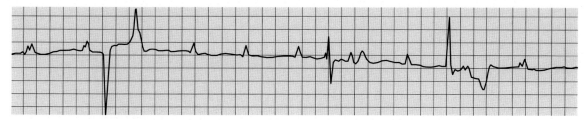

Figure 13.3 Lead II ECG obtained from a horse with complete heart block. Notice the large wide QRS complexes of differing configurations that are not associated with the preceding P waves. There is complete AV dissociation with a rapid regular atrial rate of 70/minute and a slow irregular ventricular rate of 30 bpm. The P–P interval is regular and the R–R interval is irregular. Recorded at paper speed of 25 mm/second, sensitivity of 10 mm = 1 mV.

indicated because the most common treatable cause of complete heart block is inflammatory disease in the region of the AV node. If an active viraemia is suspected, corticosteroids should be used with care. The small risk of the horse developing laminitis associated with prolonged administration of high doses of corticosteroids must also be weighed against the risk of the horse remaining in third-degree AV block, requiring the implantation of a cardiac pacemaker for long-term survival.[23,26] As emergency measures, vagolytic drugs, atropine or glycopyrrolate, can be administered (see Table 7.1). If ventricular ectopy is present, sympathomimetic drugs should be used with care, or not at all, because these drugs may exacerbate ventricular dysrhythmias. If no concurrent ventricular ectopy is present sympathomimetic drugs may be effective. Dopamine has β_1-adrenergic effects at moderate doses (3–5 μg/kg/minute) and has been effective in treating advanced AV block.[25,28] Alternatively, isoproterenol can be administered as continuous rate infusion (CRI; see Table 7.1). However, rapid tachydysrhythmias can occur with the administration of sympathomimetic drugs. If pharmacological intervention is not successful in restoring sinus rhythm, a temporary transvenous pacemaker may be necessary until a permanent transvenous pacemaker can be inserted[23,26] (see Chapter 14).

Sinus bradycardia, sinus arrhythmia, SA block and SA arrest

(SBR)

Sinus bradycardia, sinus arrhythmia, SA block and SA arrest occur in normal fit horses associated with high vagal tone but are less common than second-degree AV block (Fig. 13.4).[21] These dysrhythmias can occur in combinations: sinus arrhythmia is usually also present in horses with sinus bradycardia, SA block can occur in conjunction with second-degree AV block[29] and on resting ambulatory ECG, many normal horses will display a variety of physiological bradydysrhythmias throughout a 24-hour period. Auscultation reveals regular S1 and S2 with a pause in the rhythm (SA block or arrest) or rhythmic variation of diastolic intervals (sinus bradycardia and sinus arrhyth-

mia) with heart rates of 20–30 bpm. An S4 precedes each S1 and there are no isolated S4 in the diastolic pauses representing the period of SA block.

The atrial and ventricular rates are slow or low normal and normal QRS complexes are detected associated with the preceding P waves, evidence of AV conduction. The P–P and R–R intervals are rhythmically irregular with sinus arrhythmia. SA blocks are characterized by pauses of less than or equal to two P–P intervals, whereas sinus arrest is present if SA activity ceases for longer than two P–P intervals. These rhythms are normal manifestations of high vagal tone and disappear with exercise or the administration of a vagolytic drug, for example, atropine or glycopyrrolate (see Table 7.1).

Sick sinus syndrome

Prolonged periods of SA arrest, profound sinus bradycardia or high-grade SA block may be indicative of sinus node disease, termed sick sinus syndrome.[30] Ventricular escape rhythms may occur during prolonged pauses. Sinus node disease is rare in horses but inflammatory and degenerative changes must be considered possible aetiologies. Affected horses may have a history of collapse or weakness. These horses should be carefully evaluated with exercising electrocardiography and the response of the horse to vagolytic and sympathomimetic drugs determined. It may be possible to increase the heart rate and abolish the dysrhythmia during exercise tests, although the maximal heart rate may be reduced and the dysrhythmia may recur shortly after cessation of exercise.[30] Corticosteroids should be initiated for horses with life-threatening abnormalities of sinus rhythm, in the hope that pacemaker implantation will not be necessary. Definitive treatment of sick sinus syndrome is pacemaker implantation[30] (see Chapter 14).

Tachydysrhythmias

Tachydysrhythmias can be defined as either supraventricular or ventricular. Various forms exist including premature depolarizations, tachycardia, fibrillation and

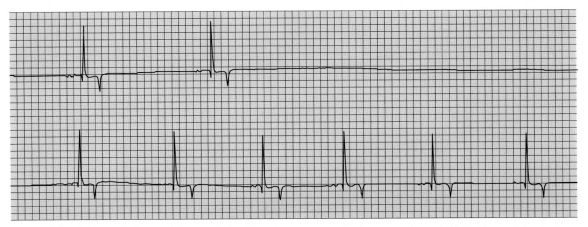

Figure 13.4 Modified base-apex ambulatory ECG recorded at rest in a healthy and fit 5-year-old Thoroughbred racehorse. There is a sinus pause of over 10 seconds. Each strip displays 13 seconds and the two strips are continuous.

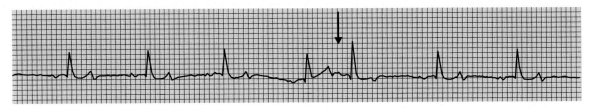

Figure 13.5 An ECG recorded on lead Y from a pony in which a dysrhythmia was auscultated during a routine examination. Supraventricular premature depolarizations (arrow) are represented by bizarre P waves followed by normal QRS–T complexes. Recorded at paper speed of 25 mm/second, sensitivity of 5 mm = 1 mV.

pre-excitations syndromes. Isolated supraventricular (SVPD) and ventricular (VPD) tachydysrhythmias are found in low numbers in horses without organic heart disease, particularly in prolonged resting ECG recordings (see Chapter 10), but these "normal" dysrhythmias are less common than second-degree AV block and other bradydysrhythmias. Persistent and frequent tachydysrhythmias are more commonly associated with cardiac and noncardiac pathology. Ambulatory ECG monitoring is very useful in documenting the frequency of dysrhythmic episodes in horses with intermittent tachydysrhythmias (see Chapter 10) and is invaluable in monitoring and assessing the effects of any treatment.

Supraventricular premature depolarizations and tachycardia

(AF, SFP)

SVPD originate in the atria before SA nodal discharge.[21] There is often an underlying regular rhythm and the SVPD may or may not be conducted to the ventricles. On auscultation, beats occurring earlier than normal are detected. Electrocardiography reveals a normally configured QRS–T complex, occurring prematurely. A bizarre P wave may be visible or may be hidden in the preceding T wave (Figs. 13.5 and 13.6). Supraventricular or atrial tachycardia is defined as more than four SVPD occurring in sequence.[21] Horses with frequent SVPD or supraventricular tachycardia are often able to maintain a normal ventricular response rate as some of the SVPD are blocked at the level of the AV node (see Fig. 13.6).

Infrequent SVPD can be detected in normal horses. However, frequent SVPD and atrial tachycardia may be indicative of myocardial disease (Fig. 13.7), or occur in association with atrial enlargement due to AV valvular disease or congenital heart disease. If an obvious predisposing cause is identified, treatment should be directed at that. In some horses, SVPD resolve following a period of rest and therapy with corticosteroids[2] (see Table 7.1). Specific antidysrhythmic therapy is rarely necessary provided that the ventricular rate is not affected by SVPD. Digoxin[31,32] or diltiazem[33,34] can be used to control the ventricular rate with rapid supraventricular tachycardia (see Table 7.1). Digoxin has a very narrow therapeutic to toxic range and therefore horses should be monitored for any signs of digoxin toxicity. Serum or plasma samples should be obtained for digoxin concentrations after several days of

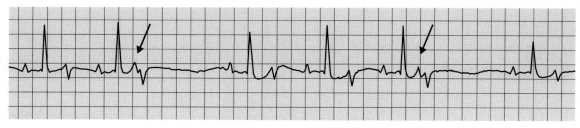

Figure 13.6 An ECG recorded on lead Y from a 10-year-old riding horse with a history of exercise intolerance. Blocked supraventricular premature depolarizations are located in the S–T segment of the preceding sinus beat (arrows). Recorded at paper speed of 25 mm/second, sensitivity of 5 mm = 1 mV.

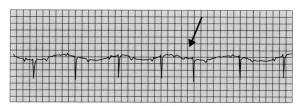

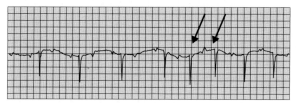

Figure 13.7 Base-apex ECGs from an 11-year-old Arabian mare with generalized myocarditis. Frequent supraventricular premature depolarizations (more than 100 per hour) were detected with 24-hour ambulatory ECG.

oral therapy to see if adjustments in the dosage are necessary (see Chapter 7). Phenytoin may also be helpful in suppressing SVPD in some cases (see Table 7.1). Horses with persistent, numerous SVPD, no performance limitations, and minimal identifiable underlying cardiac disease, can continue to be used for ridden activities as it is unlikely that these horses will collapse or represent a danger to a rider. However, numerous SVPD are a risk factor for the development of atrial fibrillation (see below) and thus, the potential for future performance-limiting problems must be considered, particularly when advising potential purchasers.

Atrial fibrillation

 AF, VMD)

Atrial fibrillation (AF) is a common arrhythmia in horses.[35-38] The estimated minimum frequency (i.e. no. of episodes per race starts) of AF in Japanese racehorses is 0.03% with an estimated minimum prevalence (i.e.

no. of horses with AF per no. of racehorses) of AF among Japanese racehorses being 0.29%.[38] A similar frequency has been reported in the UK.[39] In the vast majority of horses that develop AF during racing the dysrhythmia is paroxysmal.[38,39] There do not appear to be any gender predispositions but AF is more prevalent in racehorses >4 years of age compared to 2-year-olds. Horses racing on turf were more likely to develop AF than those racing on dirt in one study.[38] AF is also very common in large draft breeds[40] and Standardbreds have been over-represented compared to hospital populations in some studies.[35-37]

AF is due to re-entry (see Chapter 6). Shortening of the effective refractory period, atrial inhomogeneity and SVPD set the stage for the development of AF and normal horses are predisposed to the development of AF in the absence of structural heart disease due to their high resting vagal tone and large atrial mass. Most horses with AF have little or no underlying cardiac disease and in this situation, the term "lone AF" is applied. However, AF can also be related to atrial enlargement and horses with congestive heart failure due to congenital or acquired cardiac disease frequently develop AF. Transient potassium depletion, such as can occur with the administration of furosemide or with the loss of large amounts of potassium in the sweat of exercising horses, is also thought to be a predisposing factor in the development of AF.

Presenting complaints for horses with AF include poor performance in horses engaged in athletic activities, tachypnoea, dyspnoea, exercise-induced pulmonary haemorrhage, myopathy and colic. AF can also be an incidental finding during a routine examination, particularly in horses that do not routinely perform vigorous exercise. Horses with lone AF usually have normal resting heart rates (<44 bpm), although the rhythm is irregularly irregular and no S4 is produced. The intensity of the peripheral arterial pulses is also irregularly irregular. Pulse deficits may be present, particularly in horses with two conducted beats occurring in rapid succession. Increased resting heart rates (>50 bpm) and loud cardiac murmurs and signs consistent with congestive heart failure should alert the clinician to the possibility that significant underlying heart

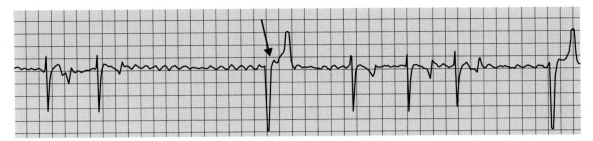

Figure 13.8 Base-apex ECG obtained from a horse with atrial fibrillation. Notice the irregularly irregular R–R intervals, the absence of P waves and the presence of baseline "f" waves. A ventricular complex is present (arrow) and the remainder of the QRS configurations are normal, as is the ventricular rate (30 bpm). Recorded at a paper speed of 25 mm/second, sensitivity of 5 mm = 1 mV.

disease is present. Clinical signs of left-sided heart failure (pulmonary oedema, coughing, tachypnoea) and/or right-sided heart failure (generalized venous distention, jugular pulsations and peripheral oedema) may be present (see Chapter 16).

The ECG reveals irregularly irregular R–R intervals, no P waves and normal appearing QRS complexes (Fig. 13.8). Rapid baseline fibrillation "f" waves are usually present, which may be small (fine) or large (coarse). In approximately 10% of horses with AF, QRS complexes originating from the ventricle will also be detected (see Fig. 13.8) while with congestive heart failure, tachycardia is confirmed.

AF may be paroxysmal and spontaneous conversion to normal sinus rhythm may occur in otherwise normal horses. Spontaneous conversion usually occurs within 24–48 hours of the onset of AF.[38] Paroxysmal AF (PAF) most often occurs during strenuous exercise and the horse will often pull up abruptly, displaying signs of distress. In these cases, it is extremely helpful if the dysrhythmia can be documented to be AF at the time of the initial episode. However, if this is not achieved, frequent SVPD documented on subsequent 24-hour ambulatory ECGs provides supportive evidence that the episode of distress was due to PAF (see Chapter 11). However, very similar clinical signs can be seen with exercise-associated ventricular dysrhythmias and this possibility should be explored with 24-hour ambulatory and exercising ECG if it has not been possible to obtain an ECG at the time of the initial episode. Where PAF is confirmed, or suspected, echocardiography, haematology and blood biochemistry including cardiac troponin I concentrations should be assessed. Whole body potassium and/or magnesium depletion may be a predisposing factor in PAF, and these can be investigated using red cell electrolyte concentrations or by calculating a fractional excretion of potassium and magnesium in the urine. A urine and serum sample must be obtained simultaneously, preferably before exercise and morning feeding, and serum and urinary creatinine and electrolyte concentrations meas-

ured. The fractional excretion (FE) of electrolytes is calculated using the following equation:

$$FE = \frac{urine\,(electrolyte) \times serum\,(creatinine) \times 100}{serum\,(electrolyte) \times urine\,(creatinine)}$$

A low fractional excretion of potassium or magnesium indicates renal conservation and a probable low total-body potassium or magnesium status. Although PAF can be a recurrent condition, this is not typically the case, but exercising ECG should be obtained when training resumes to ensure that there is no persistent, exercise-associated arrhythmia.

Horses with little or no underlying cardiac disease are candidates for conversion to sinus rhythm either with pharmacological or electrical cardioversion. Factors likely to influence the success of treatment include the presence of AV valvular regurgitation, atrial enlargement and primary myocardial disease[36,37] and thus echocardiography is an important component of the pretreatment assessment in horses with sustained AF. In particular the diameter of the left atrium and the presence of valvular regurgitation should be noted. Horses with AF often have mild reductions in fractional shortening and Doppler echocardiographic indices of systolic function that can be expected to improve after successful conversion and should not be mistaken for evidence of global myocardial disease.[41,42] Echocardiographic findings will vary depending on the underlying cause in horses with AF and congestive heart failure.

The atria undergo electrical remodelling in response to AF[43] and the likelihood of successful conversion decreases and recurrence rate increases with increased duration. In one study, in horses with AF of less than 3 months' duration the recurrence rate was 15%, whereas if AF had been present for longer, the recurrence rate was 65%.[36] It can be difficult to determine the onset of the AF but the horse's caretakers should be questioned closely on the horse's performance history. All available treatment options carry some risk, and in horses with no performance limitations, particularly those in which the AF has likely been present for a considerable period, owners should be counselled to consider the risks and benefits of treatment carefully. It may be more appropriate to evaluate such horses' exercising heart rates and rhythms and continue to use them for ridden activities, provided the exercising ECG reveals no further abnormalities.

Quinidine remains the most widely used drug for treatment of AF due to its action of prolonging the effective refractory period (see Chapter 7). However, it is also proarrhythmic and has a wide range of cardiovascular and noncardiac side-effects and therefore must be used with care. Physical examination and laboratory assessment prior to treatment should ensure that the horse is healthy, and in particular any electrolyte disturbances should be ruled out. An intravenous catheter should be inserted prior to beginning the quinidine treatment so that rapid venous access is available if severe dysrhythmias develop. A continuous ECG should be obtained throughout the entire treatment period to monitor cardiac rhythm and conduction times. The QRS duration should be measured from the ECG prior to each planned administration of quinidine and compared to the pretreatment duration. Increases of >25% are suggestive of quinidine toxicity.

The duration of the AF prior to treatment and the presence and severity of any underlying cardiac disease detected help to determine the ideal treatment regimen. If the duration of the arrhythmia is recent, ideally less than 2 weeks' duration, quinidine gluconate can be administered intravenously to effect[44] (see Table 7.1). If the AF is of more longstanding duration (>2 weeks) and/or there is mild to moderate, but not severe, underlying cardiac disease (mild to moderate tricuspid, mitral or aortic regurgitation or mild myocardial dysfunction), quinidine sulphate can be administered at 22 mg/kg via nasogastric intubation every 2 hours until the horse converts to sinus rhythm, experiences adverse reactions or toxic side effects to quinidine sulphate treatment (Table 13.2) or has received four treatments at 2-hour intervals.[36,37,45] The majority of horses with AF can only tolerate four treatments every 2 hours before exhibiting adverse or toxic side effects. If no adverse reactions or toxic side effects are experienced by the horse and the horse has not converted to sinus rhythm after the first four treatments ideally therapeutic drug monitoring should begin. The therapeutic plasma concentration of quinidine is 2–5 µg/mL. Provided that the plasma quinidine concentrations are in this range, or where quinidine concentrations cannot be measured, after four to five doses, treatment intervals should be prolonged to every half-life, approximately every 6 hours. Treatment intervals should be maintained at every 6 hours until conversion to sinus rhythm, adverse reactions or toxic side effects develop or the owner elects to discontinue treatment.[37] If conversion has not occurred by day 2, oral digoxin (0.011 mg/kg twice daily) appears to be helpful in the conversion of some horses that do not convert with quinidine alone. However, digoxin should not be administered beyond

day 2 without monitoring serum digoxin concentrations. Digoxin and quinidine compete for binding to plasma proteins and the administration of digoxin and quinidine together results in rapid elevations of serum digoxin concentrations (nearly double) and the possible development of digoxin toxicity.[46] Horses with digoxin toxicity may be anorexic, depressed, colicky and/or have other cardiac dysrhythmias.

Horses being treated for AF with quinidine should be monitored carefully for adverse reactions and signs of quinidine toxicity. The adverse reactions or toxic side effects are primarily cardiovascular, neurological or gastrointestinal. The detection of any significant adverse reactions or signs of quinidine toxicity (see Table 13.2) should prompt discontinuation of quinidine administration and may require additional treatment if the induced problem is serious (Tables 13.2, 13.3).

The cardiovascular side effects or adverse reactions of quinidine administration include hypotension, decreased cardiac contractility, congestive heart failure, prolongation of the QRS complex (Fig. 13.9), a rapid supraventricular tachycardia (Fig. 13.10), ventricular dysrhythmias (Figs. 13.11 and 13.12) and sudden death (see Table 13.3). Horses being treated with quinidine should have their blood pressure monitored during treatment for quinidine-induced hypotension. If the pulse pressure becomes very weak and severe hypotension develops, quinidine administration should be discontinued. Polyionic fluids and CRI of phenylephrine are used to restore blood pressure in horses with severe hypotension. Prolongation of the QRS duration to greater than 25% of the pretreatment QRS duration is an indication of quinidine toxicity and quinidine sulphate administration should be discontinued (see Fig. 13.9). QT interval prolongation also occurs with quinidine administration.

Rapid supraventricular tachycardia occurs in horses being treated for AF with quinidine caused by a sudden removal of vagal tone at the AV node (see Fig. 13.10). This very rapid heart rate is an idiosyncratic reaction and is not necessarily associated with high plasma quinidine concentrations. Sustained ventricular response rates greater than 100 bpm in horses being treated for AF with quinidine should be treated and controlled, before continuing quinidine administration, to prevent further deterioration of the cardiac rhythm (see Table 13.3). Digoxin should be administered intravenously if the heart rate is rapidly increasing and does not return to normal rapidly. Oral digoxin may be administered if the heart rate is rapid but readily returns to a more normal value. Heart rates greater than 200 bpm are potentially life-threatening (see Fig. 13.10) and require immediate therapy (see Table 13.3) to slow the ventricular response rate and prevent deterioration of the horse's cardiovascular status. Intravenous sodium bicarbonate is also indicated and should bind any free circulating quinidine, helping to prevent a further increase in heart rate and deterioration of the cardiac

Table 13.2 Adverse reactions and toxic side effects of quinidine sulphate/gluconate treatment

1. Depression
R$_x$: Seen in all treated horses, no R$_x$ indicated

2. Paraphimosis
R$_x$: Seen in all treated stallions or geldings, no R$_x$ indicated

3. Urticaria and/or wheals
R$_x$: Discontinue quinidine; if severe, administer corticosteroids and/or antihistamines

4. Nasal mucosal swelling
Snoring
R$_x$: Monitor degree of airflow; discontinue quinidine if significant decrease in air flow through nares
Upper respiratory tract obstruction
R$_x$: Discontinue quinidine; if severe administer corticosteroids and/or antihistamines, insert nasotracheal tube preferably, or perform emergency tracheotomy

5. Laminitis
R$_x$: Discontinue quinidine; administer analgesics and shoeing changes as needed

6. Neurological
Ataxia
R$_x$: Discontinue quinidine; sign of quinidine toxicity
Bizarre behaviour – hallucinations?
R$_x$: Discontinue quinidine; sign of quinidine toxicity
Convulsions
R$_x$: Discontinue quinidine; sign of quinidine toxicity; administer anticonvulsants as indicated

7. Gastrointestinal
Flatulence
R$_x$: Seen in many treated horses; R$_x$ not indicated
Diarrhoea
R$_x$: Usually resolves with discontinuation of R$_x$; discontinue R$_x$ if diarrhoea severe
Colic
R$_x$: Usually resolves with administration of dipyrone; use other analgesics as needed

8. Cardiovascular
Tachycardia – supraventricular or ventricular – uniform, multiform, torsades de pointes
R$_x$: See Table 7.1
Prolongation of the QRS duration (>25% of pretreatment value)
R$_x$: Discontinue quinidine
Hypotension
R$_x$: Discontinue quinidine; administer phenylephrine if needed (0.1–0.2 µg/kg/minute)
Congestive heart failure
R$_x$: Discontinue quinidine; administer digoxin if not already given
Sudden death
R$_x$: CPR

rhythm. If the horse's heart rate remains increased, propranolol should be administered to help slow the ventricular response rate. Diltiazem can also be effective in controlling the ventricular rate in quinidine-induced supraventricular tachycardia.[33,34]

Quinidine can also produce life-threatening ventricular dysrhythmias (see Figs. 13.11 and 13.12). If a large number of VPD, ventricular tachycardia or polymorphic VPD are detected, quinidine administration should cease. If these ventricular dysrhythmias persist or there are clinical signs associated with these dysrhythmias, the intravenous administration of antiarrhythmic drugs should be instituted (see Table 13.3). Torsades de pointes, a wide ventricular tachycardia (see Figs. 13.11 and 13.12), is a dysrhythmia induced by quinidine administration that is more likely to occur in hypokalaemic horses (see Fig. 13.12). Therefore, every effort should be made prior to quinidine treatment to be sure that horses have an adequate whole-body potassium status. Intravenous magnesium sulphate should be started immediately in horses with quinidine-induced torsades de pointes. Sudden death in horses with AF treated with quinidine is probably associated with the deterioration of rapid supraventricular or ventricular tachycardia to ventricular fibrillation or cardiac arrest. The possibility of sudden death occurring underscores the importance of continuous electrocardiographic monitoring and rapid treatment of any dysrhythmias that do occur.

Table 13.3 Treatment of quinidine-induced dysrhythmias and hypotension

Determine if dysrhythmia is supraventricular or ventricular

a. Obtain another ECG lead if unable to make this determination from the base-apex lead; look for changes in QRS configuration from normal or preceding QRS configuration. Record ECG during entire treatment with radiotelemetry, if possible
b. Obtain blood pressure if possible
c. Don't panic

If dysrhythmia is supraventricular

1. If rate is sustained in excess of 100 bpm
    a. Administer digoxin at 0.0022 mg/kg IV (1 mg/450 kg) or 0.011 mg/kg orally (5 mg/450 kg)
2. If rate is sustained in excess of 150 bpm and/or blood pressures are poor
    a. Administer digoxin at 0.0022 mg/kg IV (1 mg/450 kg); can repeat dose once in a relatively short period of time if necessary
    b. Administer sodium bicarbonate IV at 1 mmol/kg
3. If rate is still high
    a. Administer propanolol at 0.03 mg/kg IV (13.5 mg/450 kg) to slow heart rate
    b. Administer diltiazem at 0.125 mg/kg IV over 2 min repeated every 12 min
    c. Administer verapamil at 0.025–0.025 mg/kg IV every 30 min, can repeat up to 0.2 mg/kg total dose

If dysrhythmia is ventricular

1. If wide QRS tachycardia (torsade de pointes)
    a. Administer magnesium sulphate at 2.2–5.5 mg/kg/min IV to effect up to 55 mg/kg total dose
2. If ventricular tachycardia is unstable
    a. Administer propanolol at 0.03 mg/kg IV
    b. Administer lignocaine HCl at 20–50 µg/kg/min or 0.25–0.5 mg/kg very slowly IV, can repeat q 5–10 min
    c. Administer magnesium sulphate at 2.2–5.5 mg/kg/min IV to effect up to 55 mg/kg total dose
    d. Administer propafenone at 0.5–1 mg/kg in 5% dextrose IV over 5– 8min
    e. Administer bretylium at 3–5 mg/kg IV. Can repeat up to 10 mg/kg total dose.

If blood pressure is poor

a. Administer polyionic fluids IV as rapidly as possible
b. Administer phenylephrine to effect at 0.1–0.2 µg/kg/min IV up to 0.01 mg/kg total dose to improve blood pressure

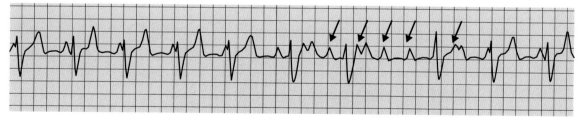

Figure 13.9 Base-apex ECG obtained from a horse with atrial fibrillation that was then treated with quinidine sulphate and developed prolongation of the QRS complex. Following treatment with four doses of 22 mg/kg of quinidine sulphate the QRS complexes prolonged to 140 ms and the ventricular rate has increased to 60 bpm. There are now large P waves (arrows) occurring regularly and buried in many of the QRS and T complexes associated with an atrial tachycardia (atrial rate of 150/minute) with block. A quinidine plasma concentration obtained at this time was elevated. Recorded at paper speed of 25 mm/second, sensitivity of 5 mm = 1 mV.

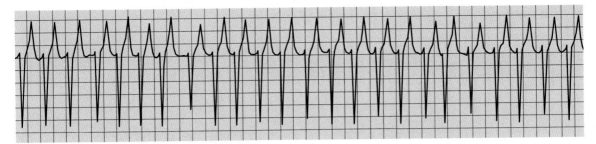

Figure 13.10 Base-apex ECG obtained from a horse with atrial fibrillation that developed a rapid supraventricular tachycardia with a heart rate of 210 bpm following the second dose of quinidine sulphate at 22 mg/kg. Notice the slightly irregular R–R intervals, the absence of P waves and the normal orientation of the QRS complex for the base-apex lead. The "f" waves are not visible due to the rapid ventricular response rate. Recorded at paper speed of 25 mm/second, sensitivity of 5 mm = 1 mV.

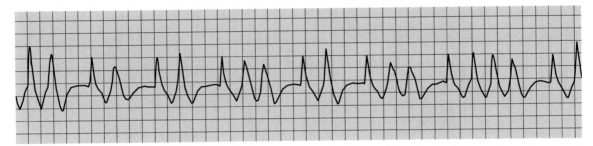

Figure 13.11 Base-apex ECG obtained from a horse with atrial fibrillation that had received 2 doses of quinidine sulphate and developed a wide ventricular tachycardia (torsades de pointes). Notice how the QRS complexes and T waves twist around the baseline and are difficult to distinguish from one another. Recorded at paper speed of 25 mm/s, sensitivity of 2 mm = 1 mV.

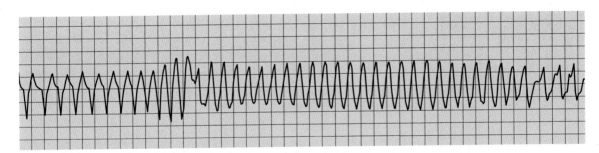

Figure 13.12 Base-apex ECG obtained from a horse with atrial fibrillation that had received six doses of quinidine sulphate and developed torsades de pointes, which was immediately treated with an intravenous infusion of magnesium sulphate. Notice the widened QRS complexes and T waves. Notice also the twisting of the QRS complexes and T waves around the baseline, which is still present although the torsades de pointes is resolving at this time. This horse was hypokalaemic (2.4 mEq/L). The wide QRS tachycardia resolved with magnesium and potassium replacement fluids. Recorded at paper speed of 25 mm/second, sensitivity of 5 mm = 1 mV.

All horses receiving quinidine should be closely monitored for quinidine-induced upper respiratory tract obstruction secondary to nasal mucosal swelling. If airflow through the external nares decreases significantly quinidine administration should be discontinued. A nasotracheal tube should be inserted if airflow continues to decrease. Corticosteroids and/or antihistamines should be administered if the upper respiratory tract obstruction is severe. An emergency tracheotomy may be necessary in some horses if a nasotracheal tube is not inserted when a significant decrease in airflow is detected. Urticaria and/or wheals occur infrequently in horses receiving quinidine, but the every 2 hour administration of quinidine sulphate should be discontinued if urticaria and/or wheals develop. If the urticaria and wheals are severe antihistamines and corticosteroids may be indicated.

Paraphimosis is a common transient problem in all geldings and stallions and disappears with a return of plasma quinidine concentrations to negligible levels. Therefore, it is not necessary to discontinue quinidine administration if the horse develops paraphimosis. Laminitis, a serious potential complication of quinidine treatment, is extremely rare. However, if the horse's digital pulses are increased, quinidine administration should be discontinued. If the horse is uncomfortable because of the laminitis, aggressive treatment for laminitis should begin. Neurological signs are indicative of quinidine toxicity and quinidine treatment should be discontinued if the horse exhibits any bizarre behaviour, ataxia or has a seizure. If seizures occur anticonvulsants may be indicated until the plasma quinidine concentrations have decreased and the seizures resolve.

Quinidine is very irritating to the gastrointestinal tract and some evidence of this is usually detected in every horse receiving quinidine. Flatulence is very common and is seen in nearly all horses after several doses of quinidine sulphate but is not associated with any adverse reactions, and thus the administration of quinidine should not be discontinued. Diarrhoea often occurs in horses receiving multiple doses of quinidine and usually resolves with discontinuation of quinidine treatment. If the horse's faeces are just loose, but not pipe-stream, quinidine administration can be continued. However, if the diarrhoea worsens with continued quinidine treatment, quinidine sulphate administration should be discontinued. Quinidine administration should be discontinued in horses with colic. Analgesics should be administered if needed for abdominal pain. Oral ulcerations are associated with oral administration of the drug and can be severe; therefore, the oral administration of quinidine sulphate is contraindicated.

Electrical cardioversion (see Chapter 14) appears to be the most viable alternative to treatment with quinidine sulphate at this time.[47-50] But, alternative, more modern antidysrhythmic drugs are currently under investigation. Amiodarone, a class 3 antidysrhythmic and β-adrenergic drug that increases the refractory period by blocking potassium and sodium channels has a good conversion rate and few side effects in human AF. Amiodarone has low oral bioavailability in horses.[51] To date, two different treatment regimens have been reported and 4 of 6 and 3 of 6 cases converted to sinus rhythm with these protocols.[52,53] In the horses that did not convert, treatment had to be abandoned due to adverse effects of hindlimb weakness or depression and diarrhoea.

Flecainide is a class 1c antidysrhythmic drug. It slows intracardiac condition and prolongs the refractory period. Intravenous flecainide is unsuccessful in treating chronic AF and has an unacceptable number of side effects, including dangerous tachydysrhythmias.[54] However, a protocol for oral administration of flecainide has been used successfully in an experimental AF model,[55] and at the current time, in one naturally occurring case.[56] Feed is withdrawn overnight and flecainide is administered orally at 4.1 mg/kg at 2-hour intervals for a maximum of 4–6 doses then the dosing interval is extended to 4–6 hours. Side effects include depression, agitation, mild abdominal pain, reduced gastrointestinal sounds, hypotension, and prolongation of the QRS and QT intervals.[55,56] There are also two reported cases of sudden death in horses given flecainide orally within 24 hours of unsuccessful attempts at conversion with quinidine sulphate.[57] Further work is required to confirm the optimal dosage regimens and the safety and efficacy of flecainide, but when used orally, it may offer a potential alternative to quinidine sulphate.

Following treatment of AF, it is prudent to perform a 24-hour ambulatory ECG to confirm that there are no residual dysrhythmias. AF leads to left atrial mechanical dysfunction[43,58] and over time, electrical remodelling associated with a progressive shortening of the atrial effective refractory period, attenuation of the atrial refractory period rate adaptation and decrease in the AF cycle length.[43] These changes are likely to be more pronounced with long-standing AF. Consequently, following conversion to sinus rhythm, a period of reduced workload of up to 4 weeks is recommended.

Cardioversion is not indicated in AF associated with congestive heart failure, and the aim of treatment is rate control, rather than rhythm control, thus treatment of horses with congestive heart failure and AF should be directed towards slowing the ventricular response rate and supporting the failing myocardium.[1,59,60] These are also inappropriate patients for conversion with quinidine because of its negative inotropic effect (see Chapter 19).

Ventricular pre-excitation

Ventricular pre-excitation syndrome is very rare in horses.[61-64] It is characterized by a shortened P–R interval (<0.22 seconds) and is the result of accelerated conduction from the atria to the ventricle through an accessory conduction pathway. There may be a δ wave, a slurring of the R wave due to abnormal ventricular activation. Pharmacological testing can be used to confirm the presence of the accessory pathway: isoprotenerol accelerates conduction through the AV node while quinidine inhibits conduction through the AV node.[64] Pre-excitation syndrome may be an incidental ECG finding, or if rapid tachycardia develops, may present with clinical signs of weakness and distress. The accessory pathway may allow the establishment of a circus movement with antegrade movement from the atria to the ventricles through the pathway and retrograde movement from the ventricles to the atria through the bundle of His and AV node.[65] Although this is a form of supraventricular tachycardia, it appears electrocardiographically very similar to ventricular tachycardia, with broad QRS complexes (Fig 13.13).

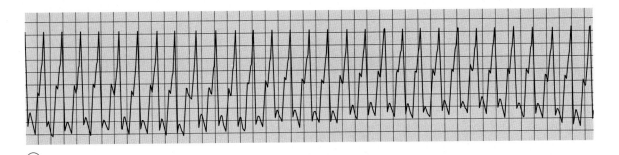

(A)

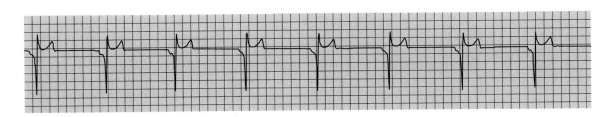

(B)

Figure 13.13 (A) Supraventricular tachycardia with wide and bizarre complexes in a 15-year-old Warmblood gelding with pre-excitation. This horse was usually asymptomatic with a normal resting heart rate but on two occasions over a 4-year period developed weakness and distress due to this tachycardia that resolved in response to treatment with procainamide on both occasions. Base-apex lead, recorded at paper speed of 25 mm/second, sensitivity of 5 mm = 1 mV. (**B**) When the heart rate is normal, the P–R interval is absent as conduction from the atria to the ventricles is through an accessory pathway and a delta wave is evident on the downstroke of the R wave. Modified base-apex lead, each strip displays 13 seconds and the two strips are continuous.

Procainamide is the treatment of choice in this form of supraventricular tachycardia[65] (see Table 7.1).

Ventricular premature depolarizations

Ventricular premature depolarizations (VPD) originate within the ventricular myocardium.[19] Auscultation reveals a beat occurring earlier than normal, loud first heart sound and loud sounds produced when two heart sounds are occurring simultaneously. There may be pulse deficits. On electrocardiography, VPD occur early, have abnormal QRS–T complexes and are not preceded by P waves. The most common form is a wide QRS complex that is followed by a T wave orientated in the opposite direction (Fig. 13.14). If all the VPD have the same configuration, they are described as monomorphic whereas VPD with more than one configuration are defined as polymorphic, and implies that they are originating from more than one site within the ventricles.

Infrequent VPD can be detected at rest, and during and following exercise in normal horses (see Fig. 13.14). However, if they are frequent, polymorphic or occur frequently during exercise, they are considered to be abnormal. Potential causes include myocardial inflammation,

degeneration, necrosis or fibrosis, electrolyte abnormalities, hypoxia and endotoxaemia.[21] VPD are common in horses with severe mitral insufficiency and heart failure.[18] Again, if an underlying cause can be identified, treatment is directed at that. In some horses, VPD resolve following a period of rest and therapy with corticosteroids such as dexamethasone at a dose of 0.05–0.2 mg/kg IV.[4] (*RCT, CN, AF*)

Ventricular tachycardia

(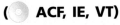 **ACF, IE, VT)**

Ventricular tachycardia is defined as four or more VPD occurring in sequence and it is often indicative of primary myocardial disease.[2–4,7,8,18] However, the horse should be carefully examined for other causes of ventricular tachycardia such as hypoxia, electrolyte imbalances[11,12] or drug-induced ventricular dysrhythmias. Aorto-cardiac fistula occurs in older (usually >10 years) horses, often stallions, with acute onset of distress that may be interpreted initially as colic and monomorphic ventricular tachycardia (usually with rapid regular heart rates >120 bpm).[66] Infective endocarditis involving the mitral or aortic valves is also associated with ventricular tachycardia caused by septic embolization of the ventricular myocardium

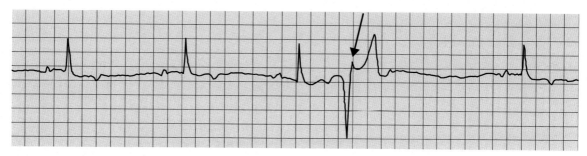

Figure 13.14 An ECG recorded on lead Y from a normal horse. A ventricular premature depolarization (arrow) is represented by a large, wide QRS complex with the T wave orientated in the opposite direction. Recorded at paper speed of 25 mm/second, sensitivity of 5 mm = 1 mV.

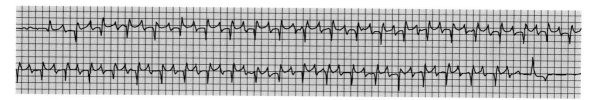

Figure 13.15 An ECG showing paroxysmal monomorphic ventricular tachycardia in a 7-year-old hunter gelding. After one sinus beat there is a run of ventricular tachycardia before sinus rhythm is restored. Recorded on lead Y at paper speed of 25 mm/second, sensitivity of 5 mm = 1 mV.

through the coronary circulation (see Chapter 17). Rattlesnake envenomation,[5] severe metabolic disturbances,[11] endotoxaemia,[15,16] septic shock[14] and severe haemoperitoneum[67] can lead to ventricular tachycardia. Life-threatening dysrhythmias can also occur following subarachnoid haemorrhage and head trauma which can lead to markedly increased sympathetic and parasympathetic output. Clinical signs of congestive heart failure develop rapidly in horses with shorter cycle lengths and higher heart rates and when the ventricular rhythm is polymorphic. Clinical signs of congestive heart failure become more severe, the longer ventricular tachycardia is present. Generalized venous distention, jugular pulsations, ventral oedema and pleural effusion will typically develop in horses with sustained ventricular tachycardia at a rate of equal to or greater than 120 bpm. Occasionally, these horses will also develop pericardial effusion, pulmonary oedema and ascites. Syncope has been detected in horses with monomorphic ventricular tachycardia and a heart rate equal to or greater than 150 bpm.

Auscultation reveals a rapid rhythm that can be fairly regular if monomorphic ventricular tachycardia is present and irregular with polymorphic ventricular tachycardia. Heart sounds are often loud and vary in intensity. Loud booming heart sounds (bruit de cannon) can be detected in some horses associated with the simultaneous production of two heart sounds during periods of AV dissociation. The ventricular rate in horses with ventricular tachycardia is usually increased (>60 bpm) with a slower independent atrial rate. Jugular pulsations occur in association with the AV dissociation.

The ECG is important in determining the frequency severity of the ventricular dysrhythmias detected.[18,19] The configuration of the QRS complex and T wave is abnormal and the QRS complex is unrelated to the preceding P wave. The P–P interval is regular but the P waves are often buried in QRS and T complexes (AV dissociation). Monomorphic ventricular tachycardia occurs when the ectopic focus originates from one place in the ventricle, creating only one abnormal QRS and T wave configuration and usually the R–R interval is regular (Fig. 13.15). Polymorphic ventricular tachycardia occurs when the VPD originate from more than one focus in the ventricle, creating abnormal QRS and T complexes of different orientations (Fig. 13.16). Polymorphic VPD are associated with increased electrical inhomogeneity and instability and an increased risk of a fatal ventricular rhythm developing. The R on T phenomenon, a QRS complex occurring within the preceding T wave, also indicates marked electrical inhomogeneity and instability and increases the chance for ventricular fibrillation to develop (Fig. 13.17). Wide QRS tachycardia or torsades de pointes (see Figs. 13.11 and 13.12), in which the QRS and T complexes twist around the baseline, is another ventricular rhythm which may rapidly deteriorate into ventricular fibrillation and result in sudden death.

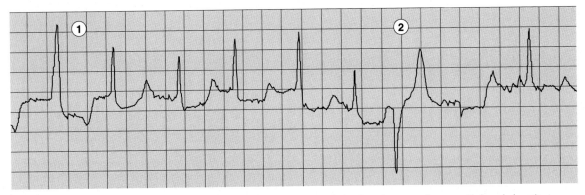

Figure 13.16 An ECG showing polymorphic ventricular premature depolarizations in an aged pony with hypokalaemia, hypocalcaemia, hypomagnesaemia and disseminated intravascular coagulation following surgery for small intestinal strangulation. Two abnormal QRS–T complexes (1 and 2) are present on this strip. Recorded on lead Y at paper speed of 25 mm/second, sensitivity of 5 mm = 1 mV.

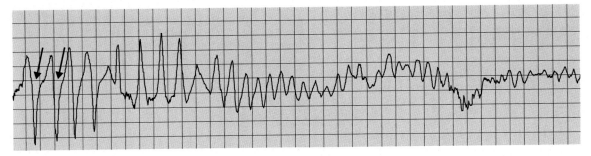

Figure 13.17 ECG showing R on T phenomenon (arrows) in the pony shown in Figure 13.16 with polymorphic ventricular tachycardia which progresses to fatal ventricular fibrillation. Recorded on lead Y at paper speed of 25 mm/second, sensitivity of 5 mm = 1 mV.

The echocardiogram in horses with monomorphic ventricular tachycardia is usually normal other than the presence of wall motion abnormalities associated with the rhythm disturbance. (VT) Severe myocardial dysfunction is usually detected in horses with polymorphic ventricular tachycardia, indicating possible myocardial disease.[2] The aortic root should be carefully examined in horses with colic and monomorphic ventricular tachycardia, particularly older stallions, as these horses may have intracardiac aortic root rupture. (ACF, VT)

Treatment of ventricular tachycardia is indicated if the horse is showing clinical signs at rest attributable to the dysrhythmia, the rate is excessively high, the rhythm is polymorphic or R on T complexes are detected. If pulmonary oedema is present emergency treatment should be instituted as soon as possible and should include furosemide (1–2 mg/kg IV), intranasal oxygen and drugs to reduce anxiety, if needed.[60] The selection of an appropriate antidysrhythmic for a horse with ventricular tachycardia depends upon the severity of the dysrhythmia, the associated clinical signs, the suspected aetiology and the availability of appropriate antiarrhythmic drugs (see Table 7.1). All antiarrhythmic drugs may have adverse effects and can also be proarrhythmic (Table 13.4) and therefore they should be administered with care, ideally while the ECG is monitored continuously. (ACF, VT)

A number of antidysrhythmic drugs are appropriate for treatment of unstable ventricular tachycardia in the horse, with no specific one emerging as the drug of first choice when availability, efficacy and adverse effects are considered (see Tables 7.1 and 13.4). Lignocaine is readily available and is the most rapidly acting drug but must be administered carefully and in small doses due to the excitement and seizures associated with larger doses.[31,32,59] Diazepam (0.05 mg/kg IV) may be used to control the excitability or seizures that may result from lignocaine.[32] The therapeutic plasma concentration of lignocaine is 1.5–5 µmg/mL. Quinidine gluconate,[45] procainamide,[69] amiodarone[70] and propafenone[71] are either administered intravenously slowly, in graded doses, or as CRI (see Table 7.1). The principal metabolite of procainamide is *N*-acetylprocainamide (NAPA), which is also pharmaco-

Table 13.4 Adverse effects of antidysrhythmic drugs

DRUG	ADVERSE EFFECTS	CARDIOVASCULAR EFFECTS
Amiodarone	Hindlimb weakness, depression, Diarrhoea	Bradycardia and VT in human beings
Atropine	Ileus, mydriasis	Tachycardia, arrhythmias
Bretylium tosylate	GI	Hypotension, tachycardia, arrhythmias
Digoxin	Depression, anorexia, colic	SVPD, VPD, SVT, VT
Flecanide	Collapse, depression, agitation, Colic	VT, life threatening if used IV, sudden death, hypotension, prolongs QRS and QT intervals
Lignocaine (lidocaine)	Excitement, seizures	VT, sudden death
Quinidine	Depression, paraphimosis, urticaria, wheals, nasal mucosal swelling, laminitis, neurological, GI	Hypotension, SVT, VT, prolongs QRS, sudden death, neg. inotrope
Phenytoin	Sedation, drowsiness, lip and facial twitching, gait deficits, seizures	Arrhythmias
Procainamide	GI, neurological – similar to quinidine	Hypotension, SVT, VT prolongs QRS, sudden death, neg. inotrope
Propafenone	GI, neurological – similar to quinidine, bronchospasm	CHF, AV block, arrhythmias, neg. inotrope
Propranolol	Lethargy, worsening of chronic obstructive pulmonary disease	Bradycardia, third-degree AV block, arrhythmias, CHF, neg. inotrope
Verapamil		Hypotension, bradycardia, AV block, asystole, arrhythmias, neg. inotrope

CHF, congestive heart failure; GI, gastrointestinal; neg., negative; SVPD, supraventricular premature depolarizations; SVT, supraventricular tachycardia; VPD, ventricular premature depolarizations; VT, ventricular tachycardia.

logically active. The half-life for procainamide administered intravenously is 3.5 + 0.6 hours and for N-acetylprocainamide is 6.3 + 1.5 hours. The therapeutic plasma concentration for procainamide is thought to be 4–10 µg/mL, for N-acetylprocainamide 7–15 µg/mL and for procainamide and NAPA together 10–30 µg/mL.[69] Intravenous propafenone, if available, should be reserved for horses with refractory ventricular tachycardia. Therapeutic plasma concentrations appear to be between 0.2 and 3.0 µg/mL in horses. Propranolol has negative inotropic effects and is rarely successful in converting horses with ventricular tachycardia. Propranolol should be tried, however, in horses that do not respond to other antiarrhythmics. Therapeutic plasma concentrations of propranolol are 20–80 ng/mL in horses.[31] Magnesium sulphate can be effective in refractory ventricular tachycardia in horses, particularly when used in conjunction with other antidysrhythmic agents.[72] Bretylium tosylate, if available, should be reserved for horses with severe, life-threatening ventricular tachycardia or ventricular fibrillation. Phenytoin, administered orally, can be effective in horses with ventricular tachycardia that is refractory to treatment with lignocaine and/or procainamide (see Table 7.1). The therapeutic plasma concentrations are 5–10 mg/L while sedation, recumbency and excitement can occur at higher plasma concentrations; thus, ideally, therapeutic drug monitoring is used to modify the dosage regimen in individual horses.[73] Amiodarone is indicated in human ventricular tachycardia and has been used successfully in one horse given 5 mg/kg/hour for 1 hour then 0.83 mg/kg/hour for 23 hours. Sinus rhythm was initially achieved within 24 hours; however, the ventricular tachycardia recurred, despite on-going treatment with phenytoin. For a second time, amiodarone successfully converted the horse to normal sinus rhythm.[70] No major side effects were noted in that horse but horses receiving amiodarone may develop hindlimb weakness, depression and diarrhoea.[51-53] (ACF, AF, VT)

REFERENCES

1. Reef VB, Bain FT, Spencer PA. Severe mitral regurgitation in horses: clinical, echocardiographic and pathological findings. Equine Vet J 1998;30:18–27.

2. Reef V. Pericardial and myocardial disease. In: Koblick C, Ames TR, Geor RJ, Trent AM, editors. The Horse: Diseases and Clinical Management. Edinburgh: Churchill Livingstone; 1993, p. 185–197.

3. Diana A, Guglielmini C, Candini D, et al. Cardiac arrhythmias associated with piroplasmosis in the horse: a case report. Vet J 2007;174:193–195.

4. Coudry V, Jean D, Desbois C, et al. Myocardial fibrosis in a horse with polymorphic ventricular tachycardia observed during general anesthesia. Can Vet J 2007;48:623–626.

5. Dickinson CE, Traub-Dargatz JL, Dargatz DA, et al. Rattlesnake venom poisoning in horses: 32 cases (1973–1993). J Am Vet Med Assoc 1996;208:1866–1871.

6. Wijnberg ID, van der Kolk JH, van Garderen E, et al. Atrial fibrillation associated with central nervous symptoms and colic in a horse: a case of equine cardiomyopathy. Vet Q 1998;20:73–76.

7. Aleman M, Magdesian KG, Peterson TS, et al. Salinomycin toxicosis in horses. J Am Vet Med Assoc 2007;230:1822–1826.

8. Bezerra P, Driemeier D, Loretti AP, Riet-Correa F, Kamphues J, de Barros CS. Monensin poisoning in Brazilian horses. Vet Hum Toxicol 1999;41:383–385.

9. Doonan G, Brown CM, Mullaney TP, et al. Monensin poisoning in horses. Can Vet J 1989;30:165–169.

10. Delesalle C, van Loon G, Nollet H, et al. Tumor-induced ventricular arrhythmia in a horse. J Vet Intern Med 2002;16:612–617.

11. MacLeay JM, Wilson JH. Type-II renal tubular acidosis and ventricular tachycardia in a horse. J Am Vet Med Assoc 1998;212:1597–1599.

12. Maxson-Sage A, Parente EJ, Beech J, et al. Effect of high-intensity exercise on arterial blood gas tensions and upper airway and cardiac function in clinically normal quarter horses and horses heterozygous and homozygous for hyperkalemic periodic paralysis. Am J Vet Res 1998;59:615–618.

13. Bright JM, Hellyer P. ECG of the month: atrial fibrillation. J Am Vet Med Assoc 2002;221:942–943.

14. Dolente BA, Seco OM, Lewis ML. Streptococcal toxic shock in a horse. J Am Vet Med Assoc 2000;217:64–67, 30.

15. Cornick JL, Seahorn TL. Cardiac arrhythmias identified in horses with duodenitis/proximal jejunitis: six cases (1985–1988). J Am Vet Med Assoc 1990;197:1054–1059.

16. Protopapas K. Studies on Metabolic Disturbances and other Post-Operative Complications Following Equine Colic Surgery. London: The Royal Veterinary College; 2000.

17. Wijnberg ID, van der Kolk JH, Hiddink EG. Use of phenytoin to treat digitalis-induced cardiac arrhythmias in a miniature Shetland pony. Vet Rec 1999;144:259–261.

18. Reimer JM, Reef VB, Sweeney RW. Ventricular arrhythmias in horses: 21 cases (1984–1989). J Am Vet Med Assoc 1992;201:1237–1243.

19. Bonagura J, Miller MS. Junctional and ventricular arrhythmias. J Equine Vet Sci 1985;5:347–350.

20. Bonagura J, Miller MS. Common conduction disturbances. J Equine Vet Sci 1986;6:23–25.

21. Miller M, Bonagura JD. Atrial arrhythmias. J Equine Vet Sci 1985;5:300–303.

22. Razavizadeh AT, Mashhadi AG, Paphan AA. The prevalence of cardiac dysrhythmias in Khozestan-Arab horses. Pak J Biol Sci 2007;10:3430–3434.

23. Reef VB, Clark ES, Oliver JA, et al. Implantation of a permanent transvenous pacing catheter in a horse with complete heart block and syncope. J Am Vet Med Assoc 1986;189:449–452.

24. Muir W. Anesthetic complications and cardiopulmonary resuscitation in the horse. In: Muir W, Hubbell JAE, editors. Equine Anesthesia Monitoring and Emergency Therapy. St Louis: Mosby; 1991, p. 461–484.

25. Whitton DL, Trim CM. Use of dopamine hydrochloride during general anesthesia in the treatment of advanced atrioventricular heart block in four foals. J Am Vet Med Assoc 1985;187:1357–1361.

26. Pibarot P, Vrins A, Salmon Y. Implantation of a programmable atrioventricular pacenaker in a donkey with complete atrioventricular block and syncope. Equine Vet J 1993;25:248–251.

27. Sugiyama A, Takeuchi T, Morita T, et al. Mediastinal lymphoma with complete atrioventricular block in a horse. J Vet Med Sci 2008;70:1101–1105.

28. Lawler JB, Frye MA, Bera MM, et al. Third-degree atrioventricular block in a horse secondary to rattlesnake envenomation. J Vet Intern Med 2008;22:486–490.

29. Rezakhani A, Godarzi M, Tabatabei Naeini I. A combination of atrioventricular block and sinoatrial block in a horse. Acta Vet Scand 2005;46:173–175.

30. van Loon G, Fonteyne W, Rottiers H, et al. Implantation of a dual-chamber, rate-adaptive pacemaker in a horse with suspected sick sinus syndrome. Vet Rec 2002;151:541–545.

31. McGuirk SM, Muir WW. Diagnosis and treatment of cardiac arrhythmias. Vet Clin North Am Equine Pract 1985;1:353–370.

32. Baggott J. The pharmacological basis of cardiac drug selection for use in horses. Equine Vet J Suppl 1995;19:97–100.

33. Schwarzwald CC, Bonagura JD, Luis-Fuentes V. Effects of diltiazem on hemodynamic variables and ventricular function in healthy horses. J Vet Intern Med 2005;19:703–711.

34. Schwarzwald CC, Hamlin RL, Bonagura JD, et al. Atrial, SA nodal, and AV nodal electrophysiology in standing horses: normal findings and electrophysiologic effects of quinidine and diltiazem. J Vet Intern Med 2007;21:166–175.

35. Deem DA, Fregin GF. Atrial fibrillation in horses: a review of 106 clinical cases, with consideration of prevalence, clinical signs, and prognosis. J Am Vet Med Assoc 1982;180:261–265.

36. Reef VB, Levitan CW, Spencer PA. Factors affecting prognosis and conversion in equine atrial fibrillation. J Vet Intern Med 1988;2:1–6.

37. Reef VB, Reimer JM, Spencer PA. Treatment of atrial fibrillation in horses: new perspectives. J Vet Intern Med 1995;9:57–67.

38. Ohmura H, Hiraga A, Takahashi T, et al. Risk factors for atrial fibrillation during racing in slow-finishing horses. J Am Vet Med Assoc 2003;223:84–88.

39. Holmes JR, Henigan M, Williams RB, et al. Paroxysmal atrial fibrillation in racehorses. Equine Vet J 1986;18:37–42.

40. Holmes J, Darker PGG, Else RW. Atrial fibrillation in the horse. Equine vet J 1968;1:212–222.

41. Marr CM, Reef VB, Reimer JM, et al. An echocardiographic study of atrial fibrillation in horses: before and after conversion to sinus rhythm. J Vet Intern Med 1995;9:336–340.

42. Gehlen H, Stadler P. Comparison of systolic cardiac function before and after treatment of atrial fibrillation in horses with and without additional cardiac valve insufficiencies. Vet Res Commun 2004;28:317–329.

43. De Clercq D, van Loon G, Tavernier R, et al. Atrial and ventricular electrical and contractile remodeling and reverse remodeling owing to short-term pacing-induced atrial fibrillation in horses. J Vet Intern Med 2008;22:1353–1359.

44. Muir WW 3rd, Reed SM, McGuirk SM. Treatment of atrial fibrillation in horses by intravenous administration of quinidine. J Am

Vet Med Assoc 1990;197:1607–1610.

45. McGuirk S, Muir WW, Sams RA. Pharmacokinetic analysis of intravenously and orally administered quinidine in horses. Am J Vet Res 1981;42:938–942.

46. Parraga ME, Kittleson MD, Drake CM. Quinidine administration increases steady state serum digoxin concentration in horses. Equine Vet J Suppl 1995:114–119.

47. McGurrin MK, Physick-Sheard PW, Kenney DG. Transvenous electrical cardioversion of equine atrial fibrillation: patient factors and clinical results in 72 treatment episodes. J Vet Intern Med 2008;22:609–615.

48. McGurrin MK, Physick-Sheard PW, Kenney DG, et al. Transvenous electrical cardioversion of equine atrial fibrillation: technical considerations. J Vet Intern Med 2005;19:695–702.

49. McGurrin MK, Physick-Sheard PW, Kenney DG, et al. Transvenous electrical cardioversion in equine atrial fibrillation: technique and successful treatment of 3 horses. J Vet Intern Med 2003;17:715–718.

50. De Clercq D, van Loon G, Schauvliege S, et al. Transvenous electrical cardioversion of atrial fibrillation in six horses using custom made cardioversion catheters. Vet J 2008;177:198–204.

51. De Clercq D, Baert K, Croubels S, et al. Evaluation of the pharmacokinetics and bioavailability of intravenously and orally administered amiodarone in horses. Am J Vet Res 2006;67:448–454.

52. De Clercq D, van Loon G, Baert K, et al. Intravenous amiodarone treatment in horses with chronic atrial fibrillation. Vet J 2006;172:129–134.

53. De Clercq D, van Loon G, Baert K, et al. Effects of an adapted intravenous amiodarone treatment protocol in horses with atrial fibrillation. Equine Vet J 2007;39:344–349.

54. van Loon G, Blissitt KJ, Keen JA, et al. Use of intravenous flecainide in horses with naturally-occurring atrial fibrillation. Equine Vet J 2004;36:609–614.

55. Ohmura H, Hiraga A, Aida H, et al. Determination of oral dosage and pharmacokinetic analysis of flecainide in horses. J Vet Med Sci 2001;63:511–514.

56. Risberg AI, McGuirk SM. Successful conversion of equine atrial fibrillation using oral flecainide. J Vet Intern Med 2006;20:207–209.

57. Robinson S, Feary DJ. Sudden death following oral administration of flecainide to horses with naturally occuring atrial fibrillation. Aust Equine Vet 2008;27:49–51.

58. Schwarzwald CC, Schober KE, Bonagura JD. Echocardiographic evidence of left atrial mechanical dysfunction after conversion of atrial fibrillation to sinus rhythm in 5 horses. J Vet Intern Med 2007;21:820–827.

59. Muir WW, McGuirk SM. Pharmacology and pharmacokinetics of drugs used to treat cardiac disease in horses. Vet Clin North Am Equine Pract 1985;1:335–352.

60. Muir W, Bednarski RM. Equine cardiopulmonary resuscitation – part II. Compend Contin Educ Pract Vet 1983;5:S287–S295.

61. Cooper S. Ventricular pre-excitation Wolff-Parkinson-White syndrome in a horse. Vet Rec 1962;74:527.

62. Delahanty D, Glazier DB. The Wolff-Parkinson-White syndrome in a a horse. Ir Vet J 1959;13:295.

63. Glazier D. The Wolff-Parkinson-White syndrome in a racing Thoroughbred. Ir Vet J 1966;22:214.

64. Muir WW, McGuirk SM. Ventricular preexcitation in two horses. J Am Vet Med Assoc 1983;183:573–576.

65. Marriott H, Conover MB. The other broads. In: Marriott H, Conover MB, editors. Advanced Concepts in Arrhythmias. 3rd ed. St Louis: Mosby; 1998, p. 261–292.

66. Marr CM, Reef VB, Brazil TJ, et al. Aorto-cardiac fistulas in seven horses. Vet Radiol Ultrasound 1998;39:22–31.

67. Arnold CE, Payne M, Thompson JA, et al. Periparturient hemorrhage in mares: 73 cases (1998–2005). J Am Vet Med Assoc 2008;232:1345–1351.

68. Groh W, Zipes DP. Neurological disorders and cardiovascular disease. In: Zipes DP, Libby P, Bonow RO, Braunwald E, editors. Braunwald's Heart Disease: A Textbook of Cardiovascular Medicine. 7th ed. Philadelphia: Elsevier Saunders; 2005, p. 2145–2160.

69. Ellis E, Ravis WR, Malloy M. Pharmacokinetics and pharmacodynamics of procainamide in horses after intravenous administration. J Vet Pharmacol Ther 1994;17:265–270.

70. De Clercq D, van Loon G, Baert K, et al. Treatment with amiodarone of refractory ventricular tachycardia in a horse. J Vet Intern Med 2007;21:878–880.

71. Puigdemont A, Riu JL, Guitart R, et al. Propafenone kinetics in the horse: comparative analysis of compartmental and noncompartmental models. J Pharmacol Methods 1990;23:79–85.

72. Marr CM, Reef VB. ECG of the month. J Am Vet Med Assoc 1991;198:1533–1534.

73. Wijnberg ID, Ververs FF. Phenytoin sodium as a treatment for ventricular dysrhythmia in horses. J Vet Intern Med 2004;18:350–353.

Chapter | 14 |

Dysrhythmias: cardiac pacing and electrical cardioversion

Gunther van Loon

INTRODUCTION

Cardiac cells, due to their excitable properties, are capable of being depolarized by an external stimulus such as an electrical pulse. Such depolarization will only occur if the external stimulus has sufficient strength to reach the threshold for stimulation and provided that the stimulus is not delivered while the cell is in a refractory period.[1,2] As atria and ventricles act as a pseudosyncytium, depolarization of a few atrial or ventricular cells leads to depolarization of the whole atrium or ventricle, respectively. As such, by delivering electrical stimuli at a precise location in or around the heart, one can selectively induce atrial or ventricular contractions at a specific rate and this is called atrial or ventricular pacing. Certain pacing techniques can be performed in the standing, unsedated horse without being sensed as the required electrical stimuli are of relatively low intensity.

It is possible to depolarize nearly the whole atrium or ventricle at once using a high-energy direct current shock from a capacitor discharge. The whole myocardium is instantaneously brought into a refractory state, and this technique can be used to treat certain tachyarrhythmias such as atrial or ventricular fibrillation. This procedure is called electrical defibrillation (in case of ventricular fibrillation) or electrical cardioversion (in case of other tachyarrhythmias). Required energy levels are high and render the technique impossible to be performed without general anaesthesia. It is critical that the clinician is aware that delivery of an electrical pulse or shock with inappropriate amplitude, duration or timing may induce unwanted or even dangerous arrhythmias.

CARDIAC PACING

During pacing, current pulses with specific amplitude, duration and interval are transmitted to the atrium or ventricle via appropriately positioned electrodes. Only when the current is able to reduce the resting potential of the cardiac cell by a critical amount and within a critical time, will "capture" be achieved, which means that a depolarization of that chamber will follow. The intensity of the electrical pulse required to reach the threshold for stimulation is determined mainly by the position of the electrodes in relation to the heart. This intensity is expressed by the pacing amplitude (strength, V) and the pulse width (duration, ms) of the electrical stimulus. A stimulus that is large in amplitude requires a shorter duration to reach threshold, and vice versa. At a given pulse duration, the corresponding threshold amplitude can be easily determined by the stimulus reduction method. With a fixed pulse duration, pacing is started at a high amplitude, which results in consistent capture. Every few beats the amplitude is gradually reduced until, finally, capture is lost. The

© 2010 Elsevier Ltd.
DOI: 10.1016/B978-0-7020-2817-5.00019-5

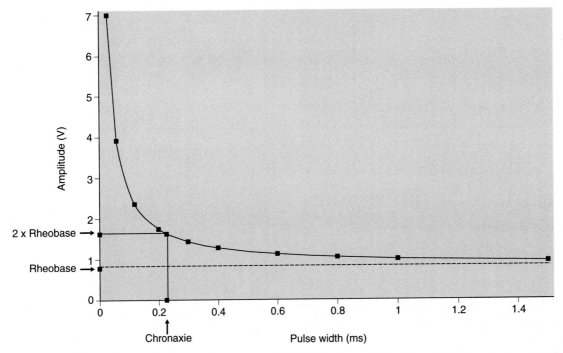

Figure 14.1 A strength-duration curve from a temporary atrial lead in a horse displays the combinations of pulse strength and duration above which consistent capture is achieved. The rheobase is the lowest voltage at (infinitely) long pulse duration that results in capture. The chronaxie is the threshold pulse width at twice rheobase.

lowest amplitude resulting in capture represents the threshold value for that pulse duration. Similarly, the threshold pulse duration can be determined for a fixed pulse amplitude. Threshold values describe a hyperbolic-like strength-duration curve (Fig. 14.1), which is a means of verifying that a given electrode position is likely to achieve safe and effective cardiac pacing.[2] Two important features of the strength-duration curve are the rheobase and chronaxie. The rheobase is the lowest voltage that results in capture at "infinitely" long pulse duration (usually less than 1.5 ms). The chronaxie is the required pulse width when pacing at two times the rheobase voltage. When two random points of the strength-duration curve are determined, the rheobase, the chronaxie and the remaining points of the curve can be calculated using the following equation[3]:

$$I = Ir(1 + tc/t)$$

where I is the stimulus intensity (voltage or current), t the pulse width, Ir the rheobase and tc the chronaxie.

It is critical that a stimulus is not delivered near the end of the refractory period, i.e. the "vulnerable" period, because this might initiate fibrillation[4] and is extremely dangerous in case of ventricular stimulation. For this reason, most pulse generators (pacemakers) are able to "sense" each cardiac depolarization, thereby temporarily inhibiting the pacing function.

ELECTRODES

Cardiac pacing techniques can be subdivided depending on: (1) the polarity of the electrodes (unipolar or bipolar), (2) the location of the electrodes (transcutaneous, trans-oesophageal, epicardial, endomyocardial) and (3) the duration of pacing (temporary or permanent).

An electrical current flows between two electrodes, the cathode and the anode. The number of electrodes in contact with or close to the heart determines whether unipolar or bipolar pacing is performed. The electrode nearest to the myocardium should be the cathode (negative) because cathodal stimulation is less likely to induce arrhythmias.[5] For unipolar pacing, one electrode, the cathode, is in contact with the heart while the second electrode is at a remote site of the heart. In case of bipolar pacing, cathode and anode are, within a short distance of each other, in contact with the heart. Unipolar pacing results in a much larger pacing artifact on the surface ECG and is more likely to induce skeletal muscle stimulation (near the anode) than bipolar pacing. Finally, recording an intracardiac ECG through a unipolar lead is more susceptible to muscle potential artifacts than bipolar recordings.

Electrode size and especially location determine which cardiac chamber will be stimulated and which pulse inten-

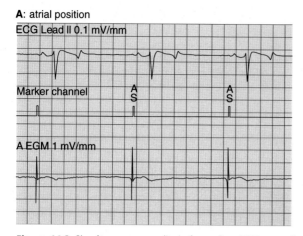
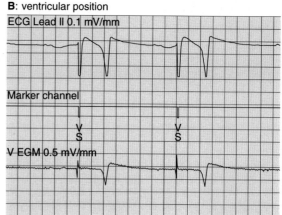

Figure 14.2 Simultaneous recording of a surface ECG, a marker channel and an intracardiac electrogram in a horse. With an atrial (**A**) or ventricular (**B**) position of the electrode, the largest deflection on the intra-atrial (A-EGM) or intraventricular (V-EGM) electrogram coincides with a P wave or QRS complex on the surface ECG, respectively. The marker channel indicates when atrial (AS) or ventricular (VS) sensing occurs.

sity will be required to reach the threshold for stimulation. Electrodes at remote distance from the heart, such as transcutaneous electrodes, will require a rather high pulse intensity. As such, pacing will be sensed by the patient rendering the technique inapplicable in conscious horses. There is no available information regarding transoesophageal pacing in horses, but most likely, the technique is not applicable in the conscious horse, due to the larger distance between oesophagus and atrium or ventricle compared to humans. Electrodes in close contact with the heart (epicardial or endomyocardial) will require such little intensity to achieve consistent capture that stimulation is not sensed by the patient and this method has been most widely applied in equine cardiology.

During right atrial pacing, electrodes located near the phrenic nerve can result in hiccups during atrial pacing, especially at higher pacing thresholds. As the nerve cannot be easily identified by ultrasonography, testing stimuli should be applied at higher strength-duration values to determine whether diaphragmatic stimulation occurs, and if so, the right atrial electrode must be repositioned.

The most suitable and safest approach for atrial and ventricular pacing in horses utilizes a lead or catheter with electrodes on its tip, inserted transvenously and positioned in the respective right cardiac chambers, to allow stimulation of the endomyocardium.[6] Due to the close contact between electrode and myocardium, a minimal amount of energy, usually between 0.5 and 7.5 V and 0.3 and 1.2 ms, is sufficient to achieve consistent capture. Therefore, pacing will not be sensed by the patient. Positioning of the electrode is guided by fluoroscopy and echocardiography. In addition, the electrode position is verified by recording the intracavitary electrogram from the lead simultaneously with a surface ECG.[6] During trans-

venous insertion of the lead the intracavitary electrogram will successively show: (1) no or minimal deflections during passage through the vein, (2) a deflection simultaneous with the P wave from the surface ECG during right atrial positioning (Fig. 14.2A) and (3) a deflection simultaneous with the QRS complex when located in the right ventricle (see Fig. 14.2B). Additionally, electrode position is verified by connecting the lead with a pacing device and applying testing stimuli of sufficient strength. An intravenous position will not result in capture, while an atrial or ventricular position will produce a P wave or QRS complex, respectively.

Temporary pacing is achieved with a temporary lead or catheter that possesses (at least) two closely spaced electrodes at the tip to obtain bipolar pacing. The lead is transvenously inserted and the external part of the lead is connected with an external pacing device from which pacing rate and pulse strength and duration can be adapted. On the other hand, permanent pacing requires permanently implanted pacing device (pacemaker) and leads. It is crucial for this system that the electrodes remain in a secure position. To maintain transvenously inserted endocardial electrodes in a stable position, implantable leads have a fixation mechanism to preserve endocardial contact. Available options are either active fixation leads that invade the endomyocardium with a screw or small jaw or passive fixation leads that have little tines of fins to enhance entanglement in trabeculae of the myocardium. In horses, the atrial lead should have active fixation because in the large equine right atrium, a passive fixation lead is very likely to drop ventrally towards the right ventricle, resulting in loss of atrial capture. Although it is also advisable to use an active fixation lead for the equine ventricle, the ventrally located lead tip in the right ventricular apex can remain in position even with a passive fixation tip.

THERAPEUTIC USE OF PACING

Permanent pacing

Bradydysrhythmias such as third-degree AV block and sick sinus syndrome are the major indications for permanent pacing, requiring implantation of an artificial pacemaker.[7] The pacemaker is a multi-programmable and implantable battery-powered pacing device. It is connected with one or more leads towards the right atrium or ventricle (single chamber pacemaker) or towards both (dual chamber pacemaker) to stimulate a specific chamber at a specific rate (e.g. 35 bpm) so that symptomatic bradycardia is avoided. However, because an intrinsic atrial and/or ventricular rhythm might still be present, pacemakers have the ability to sense this intrinsic rate via the implanted leads and can be programmed to respond in a specific way to an intrinsic beat. Besides the treatment of bradydysrhythmias, in humans, pacemaker implantation is also used to prevent induction of certain tachydysrhythmias.[8] However, this technique has never been used in horses.

Pacemaker types are described using a three-letter code, with an optional fourth or even fifth letter. The first and second position indicate the chamber being paced and sensed, respectively: A (atrium), V (ventricle), D (double, both) or O (none). Manufacturers occasionally use the S to indicate that the device is capable of pacing/sensing only a single chamber. The third position denotes the reaction of the pacemaker when an intrinsic beat is sensed: I (inhibited) when pacing is inhibited by a sensed beat, T (triggered) when pacing is triggered, D (dual, both) for a dual mode of response, or O (none) when the pacemaker does not react on a sensed signal. The fourth position of the code may reflect the programmability of the device but is most frequently used to indicate that the pacemaker incorporates a sensor for rate modulation (R). Such a sensor detects changes in pressure, temperature, oxygen saturation, ventilation or detects patient activity and is capable of adapting the pacing rate towards an upper or lower limit. The fifth letter is rarely used and is restricted to antitachycardia functions: P (antitachycardia pacing), S (direct current shock), D (dual, P+S), or O (none). After implantation multiple pacing and sensing parameters can be adapted by telemetric (transcutaneous) programming of the pacemaker. Telemetric access requires the pacemaker to be implanted at a short distance from the skin at a location where it does not get damaged or hamper the animal to move or lie down.

Depending on the kind of dysrhythmia, different types of pacemakers can be applied. If the cause of bradycardia is a depressed or absent AV node conduction, a "simple", single chamber (ventricular) pacemaker can be implanted. When this pacemaker is programmed to the VVI mode, with a minimal ventricular rate of, for example, 35 beats per minute, syncope will be prevented by preserving this minimal heart rate. However, no adaptation of heart rate to the physical needs (e.g. exercise) will occur. Rate-modulation, for example, based upon an activity sensor, is achieved with a VVIR pacemaker. However, much more efficient in case of a third-degree AV block, is to implant a dual chamber pacemaker. Such a pacemaker can be programmed to prevent a too slow atrial and ventricular rate but also to "look for" (sense) an intrinsic atrial depolarisation and to deliver (trigger) a ventricular stimulus for each sensed atrial signal, which is achieved in the DDD function (Fig. 14.3). As sinus node function in an animal with third-degree AV block is usually intact, a fairly normal paced ventricular rate, which adapts with stress or exercise, can then be obtained. If bradycardia is caused by an abnormal sinus node function, adaptation of pacing rate with exercise can only be achieved by using a pacemaker with an incorporated sensor (e.g. VVIR, DDIR).

In horses, both epicardial and transvenous lead placement has been described. The epicardial lead placement requires general anaesthesia and thoracotomy, which implies a risk, especially in an animal with a compromised cardiovascular system.[9,10] This method has successfully been applied in a healthy pony and in two donkeys with third-degree AV block for implantation of a single chamber or dual chamber pacemaker.[11,12,13] The pacemaker device was inserted underneath the pectoral muscle or, subcutaneously, caudal to the left elbow. In the donkeys, successful pacing was obtained for 6 weeks in one and more than 1 year in the other. During an attempt to place an epicardial lead in a mature horse with third-degree AV block, the horse developed ventricular fibrillation during general anaesthesia and died.[14]

Transvenous lead placement is a much safer and simpler procedure to achieve cardiac pacing and is widely used in human and small animal medicine. It requires a vein that is located relatively close to the heart (maximal lead length is around 110 cm), that is large enough to introduce one or two leads and that can be ligated permanently. A standardized approach has been described to implant a dual chamber pacemaker via the cephalic vein.[6] As the whole procedure can be performed in the standing, sedated horse, the additional risk of anaesthesia can be avoided. During the implantation procedure, an atrial and a ventricular active fixation lead are inserted through a surgically exposed cephalic vein. Lead placement is guided by both echocardiography and by measuring the electrical characteristics of the lead. After permanent ligation of the vein a pacemaker pocket is created between the lateral pectoral groove and the *manubrium sterni*. Successful clinical application of transvenous lead placement was first

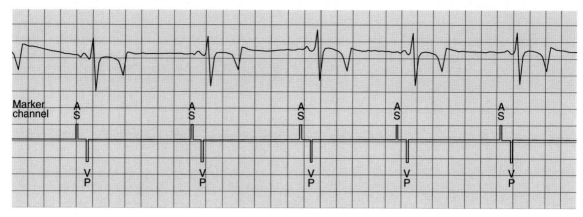

Figure 14.3 During DDD pacing, every atrial spontaneous depolarization is sensed (AS), which triggers a ventricular paced beat (VP).

reported by Reef et al.,[15] implanting a single chamber (ventricular) pacemaker in a horse with third-degree AV block. Under general anaesthesia, a passive fixation lead was inserted in the jugular vein and placed in the right ventricular apex under echocardiographic guidance. The pacemaker pocket was created dorsal to the jugular vein. Although the horse remained asymptomatic, 16 months later, a second lead with active fixation was implanted in the right atrium and the pacemaker was updated to a dual chamber model, allowing AV sequential pacing of the ventricles. Consequently, a physiological rate response to exercise and stress occurred. With the dual chamber pacemaker the horse was able to perform exercise with a maximal achievable heart rate of 150 beats per minute. About 3 years after the initial implantation, however, the horse suddenly died due to a suppurative endocarditis and suspected terminal bacteraemia.[16] Implantation of a dual chamber rate-adaptive pacemaker has also been used in a horse with post-exercise bradycardia and syncope due to sinus node dysfunction.[17] At 7-year follow-up, proper dual chamber pacing was still achieved.

Temporary pacing

Short-term therapeutic pacing is generally applied as a temporary solution for bradydysrhythmias, e.g. prior to the implantation of a permanent pacemaker and during neonatal cardiopulmonary resuscitation. On rare occasions, it can also be used to terminate certain tachydysrhythmias. Temporary pacing is achieved with an external, temporary pacing device, connected to two electrodes (bipolar pacing) which are positioned near the heart, usually near the ventricles, in order to accelerate ventricular rate. The closer the electrodes are positioned to the heart, the smaller the pulse intensity required to elicit a ventricular depolarization, and thus the better pacing will

be tolerated. Although little information is available in equine medicine, transcutaneous and transoesophageal pacing are likely to be poorly tolerated in the conscious adult horse and therefore only applicable during general anaesthesia, but transcutaneous temporary pacing can be used successfully in sick, obtunded foals. (SBR)

A transvenously inserted catheter, electrode or lead within the right atrium or right ventricle can directly stimulate the endomyocardium, requiring only low pulse intensity, and is a safe and effective means to obtain consistent cardiac pacing. As the pacing stimuli are not sensed by the horse the technique can be used without sedation or anaesthesia. Temporary transvenous pacing has been used in horses with symptomatic bradycardia to avoid syncope prior to the permanent implantation of a pacemaker.[13–15,17,18] Transvenous temporary pacing has also been used to treat transient asystole following electrical cardioversion of atrial fibrillation (AF) in a horse.[19]

In human beings, temporary pacing is also used to terminate tachydysrhythmias such as atrial flutter, AV node tachycardia and sustained ventricular tachycardia.[7] During such a transvenous overdrive pacing procedure, a train of electrical pulses is repeatedly given at a fixed rate in excess of the basic natural rhythm. The purpose is to entrain and interrupt the tachydysrhythmia by depolarizing regions of the excitable gap of the re-entry cycle.[8,20] This technique has been successfully applied in a horse with persistent, medically resistant atrial flutter.[21] In this horse, right atrial pacing at a rate slightly higher (300 ms cycle length) than the atrial flutter rate (365 ms cycle length) terminated the re-entry phenomenon and re-established sinus rhythm. The procedure was performed in the standing unsedated horse and was well tolerated. However, because overdrive pacing can accelerate tachycardia and result in fibrillation, the technique is not recommended for ventricular tachycardia in horses.

NONTHERAPEUTIC USE OF PACING

Nontherapeutic pacing in horses has been applied to study atrial and ventricular electrophysiological properties and to investigate the pathophysiology and treatment of cardiac dysrhythmias. Short-term or long-term research studies have been carried out using temporary pacing or permanent pacemaker implantation, respectively.

Specific pacing protocols can be used to investigate electrophysiological properties of the heart. Atrial pacing at a constant, regular rate documents the ventricular response, and thus AV node conduction,[22,23] and can be used to determine the sinus node recovery time (SNRT), defined as the longest time it takes for the first spontaneous P wave to occur after termination of atrial pacing.[24,25] Because the SNRT largely depends on the basic sinus cycle length (BCL), a correction (c) can be made: cSNRT = SNRT − BCL.

Programmed electrical stimulation protocols estimate the atrial effective refractory period (AERP) or ventricular effective refractory period (VERP). Because the ERP changes at different rates, regular atrial (or ventricular) pacing (S1–S1) is first started at a specific rate, e.g. 75 stimuli per minute representing a pacing cycle length of 800 ms (S1–S1 = 800 ms). Subsequently, a premature atrial or ventricular stimulus (S2) at two or three times threshold is delivered with a coupling (S1–S2) interval shorter than the expected refractory period. If stimulation occurs during the atrial or ventricular refractory period, "capture" will not occur (Figs.14.4A, 14.5A). Subsequently, the S1–S2 interval is increased in a stepwise manner until S2 produces a following P' or QRS' complex, i.e. capture occurs (see Figs. 14.4B, 14.5B). The longest S1–S2 interval without capture is taken as the AERP or VERP. In normal horses and ponies, at a basic pacing cycle length of 1000 ms, the right AERP is around 200–300 ms[24,25] and the right VERP is around 270–440 ms (G. van Loon, unpublished results). Both AERP and VERP display physiological rate adaptation, whereby the ERP shortens at higher rates. For example, at a pacing CL of 500 ms (120 bpm), AERP and VERP are 170–300 ms and 220–300 ms, respectively (G. van Loon, unpublished results).

The extrastimulus method, applied during the ERP measurement, may result in rapid responses, such as tachycardia, flutter or fibrillation. The S1–S2 interval at which these rapid responses occur indicates the vulnerable period. For the atria, this vulnerable period is between 140 and 420 ms.[26] In healthy horses, application of the extrastimulus method at different pacing rates in the right ventricle did not result in any repetitive responses (G. van Loon, unpublished data).

Atrial pacing at a very rapid rate (e.g. at 20–30 Hz), which is called burst pacing, can result in a short-lasting, self-terminating episode of AF. In healthy horses such

A: no atrial capture

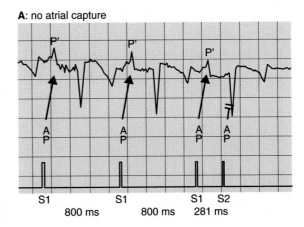

B: atrial capture

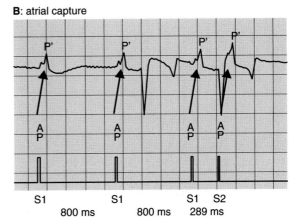

Figure 14.4 During atrial pacing (AP) at a driving cycle length (S1–S1) of 800 ms (75 bpm), an extrastimulus (S2) at 281 ms does not result in atrial capture (**A**), while an extrastimulus at 289 ms results in capture (**B**). AERP$_{800}$ in this horse is 281 ms.

acutely induced AF will generally last for a few seconds to a few hours. Determining the inducibility and duration of this short-term AF episode provides information about the vulnerability and susceptibility to the arrhythmia.[25–28] Once an acute episode of AF is initiated, changes in cardiac function, such as ventricular response and cardiac output, can be studied[29] and the effect of antiarrhythmic drugs can be evaluated.[30] However, because of major differences between acute and chronic AF[31] long-term pacing models have been developed to study chronic AF in horses.[25,32] By implanting a pacemaker or pulse generator, long-term, repetitive burst pacing induces repeated bouts of AF and due to remodelling of the atria, a progressive increase in AF susceptibility will eventually lead to self-sustained, persistent AF to create a model for the study of the pathophysiology of chronic AF.

A: no ventricular capture

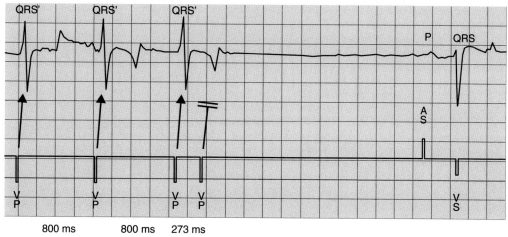

800 ms   800 ms   273 ms

B: ventricular capture

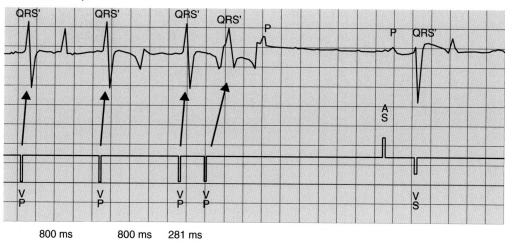

800 ms   800 ms   281 ms

Figure 14.5 Regular ventricular pacing (VP) is performed at 75 bpm (800 ms pacing cycle length). Because an extrastimulus does not result in ventricular capture (**A**) at 273 ms but produces a QRS′ complex when delivered at 281 ms, VERP$_{800}$ is 273 ms. After termination of the test spontaneous P waves and QRS complexes are sensed by the pacing device (AS, VS).

Burst pacing has also been used to induce ventricular fibrillation in horses in order to investigate different defibrillation techniques.[33,34] Although rapid ventricular pacing is frequently used in human patients and in other animal models to determine ventricular vulnerability and to investigate potential treatments for ventricular fibrillation, no further studies in equine subjects have been performed because the arrhythmia is generally fatal, whatever treatment is used.

ELECTRICAL DEFIBRILLATION/ CARDIOVERSION

Electrical defibrillation (DF) and electrical cardioversion (CV) are techniques to abolish fibrillation and certain tachycardias by means of a direct current (DC) electrical shock. The term defibrillation is used for the treatment of ventricular fibrillation, where QRS complexes are no longer discernible and shock delivery should be performed as soon as possible. The term cardioversion is used for all other, more "organised" arrhythmias, where QRS complexes are still present. In these circumstances cardioversion always has to be synchronized with the R wave to avoid shock delivery during the ventricular vulnerable period, i.e. near the T wave. Shock delivery during this vulnerable period may initiate ventricular tachyarrhythmias, such as ventricular fibrillation.[35,36] Most defibrillators use a surface ECG or an ECG via the defibrillation electrodes to detect the R wave of the QRS complex when in synchronous mode (Fig. 14.6A). In the text below the term DF will be used, unless specifically dealing with CV.

The electrical discharge, measured in joules (J) or Watt-second, is produced by a capacitor discharge from the electrical defibrillator. One joule is the amount of energy released in one second by a current of 1 ampere through a resistance of 1 ohm. In human patients, different waveforms have been used to achieve electrical DF. Historically, monophasic waveforms were used and here the electrical current flows in one direction, from the positive to negative electrode. The most commonly used monophasic damped sinusoidal (MDS) wave gradually returns to zero current flow (Fig. 14.7A), while the monophasic truncated exponential (MTE) wave is terminated before current flow reaches zero (see Fig. 14.7B). Monophasic waves, particularly MDS waves, have a high peak current that can damage

cardiac tissue or alter automaticity or conduction. Nowadays biphasic defibrillators are established as the waveform of choice because of higher efficacy at lower energy levels and lower peak currents. During a biphasic shock, the electrical current flows from one electrode to the other and then back in the opposite direction. Two main types of waveforms are used, the biphasic truncated exponential (BTE) (see Fig. 14.7C) and the rectilinear biphasic (RLB) wave (see Fig. 14.7D); both have comparable efficacy.

Although the exact mechanism is not fully understood, the underlying principle is that the electrical shock traverses the myocardium and causes total depolarization, often resulting in an instantaneous conversion of any tachydysrhythmia. The electrodes must be positioned so that the electrical current traverses as much fibrillating tissue as possible. External DF is achieved by placement of adhesive electrodes or paddles on the skin, whereas in internal DF electrodes are placed directly on the cardiac surface ("direct heart") or are inserted in the cardiac cavities, the pulmonary artery or the coronary sinus (e.g. transvenous electrical DF).

Factors that influence the success of DF include electrical resistance and resultant current flow, electrode size, energy level, current waveform, body weight, metabolic abnormalities and duration and nature of the arrhythmia.[37] The better the electrical contact with the patient, the less resistance there will be to discharge and the higher the resultant current that flows for a specific shock voltage.[38] Therefore,

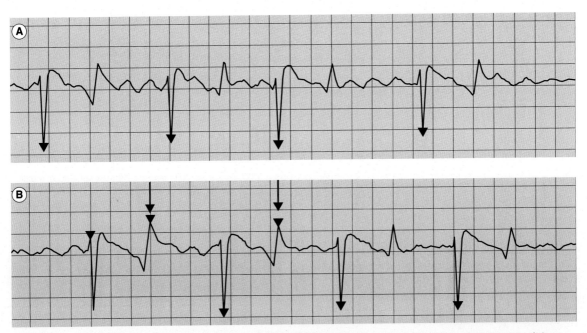

Figure 14.6 When operating in synchronous mode, the defibrillator displays marks (arrow heads) on each R wave of the surface ECG (**A**). False interpretation of a T wave (arrows) (**B**) necessitates a change in surface electrode configuration to achieve proper R wave detection in this horse with atrial fibrillation.

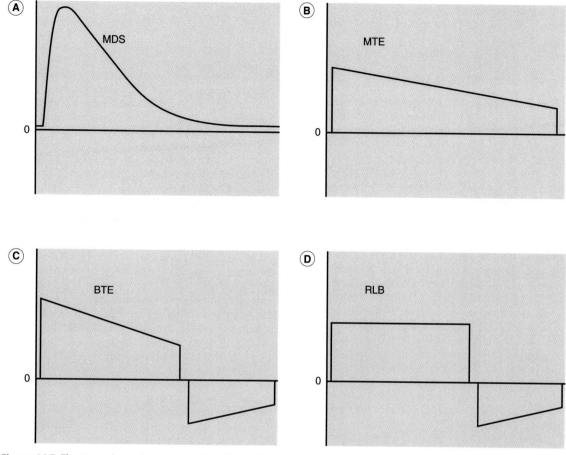

Figure 14.7 The monophasic shock can be (**A**) a damped sinusoidal wave (MDS) or (**B**) a truncated exponential wave (MTE) while the biphasic shock can be delivered as (**C**) a biphasic truncated exponential wave (BTE) or (**D**) a rectilinear biphasic (RLB) wave.

the skin is clipped and electroconductive gel is generously applied.[39] This also explains why internal DF requires much lower energy levels. Electrodes should have a large surface in order to diminish electrical resistance[40] and to reduce local peak current. One of the requirements for efficient electrode configuration is to encompass most of the fibrillating tissue between the electrodes,[41,42] so the electrical current need not pass through poorly conducting structures such as air-filled lungs, fat and bone. These insulating structures do not need to be crossed during internal DF, and therefore reduces energy requirements. In addition, the air-filled lungs may act as an insulator and confine the current to traversing the heart in internal DF.[41] Finally, a larger body weight and cardiac size of the patient requires higher energy levels to achieve DF[33,43] and this factor is clearly relevant in equine patients. Whatever technique or electrode position is used, shock delivery of this magnitude is too painful to be used in the awake horse and always necessitates general anaesthesia.

The most important risk is when a shock is delivered near the T wave, which is the most vulnerable phase of the ventricle, and can easily induce ventricular tachyarrhythmias, in particular ventricular fibrillation. Therefore, if QRS complexes are still present, the defibrillator should be switched to "synchronous mode". In this mode, the device automatically recognizes the QRS complex and ensures that the shock is delivered on the R wave of the surface ECG (see Fig. 14.6A). However, in horses, extreme care should be taken as the large T wave is easily misinterpreted by the defibrillator as an R wave (see Fig. 14.6B) which could lead to shock delivery on the T wave. In order to avoid this, surface ECG electrodes must be repositioned carefully in each patient to achieve accurate R wave detection. The device should also be activated immediately after a T wave has been observed and, therefore, in synchronous mode, it will deliver the shock on the next automatically detected complex, i.e. the R wave.

The most important arrhythmias in equine medicine in which a DC shock might be applied are ventricular fibrillation and atrial fibrillation.

Ventricular fibrillation

Ventricular fibrillation is a fatal arrhythmia that can be encountered in various situations. Although external DF is very successful in humans and small animals, it is not effective in large animals such as horses. Due to the large thorax of horses, the electrodes become further apart, thereby increasing the impedance and reducing the current flow through the heart. Because horses have a larger heart-to-body-weight ratio than other, smaller mammals, a larger cardiac mass has to be defibrillated.[33] In addition, the energy requirement for ventricular DF per kilogram of body weight in mature horses is much higher than for other species and also higher than for foals. For external DF in foals, ventricular defibrillation was achieved by delivering 1–2 J per kg body weight, using large surface paddles, placed on each side of the thorax.[44] In one report of successful DF in two "horses" with experimentally induced ventricular fibrillation, body weight was only 277 and 340 kg, shock electrodes were pre-implanted subcutaneously and the applied monophasic shock energy was 3500 and 4500 J, corresponding to more than 10 J per kg body weight.[33] Current commercially available defibrillators, with a maximal energy level of 360 J, are therefore unlikely to be efficacious in mature horses even when biphasic shocks are used.[45]

Aiming to reduce impedance and energy requirements, "direct heart" DF[34] has been studied in horses after artificial induction of ventricular fibrillation. A successful outcome was only achieved in a 140-kg pony delivering 250 J and 360 J. All attempts to defibrillate larger horses were unsuccessful.

Atrial fibrillation

 (AF)

Both external and internal CV of atrial fibrillation have been described in horses. As in ventricular DF, the external approach is less likely to be efficient because of higher energy requirements. In 1982, Deem and Fregin[46] reported external, monophasic CV attempts in three horses but all horses died. No information about their technique was reported. Buchanan reported a CV attempt using a modified oesophageal electrode but this was unsuccessful in one horse and a second horse developed ventricular fibrillation and died.[47] External CV using repeated 200 J biphasic shocks was successful in one of two cases; the successful case was a relatively small horse (393 kg) and CV could only be obtained when quinidine sulphate was concurrently administered.[48]

An internal CV technique, transvenous electrical cardioversion (TVEC), is the most efficient approach for electrical CV of AF in horses.[49-51] The procedure is performed with CV catheters that possess a large-surface electrode, positioned near the tip, for shock delivery. The large surface is necessary to minimize electrical resistance and reduce focal peak current.[52] The electrodes are positioned so as to encompass as much atrial tissue as possible. Multiple electrode positions have been reported in human patients, including caval vein, right atrium (RA), right ventricle (RV), pulmonary artery (PA) and coronary sinus. In horses, the RA to left PA appears to be the most successful combination. Two CV catheters are inserted via the jugular vein in the standing horse. This facilitates both catheter positioning and reduces anaesthesia duration. Positioning of the catheters is guided using a combination of echocardiography, pressure monitoring and radiography. On echocardiography, the catheter appears as a hyperechoic linear structure. Pressure is monitored with a fluid-filled CV catheter, allowing identification of a typical pressure profile when the catheter tip enters the RV or PA. The PA catheter is positioned first, approximately 10–20 cm into the left PA. Selective catheterization of the left PA is obtained by gentle rotation of the catheter once it enters the PA (Fig. 14.8). Although the main PA and the right PA are easily detected on ultrasound from a right parasternal image, only the origin of the left PA itself is visible. Location of the catheter into the left PA is present when the visible (main PA) part of the catheter is clearly *directed towards* the origin of the left PA (Fig. 14.9). Catheter location against the vessel wall impedes its visualization. In addition, linear artifacts frequently occur in the right PA, resembling the structure of a catheter (Fig. 14.10). Echocardiographic imaging of the pulmonary bifurcation from a

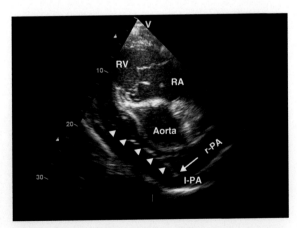

Figure 14.8 On a right parasternal image the catheter (arrow heads) enters the main pulmonary artery and the catheter tip (arrow) is directed towards the left pulmonary artery (l-PA). RA: right atrium; RV: right ventricle; r-PA: right pulmonary artery.

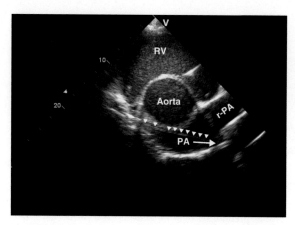

Figure 14.9 The correctly positioned cardioversion catheter (arrow heads) is visible in the main pulmonary artery (PA) and is clearly directed towards the left pulmonary artery (arrow). The left pulmonary artery itself and the catheter tip cannot be seen on ultrasound. RV: right ventricle; r-PA: right pulmonary artery.

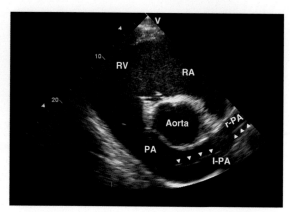

Figure 14.10 A hyperechoic, linear artifact (arrow heads) in the main (PA) and right (r-PA) pulmonary artery resembles a catheter but there is no catheter in the pulmonary artery. RA: right atrium; RV: right ventricle; l-PA: origin of the left pulmonary artery.

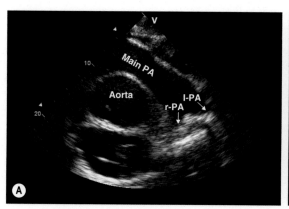

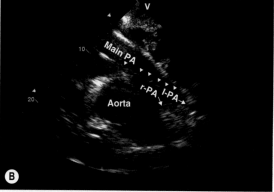

Figure 14.11 On a cranial, left parasternal view the pulmonary artery (PA) and the bifurcation towards the left (l-PA) and right (r-PA) pulmonary artery are visible (**A**). When the cardioversion catheter is correctly inserted (**B**) it is directed towards the left pulmonary artery (l-PA), away from the right pulmonary artery (r-PA).

left cranial window helps to identify the catheter position and to confirm the catheter direction towards the left pulmonary artery (Fig. 14.11). Utilizing pressure trace monitoring, the second CV catheter is inserted into the RV and then slowly pulled back into the RA. Finally, radiography is used to confirm the position of the right atrial and PA catheters and is critical to ensure that the catheter is not malpositioned within the ventricle, but the left and right branches of PA cannot be distinguished radiographically. As an additional precaution, a third temporary pacing catheter may be inserted into the right ventricular apex to allow ventricular pacing in case of post-shock asystole,[19] which has been encountered after 200–360 J monophasic shocks. However, because of a lower peak current, this arrhythmia is probably less likely to occur with biphasic shocks.

After induction of anaesthesia, catheter positions should be confirmed and repositioning performed as necessary. To facilitate this repositioning, it can be useful to insert the CV catheters deeper into the PA and into RV before anaesthesia and subsequently withdraw them after induction of anaesthesia. Subsequently, both catheters and a surface ECG are connected to a biphasic defibrillator which is operated in synchronous mode. Correct R wave detection without T wave detection (see Fig. 14.6A) is absolutely mandatory to avoid shock delivery on the T wave. If the T wave is identified as an R wave (see Fig. 14.6B), position of the surface electrodes needs to

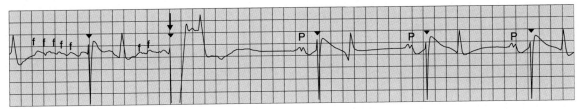

Figure 14.12 In synchronous mode, the defibrillator correctly detects R waves on the surface ECG (arrow heads) for shock delivery. A single shock of 125 J (arrow), with an impedance of 49, converts atrial fibrillation (f waves) to sinus rhythm.

be adapted. CV is started at 50 J and increased in a stepwise manner until CV is achieved[50,53] (Fig. 14.12). Shocks up to 360 J have been used without adverse effects but nevertheless the total delivered energy should be minimized. Excessive currents can have detrimental effects on the heart including post-shock arrhythmias, conduction disturbances, myocardial dysfunction and myocardial necrosis.[41,54] Furthermore, it has been postulated that cardiovascular structures might be injured by the sudden increase in intracardiac pressure that might develop when a high-energy internal shock is delivered.[55] Mean energy requirement for CV of AF in horses has been reported to be around 160 J or 0.35 J per kg body weight[50] with an impedance around 30–50. If the procedure is initially unsuccessful, shock delivery following catheter repositioning will sometimes result in CV.

Immediately following CV in human patients, the electrically remodelled atria are highly vulnerable to immediate recurrence of AF (IRAF) usually induced by atrial premature depolarizations.[56] Similarly, in horses, electrical remodelling occurs with chronic AF, and atrial premature depolarizations and IRAF have been observed immediately after electrical CV.[51,53] Protocols combining pharmacological and electrical interventions have not yet been fully explored in horses but in order to reduce IRAF pretreatment with an antiarrhythmic drug such as amiodarone has therefore been suggested.[53] In addition, after CV, catheters should be removed carefully and after an empirical 5- to 10-minute delay to reduce IRAF.

Apart from an occasional mild post-anaesthetic myopathy, the technique is safe and does not result in an increase in serum activities of cardiac enzymes. TVEC has been shown to be effective in 98% of lone AF horses.[50] Although data are currently lacking, recurrence rate is probably independent of the treatment technique and therefore is likely to be similar to that reported for pharmacological CV of AF.

REFERENCES

1. Trautwein W. Electrophysiological aspects of cardiac stimulation. In: Schaldach M, Furman S, editors. Advances in Pacemaker Technology. Berlin: Springer; 1975. p. 11–23.

2. van Loon G, Laevens H, Deprez P. Temporary transvenous atrial pacing in horses: threshold determination. Equine Vet J 2001;33:290–295.

3. Lapicque L. Considerations préalables sur la nature du phénomène par lequel l'électricité excite les nerfs. J Physiol Pathol Gener 1907;565–578.

4. Fishler MG, Thakor NV. A computer model study of the ventricular fibrillation vulnerable window: sensitivity to regional conduction depressions. Ann. Biomed Eng 1994;22:610–621.

5. Furman S, Hurzeler P, Mehra R. Cardiac Pacing and pacemakers.4. Threshold of cardiac stimulation. Am Heart J 1977;94:115–124.

6. van Loon G, Fonteyne W, Rottiers H, Tavernier R, Jordaens L, D'Hont L, et al. Dual chamber pacemaker implantation via the cephalic vein in healthy equids. J Vet Intern Med 2001a;15, 564–571.

7. Barold SS, Zipes D. Cardiac pacemakers and antiarrhythmic devices. In: Braunwald E, editor. Heart Disease, 4th ed. Philadelphia, PA: WB Saunders; 1992. p. 726–755.

8. Osborn MJ. Pacing: antitachycardia devices. In: Guiliani R, Gersh BJ,

McGoon MD, Hayes DL, Schaff HV, editors. Mayo Clinic Practice of Cardiology, 3rd ed. St. Louis: Mosby; 1996. p. 977–1016.

9. Bonagura JD, Helphrey ML, Muir WW. Complications associated with permanent pacemaker implantation in the dog. J Am Vet Med Assoc 1983;182:149–155.

10. Tilley LP. Essentials of Canine and Feline Electrocardiography, 3rd ed. Philadelphia: Lea & Febiger; 1992:1–470.

11. Berg F, Weber, Pfanzelt S, Wenzl J, Oeppert G. Use of an internal pacemaker in a donkey with the Adams-Stokes syndrome. Tierärztl Umsch 1973;28:616–618.

12. Le Nihouannen JC, Sevestre J, Dorso Y, Petit JC, Ozoux C.

Implantation of a cardiac pacemaker into horses. II. Postoperative monitoring of a pacemaker with epicardial and myocardial electrodes in a pony. Revue de Médecine Vétérinaire 1984;135:165–168.

13. Pibarot P, Vrins A, Salmon Y, Difruscia R. Implantation of a programmable atrioventricular pacemaker in a donkey with complete atrioventricular block and syncope. Equine Vet J 1993;25:248–251.

14. Brown CM. ECG of the month. J Am Vet Med Assoc 1979;175:1076–1077.

15. Reef VB, Clark ES, Oliver JA, Donawick WJ. Implantation of a permanent transvenous pacing catheter in a horse with complete heart block and syncope. J Am Vet Med Assoc 1986;189:449–452.

16. Hamir AN, Reef VB. Complications of a permanent transvenous pacing catheter in a horse. J Comp Pathol 1989;101:317–326.

17. van Loon G, Fonteyne W, Rottiers H, Tavernier R, Deprez P. Implantation of a dual-chamber, rate-adaptive pacemaker in a horse with suspected sick sinus syndrome. Vet Rec 2002;151:541–545.

18. Taylor DH, Mero MA. The use of an internal pacemaker in a horse with Adams-Stokes syndrome. J Am Vet Med Assoc 1967;151:1172–1176.

19. van Loon G, De Clercq D, Tavernier R, Amory H, Deprez P. Transient complete atrioventricular block following transvenous electrical cardioversion of atrial fibrillation in a horse. Vet J 2005;170:124–127.

20. Kantharia BK, Mookherjee S. Clinical utility and the predictors of outcome of overdrive transesophageal atrial pacing in the treatment of atrial flutter. Am J Cardiol 1995;76:144–147.

21. van Loon G, Jordaens L, Muylle E, Nollet H, Sustronck B. Intracardiac overdrive pacing as a treatment of atrial flutter in a horse. Vet Rec 1998;142:301–303.

22. Yamaya Y, Kubo K, Amada A. Relationship between atrioventricular conduction and hemodynamics during atrial pacing in horses. J Equine Sci 1997;59:149–151.

23. Yamaya Y, Kubo K, Amada A, Sato K. Intrinsic atrioventricular conductive function in horses with a second degree atrioventricular block. J Vet Med Sci 1997;59:149–151.

24. Schwarzwald CC, Hamlin RL, Bonagura JD, Nishijima Y, Meadows C, Carnes CA. Atrial, SA nodal, and AV nodal electrophysiology in standing horses: normal findings and electrophysiologic effects of quinidine and diltiazem. J Vet Intern Med 2007;21:166–175.

25. van Loon G, Duytschaever M, Tavernier R, Fonteyne W, Jordaens L, Deprez P. An equine model of chronic atrial fibrillation: methodology. Vet J 2002;164:142–150.

26. Senta T, Kubo K. Experimental induction of atrial fibrillation by electrical stimulation in the horse. Exp Rep Equine Hlth Lab 1978;15:37–46.

27. Moore EN, Spear JF. Electrophysiological studies on atrial fibrillation. Heart Vessels Suppl 1987;2:32–39.

28. Senta T, Kubo K, Sugimoto O, Amada A. Induction of atrial fibrillation by electrical stimulation in the horse. Exp Rep Equine Hlth Lab 1975;12:109–112.

29. Kubo K, Senta T, Sugimoto O. Changes in cardiac output with experimentally induced atrial fibrillation in the horse. Exp Rep Equine Hlth Lab 1975;12:101–108.

30. Ohmura H, Nukada T, Mizuno Y, Yamaya Y, Nakayama T, Amada A. Safe and efficacious dosage of flecainide acetate for treating equine atrial fibrillation. J Vet Med Sci 2000;62:711–715.

31. van Loon G, Blissitt KJ, Keen JA, Young LE. Use of intravenous flecainide in horses with naturally-occurring atrial fibrillation. Equine Vet J 2004;36:609–615.

32. van Loon G, Tavernier R, Duytschaever M, Fonteyne W, Deprez P, Jordaens L. Pacing induced sustained atrial fibrillation in a pony. Can J Vet Res 2000;64:254–258.

33. Geddes LA, Tacker WA, Rosborough JP, Moore AG, Cabler PS. Electrical dose for ventricular defibrillation of large and small animals using precordial electrodes. J Clin Invest 1974;53:310–319.

34. Witzel DA, Geddes LA, Hoff HE, McFarlane J. Electrical defibrillation of the equine heart. Am J Vet Res 1968;29:1279–1285.

35. Mazer CD, Greene MB, Misale PS, Newman D, Dorian P. Transcutaneous T wave shock: a universal method for ventricular fibrillation induction. Pacing Clin Electrophysiol 1997;20:2930–2935.

36. Sokoloski MC, Ayers GM, Kumagai K, Khrestian CM, Niwano S, Waldo AL. Safety of transvenous atrial defibrillation: studies in the canine sterile pericarditis model. Circulation 1997;96:1343–1350.

37. Tilley LP. Special methods for treating arrhythmias: cardiopulmonary arrest and resuscitation, pacemaker therapy. In: Tilley LP, editor. Essentials of Canine and Feline Electrocardiography, 3rd ed. Philadelphia: Lea & Febiger; 1992. p. 365–382.

38. Kenknight BH, Eyuboglu BM, Ideker RE. Impedance to defibrillation countershock: does an optimal impedance exist. Pace-Pacing Clin Electrophysiol 1995;18:2068–2087.

39. Pascoe PJ. Emergency care medicine. In: Short CE, editor. Principles and Practice of Veterinary Anesthesia. Baltimore: William & Wilkins; 1987. p. 581–582.

40. Benditt DG, Dunbar D, Fetter J, et al. Low-energy transvenous cardioversion defibrillation of atrial tachyarrhythmias in the canine: an assessment of electrode configurations and monophasic pulse sequencing. Am Heart J 1994;127:994–1003.

41. Cooper RA, Alferness CA, Smith WM, Ideker RE. Internal cardioversion of atrial fibrillation in sheep. Circulation 1993;87:1673–1686.

42. Ideker RE, Wolf PD, Alferness C, Krassowska W, Smith WM. Current

concepts for selecting the location, size and shape of defibrillation electrodes. Pace-Pacing Clin Electrophysiol 1991;14:227.

43. Geddes LA, Tacker WA, Rosborough J, Moore AG, Cabler P, Bailey M, et al. The electrical dose for ventricular defibrillation with electrodes applied directly to the heart. J Thorac Cardiovasc Surg 1974;68:593–602.

44. Webb AI. Neonatal resuscitation. In: Drummond AM, Kosch WH, editors. Equine Clinical Neonatology. Philadelphia: Lea & Febiger; 1990. p. 136–150.

45. Mair TS, Love S, Schumacher J, Watson E. Cardiovascular system. In: Mair TS, Love S, Schumacher J, Watson E, editors. Equine Medicine, Surgery and Reproduction. London: WB Saunders; 1998. p. 138–155.

46. Deem DA, Fregin GF. Atrial fibrillation in horses: a review of 106 clinical cases, with consideration of prevalence, clinical signs, and prognosis. J Am Vet Med Assoc 1982;180:261–265.

47. Buchanan JW. Commends successful use of electrical cardioversion in a horse. J Am Vet Med Assoc 2002;220:1777.

48. Frye MA, Selders CG, Mama KR, Wagner AE, Bright JM. Use of biphasic electrical cardioversion for treatment of idiopathic atrial fibrillation in two horses. J Am Vet Med Assoc 2002;220(7):1039–1045, 1007.

49. Bellei MHM, Kerr C, McGurrin MKJ, Kenney DG, Physick-Sheard P. Management and complications of anesthesia for transvenous electrical cardioversion of atrial fibrillation in horses: 62 cases (2002–2006). J Am Vety Med Assoc 2007;231:1225–1230.

50. McGurrin MKJ, Physick-Sheard PW, Kenney DG. How to perform transvenous electrical cardioversion in horses with atrial fibrillation. J Vet Cardiol 2005;7:109–119.

51. van Loon G. Atrial Pacing and Experimental Atrial Fibrillation in Equines, PhD thesis, Ghent University, Merelbeke, 2001.

52. Kalman JM, Power JM, Chen JM, Farish SJ, Tonkin AM. Importance of electrode design, lead configuration and impedance for successful low energy transcatheter atrial defibrillation in dogs. J Am Coll Cardiol 1993;22:1199–1206.

53. De Clercq D, van Loon G, Schauvliege ST. Transvenous electrical cardioversion of atrial fibrillation in six horses using custom made cardioversion catheters. Vet J. Published Online First: doi:10.1016/j.tvjl.2007.1008.1019.

54. Geddes LA, Tacker WA Jr. Ventricular fibrillation and defibrillation. Aust Phys Eng Sci Med 1983;6:9–19.

55. Mansourati J, Larlet JM, Salaun G, Maheu B, Blanc JJ. Safety of high energy internal cardioversion for atrial fibrillation. Pacing Clin Electrophysiol 1997;20:1919–1923.

56. Duytschaever M, Danse P, Allessie M. Supervulnerable phase immediately after termination of atrial fibrillation. J Cardiovasc Electrophysiol 2002;13:267–275.

Cardiac murmurs: congenital heart disease

Celia M Marr

PREVALENCE OF CONGENITAL CARDIAC DISEASE

Congenital cardiac defects are relatively uncommon in horses: estimates derived from pathological surveys of foals and fetuses suggest that 0.7–0.8%[1,2] that undergo post mortem examination for any reason have congenital cardiac disease while in the largest survey of equine congenital disease that has been performed to date examining 608 deformed fetuses and foals, 3.6% of all congenital organ defects were cardiac.[3] In a survey of the author's clinical population from 1993 to 1998, congenital defects were detected in 3.4% of 380 horses presented for cardiological investigation (Marr, unpublished data). Some defects are fatal before or immediately after birth and congenital cardiac defects are of particular importance in foals and young horses with loud cardiac murmurs. However, some defects (for example, small ventricular septal defects (VSD)) may not become clinically apparent

until the horse is required to perform athletic activities or may even be incidental findings in older horses.[4] Congenital cardiac defects can be classified as simple or complex. Cases with simple congenital cardiac defects greatly outnumber those with complex defects: in one survey 20 of 32 cases were classified as simple (VSD 11 cases, atrial septal defect 5 cases, patent ductus arteriosus 4 cases).[5] Congenital cardiac defects appear to be more common in certain breeds, notably Arabs,[6] Standardbreds[4] and Welsh Mountain ponies. It is likely that there are genetic factors that lead to the development of these defects but these are poorly understood in human beings and totally unexplored in the horse. Congenital cardiac disease is best considered in light of the embryological process that leads to their development.

NORMAL AND ABNORMAL DEVELOPMENT OF THE HEART

The primoirda of the heart begin as clusters of paired symmetrical mesenchymal cells that fuse into a straight tube in which the segments are arranged as follows: atria, primitive ventricle, bulbus cordis, conus and truncus. The tube becomes hollow and through differential growth characteristics the different segments expand. Very early in development, the heart adopts "sidedness" and proceeds to a pattern of asymmetrical growth. Abnormalities at this stage lead to conditions such as situs inversus where the entire body is reversed from left to right, a condition that has been reported in the horse.[7,8] Next, a process of cardiac looping occurs and the bulbus cordis migrates relative to the ventricle to take up the positions that will eventually form the right (RV) and left (LV) ventricles.

DOI: 10.1016/B978-0-7020-2817-5.00020-1

Developmental abnormalities at this stage can lead to a variety of malformations in which the ventricles fail to adopt their normal side-by-side pattern.[9]

The early looped cardiac tube has a single inlet, the common atrioventricular (AV) canal and a single outlet, the bulboventricular defect (i.e. the opening between the ventricle and the bulbus cordis) and on into the trunco-conal tube. Septation of the right (RA) and left atria (LA) involves ingrowths from several areas. The septum primum grows to meet outgrowths of the AV cushions and later the septum secundum arises near the common sinus venosus. The foramen ovale is left as a communication between the two atria throughout fetal life. Developmental abnormalities at this stage can lead to atrial septal defects (ASD) which are classifed as: (1) ostium primum ASD that is due to lack of fusion of the two medial AV cushions; (2) fossa ovalis defect that results from the resorption of the septum primum and must be distinguished from persistence of the patent foramen ovale that is a normal variant; and (3) sinus venosus ASD that is due to lack of formation or resorption of the septum secundum.[9]

Simultaneously, the AV canals remodel to align the left and right AV canals with their respective ventricles and ventricular septation ensues.[10] Septation of the ventricles is completed in the horse embryo by the 36th to 38th day.[11] This occurs through the convergence and fusion of five different components: the primitive ventricular septum, the cranial and caudal AV cushions and the dextro-dorsal and sinistro-ventral conal ridges. During this process the AV valves are formed. Failure at this stage can lead to common ventricle that is due to absence of both the primitive ventricular septum and AV cushions or, more commonly, a range of ventricular septal defects (VSD) are possible and relate to failure of individual components. Membranous or perimembranous VSD are due to inadequacy of any of the five components. This VSD is located in the LV outflow tract just between the aortic valve and is the commonest form of VSD in the horse[4,12,13] and the most common form of simple congenital cardiac defect. Supracristal or conal VSD is located in the RV outflow tract, just below the right coronary cusp of the aortic valve. This form occurs occasionally in horses. AV canal defects are the most complex and a range of abnormalities is possible. This VSD is caused by failure of the uppermost part of the septum to develop due to lack of the medial AV cushion and can also affect formation of the AV valves. The muscular VSD, which is the second commonest form in the horse,[14,15] is due to one or more defect in the primitive ventricular septum. These defects can occur in any part of the muscular septum. (⊙ CCD, VSD)

The formation of the aortic and pulmonary trunks is achieved by truncoconal septation: ridges form within either side of the truncus and grow inwards as the truncus spirals to create the aortic and pulmonary trunks. Cushions at the base of the truncus form the aortic and pulmonary valves. Septation and spiralling of the conus leads to the formation of the muscular, cranially located RV outflow tract and the shorter, fibrous LV outflow tract.[11,14] Abnormal truncoconal septation and spiralling can lead to a wide range of malformations[9] of which the most commonly reported in the horse is Tetralogy of Fallot.[16–22] Thus, it appears that conotruncal developmental abnormalities account for the majority of complex congenital cardiac defects in horses.

ADAPTATION FROM FETAL TO NEONATAL CIRCULATION

The fetal circulation is adapted to direct oxygenated blood entering the RA via the caudal vena cava towards the left side from where it can supply the body and to divert some of the RV output away from the noninflated lung. In the neonatal period, these processes must be reversed to adapt to extrauterine life. In the fetus, the foramen ovale is a tube-like flap of tissue, with fenestrations at its distal end, which extends from the RA near the aperture in the caudal vena cava to the lumen of the LA. Oxygenated blood from the placenta, returning to the RA from the caudal vena cava, passes though the foramen ovale to the LA, and then leaves the left heart via the aorta to preferentially supply the brain. Flow can be visualized through the foramen ovale in some foals for several weeks after birth (Fig. 15.1) and obliteration of the foramen ovale takes place during the first few weeks of life.[23] The fetal uninflated lung has high vascular resistance and a proportion of blood leaving the pulmonary artery (PA) bypasses the lung, by flowing through the ductus arteriosus into the aorta. When the

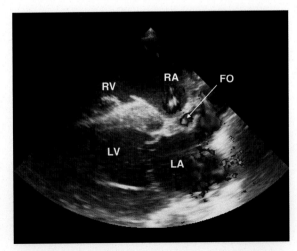

Figure 15.1 A right parasternal long-axis colour Doppler echocardiogram of the ventricles from a 12-week-old Thoroughbred foal. Blood flow is visible within the foramen ovale (arrow) towards the right ventricle (RV). RA, right atrium; LV, left ventricle; LA, left atrium. FO, foramen ovale.

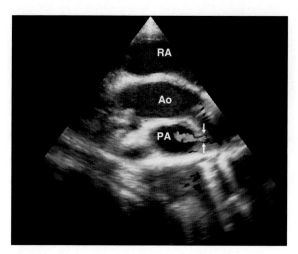

Figure 15.2 A right parasternal oblique long-axis colour Doppler echocardiogram of the aorta (Ao) and pulmonary artery (PA) from a healthy 3-day-old pony foal. Blood is flowing through the ductus arteriosus (arrows) from the descending Ao to the PA. RA, right atrium.

lungs inflate after birth, the resistance in the pulmonary circulation falls and the ductus begins to close in response to increasing arterial oxygen tension. Flow within the ductus arteriosus creates a machinery murmur high and cranially over the left heart base that usually disappears within the first few days of life and with Doppler echocardiography, ductal flow can be visualized in some foals of the same age (Fig 15.2). Ductal closure is initially physiological, due to constriction of the vessels, and subsequently becomes anatomical as closure with muscular elements occurs.[23,24] Perinatal hypoxia can delay or even reverse ductal closure, leading to persistent fetal circulation.

CLINICAL ASSESSMENT OF THE CARDIOVASCULAR SYSTEM IN FOALS

While congenital cardiac defects are rare, cardiac murmurs are extremely common in foals and the majority are physiological rather than pathological in nature. Ninety per cent of newborn Thoroughbred foals have continuous murmurs over the left cardiac base, consistent with flow in the ductus arteriosus during the first 15 minutes of life.[25] The majority of continuous murmurs have disappeared by 80 hours of age.[25] On the first day of life, 5 of 10 pony foals were found to have continuous murmurs and the remainder had systolic murmurs.[26] The continuous murmurs were not detected after 3 days of age, while systolic murmurs were more persistent, still detectable in two foals at 7 weeks of age. In that study, colour flow

Doppler echocardiography revealed that flow was frequently detected in the ductus arteriosus in the absence of continuous murmurs. Attempts to correlate the presence or absence of a systolic murmur with flow within the ductus arteriosus and foramen ovale revealed no consistent relationships.[26] This suggests that some systolic murmurs found over the left heart base in foals can be attributed to left ventricular ejection, as in adult horses.

Dysrhythmias are also common in the newborn foal. In one study, 96% of Thoroughbred foals had arrhythmias immediately after birth and these included atrial fibrillation (15/50), supraventricular tachycardia (3/50), ventricular premature depolarizations (10/50), ventricular tachycardia (4/50), idioventricular rhythm (1/50) and second-degree atrioventricular block (7/50). However, all of these neonatal dysrhythmias had disappeared within 15 minutes of birth and were attributed to high vagal tone and hypoxia.[27]

Cardiac disease should be suspected in foals with loud, widely radiating murmurs, particularly if they are associated with a precordial thrill. Foals may be stunted or fail to gain weight and have other, more specific signs of cardiovascular disease, such as dependent oedema, jugular distension and pulsation, pleural effusion, ascites, weakness and collapse.

Conventional means of clinical assessment of the cardiovascular system in foals include blood pressure measurement, electrocardiography,[28] radiography[29] and echocardiography[28,30-32] (see Chapter 9). In addition to lateral thoracic radiographs, in the smaller foals it may be possible to perform both dorsoventral thoracic radiographs, greatly adding to their diagnostic value. Radiography is less sensitive than echocardiography in estimating heart size, but large changes in cardiac dimensions may be apparent and, with left-to-right shunting, overcirculation of the pulmonary vasculature may be present (Fig. 15.3). Their smaller body size also makes angiography a feasible technique in foals and this is particularly useful in the demonstration of intra- and extracardiac shunts.[33-36] Cardiac catheterization allows pressure and oxygen tensions to be measured within various chambers to document intracardiac shunting.[37] However, as these are invasive procedures, both cardiac catheterization and angiography are now used less extensively than echocardiography, which has the great benefit of being noninvasive.[28,30-32] Nuclear angiography is an alternative noninvasive means of demonstrating left-to-right shunts.[38,39]

The echocardiographic examination should begin with a systematic evaluation of each cardiac structure individually to determine its position in relation to other structures,[31,32] and a more detailed description of the echocardiographic approach to congenital cardiac defects is given in Chapter 9. Spectral and colour Doppler echocardiography can be used to identify intra- or extracardiac shunts while contrast echocardiography is particularly

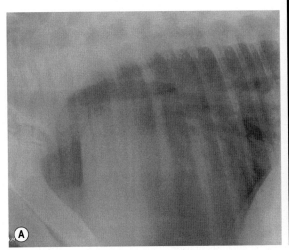
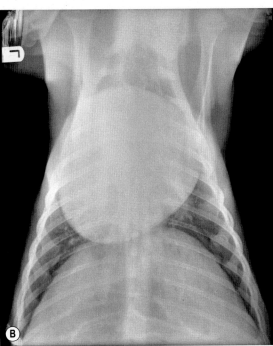

Figure 15.3 Lateral (**A**) and dorsoventral (**B**) radiographs of the thorax from a 6-week-old Thoroughbred with a large VSD. (A) There is marked cardiomegaly with tracheal elevation and overcirculation of the pulmonary vessels produces a pronounced vascular pattern. (B) The dorsoventral projection confirms biventricular enlargement.

applicable in congenital cardiac disease.[40,41] This involves the administration of a microbubble-laden solution via the jugular vein, rendering the blood echogenic and allowing the path of blood flow to be demonstrated. A suitable solution can be made by mixing equal volumes of the patient's blood and saline with a small volume of air. More contrast is achieved by holding off the jugular veins during administration and then releasing all the contrast, once injection is complete. With right-to-left shunting, bubbles can be seen entering the left side of the circulation. With left-to-right shunting, or lesions such as intact aortic aneurysms, a negative contrast effect is observed as anechoic blood is visible within an echogenic chamber. (*ACF, CCD, VSD*)

SPECIFIC CONGENITAL CARDIAC DEFECTS

Ventricular septal defect (VSD)

The VSD is the commonest congenital cardiac defect in horses[4,12–15,37,42–44]. In the author's clinical population;

simple VSDs are diagnosed approximately six times more often than any other congenital cardiac defect. VSDs are also frequently a component of complex defects.[6,35,42,43,45–49] VSDs have been documented in a wide variety of breeds. The lesion is particularly common in Welsh Mountain ponies. Welsh Section A ponies are many times more likely to have a VSD than Thoroughbreds (relative risk: 27.4, 6.16–122.01, P < 0.0000). Four per cent of 200 Welsh Mountain ponies had cardiac murmurs consistent with VSD in an auscultatory survey (H. Whishart and C. M. Marr, unpublished data).

VSDs are usually located in the membranous (nonmuscular) portion of the septum in the left ventricular outflow tract (subaortic) immediately below the right coronary cusp of the aortic valve and the tricuspid valve[4,12,13] (Figs. 15.4–15.6). In this location, defects are usually single but can be fenestrated (Fig. 15.7). Less commonly, defects are found in the right ventricular outflow tract (subpulmonic) and the perimembranous or muscular portions of the septum where they may be single, multiple or fenestrated.[14,15] Defects may also be present in more than one location. In the left ventricular outflow tract, larger defects can lead to moderate to severe aortic insufficiency as the cusps of the aortic valve are sucked into the defect (see Fig. 15.6) and, ultimately, may rupture.[4,50] The shunt direction is usually left to right with simple VSDs; however, with additional lesions, such as bicuspid pulmonary valve, bidirectional shunting may exist.[42]

The VSD is usually associated with at least two murmurs (see Chapter 8). The shunt itself causes a loud, pansystolic band-shaped or coarse murmur with its point of maximal intensity over the right fourth intercostal space. There is often also a murmur of relative pulmonic steno-

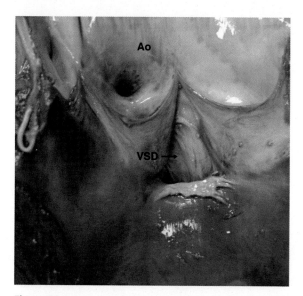

Figure 15.4 A post-mortem specimen from an 8-month-old Thoroughbred colt with a large membranous ventricular septal defect (VSD) below the aortic valve. Ao, aorta.

sis.[4] The right ventricular outflow tract is anatomically normal but, because of the increased volume of blood leaving the right ventricle, a loud holosystolic crescendo–decrescendo murmur is auscultated over the pulmonary valve area in the left third intercostal space. This murmur of relative pulmonic stenosis is typically at least one grade less than the VSD murmur. If there is concurrent aortic regurgitation, a holodiastolic decrescendo murmur will be present over the aortic valve area in the left fourth intercostal space.[50]

The integrity of the septum is assessed with two-dimensional echocardiography.[4] A membranous VSD is typically best visualized in an image of the left ventricular outflow tract (see Figs. 15.5, 15.6). The defect should be measured in two mutually perpendicular planes to determine its maximal diameter. Colour flow Doppler echocardiography demonstrates the intracardiac shunt and is particularly helpful in identifying small VSDs (Fig. 15.8). Usually, when the VSD is visualized from the right side the shunt is depicted in red and orange as it approaches the defect and then aliases to shades of blue due to the high velocities of blood flow in the VSD (see Fig. 15.8). Continuous wave Doppler echocardiography is used to document the maximal velocity of the intracardiac shunt. The maximal shunt velocity reflects the pressure difference between the left and right ventricles. If the right ventricular pressure rises, the pressure difference will fall and therefore the shunt velocity will be low. The echocardiogram should also be assessed for signs of left ventricular volume overload, dilatation of the left ventricle, rounding of the apex, right ventricular hypertrophy and dilatation, and concurrent valvular insufficiency.

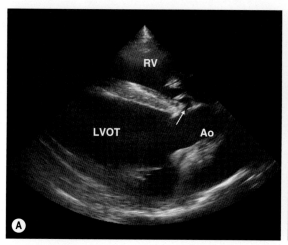
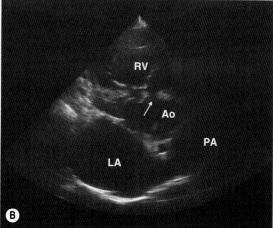

Figure 15.5 Right parasternal long-axis (**A**) and short-axis (**B**) echocardiograms of the left ventricular outflow tract (LVOT) from a 6-year-old Welsh mountain pony with no signs of exercise intolerance in which a membranous VSD (arrows) was detected during a routine physical examination. The defect is 1.37 cm in long axis and 1.17 cm in short axis. The diameter of the aorta (Ao) is 4.6 cm, giving a VSD:Ao ratio of 0.29. RV, right ventricle; PA, pulmonary artery; LVOT, left ventricular outflow tract; LA, left atrium.

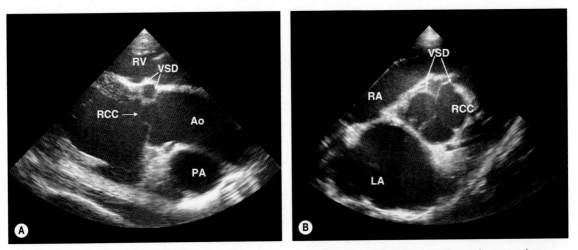

Figure 15.6 Right parasternal long-axis (**A**) and short-axis (**B**) echocardiograms of the left ventricular outflow tract from a yearling Welsh mountain pony with stunting and exercise intolerance and a membranous VSD (between arrows). The right coronary cusp (RCC) of the aortic valve is prolapsing into the defect, leading to aortic insufficiency. The VSD measures 1.26 by 1.72 cm and the aorta (Ao) measures 3.87 cm, giving a VSD:Ao ratio of 0.44. RV, right ventricle; RA, right atrium; LA, left atrium; PA, pulmonary artery.

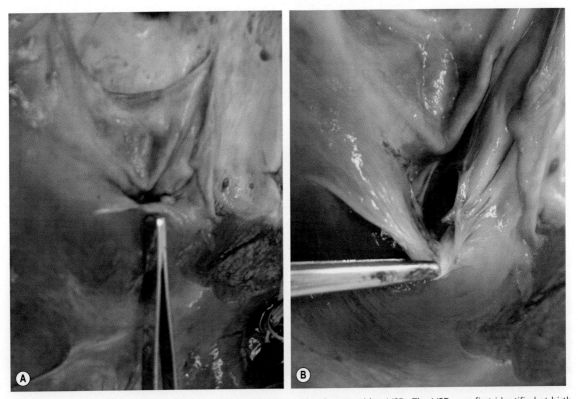

Figure 15.7 Post-mortem specimens from a 16-year-old Thoroughbred mare with a VSD. The VSD was first identified at birth but the mare had only developed signs of acute heart failure concurrently with the onset of a ventricular tachycardia 24 hours prior to euthanasia. A small VSD is visible (**A**), which when it is held apart can be seen to consist of a series of fenestrations (**B**). The chordae tendineae of the tricuspid valve

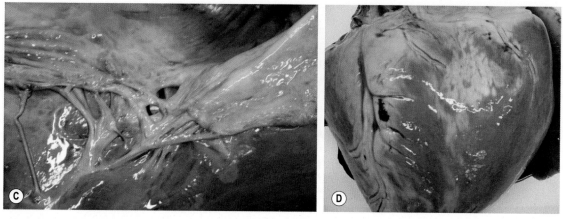

Figure 15.7 Continued (**C**) are thickened and are contributing to the series of channels. (**D**) There are large areas of pale tissue within the ventricular wall representing myocardial fibrosis that will have contributed to the cardiac arrhythmia and decompensation.

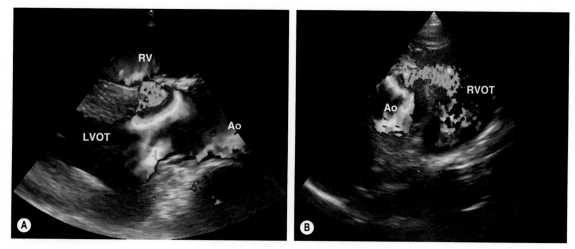

Figure 15.8 Right parasternal oblique long-axis (**A**) and short-axis (**B**) colour flow Doppler echocardiograms of the left ventricular outflow tract (LVOT) from a yearling Welsh mountain pony with stunting and exercise intolerance and a large membranous VSD. Blood in the LVOT flowing towards the defect is encoded in red and yellow; as its velocity increases it aliases to blue. Within the defect and the right ventricular outflow tract green indicates turbulence. RV, right ventricle; RVOT, right ventricular outflow tract; Ao, aorta.

There is one report of surgical correction of a VSD with the assistance of extracorporeal circulation.[51] A more straightforward approach might be to use transvenous patch closure devices designed for use in human beings. However, these are primarily designed for closure of muscular defects and require a rim of tissue around the defect into which the device is embedded; therefore, due to the high prevalence of membranous defects, many equine cases are unlikely to be suitable candidates and there are no published reports of successful closure of equine VSD using such devices currently. The athletic capability of

horses with VSD has been reported in 27 horses of a variety of breeds. Eight of 13 Standardbreds were successful racehorses, 5 of 11 horses of other breeds were successful to some degree at showing. The two racing Thoroughbreds included in the study both raced at low levels.[4] In another study, in 4 of 10 cases of VSD, it was an incidental finding in three ponies and one mixed breed horse used for light hacking; three had exercise intolerance, the youngest being 6 months of age at the time of diagnosis. Two Thoroughbreds had large VSDs with severe exercise intolerance in one broodmare and congestive heart failure in one filly of 18 months of age (H. Whishart and C. M. Marr, unpublished data). There were no Standardbreds within this group.

The prognosis in VSD depends on the size and location of the defect and the maximal velocity of the shunt. Horses with small defects in the left ventricular outflow tract can have a useful career. All horses which had a successful career had membranous or perimembranous VSDs with a maximal diameter of less than 2.8 cm in one study. Seven of 11 horses with a shunt velocity greater than 4 m/s performed successfully in vigorous types of competition, while the remainder were successful at lower levels of activity such as showing or hunting.[4] In smaller breeds of horses and ponies, it may be helpful to compare the size of the VSD with the diameter of the aortic root rather than use an absolute measurement. VSDs that are less than one-third of the aortic root are likely to be restrictive and therefore carry a more favourable prognosis.[52] These conclusions on the relationship between VSD size and athletic capability in horses with membranous VSDs have been confirmed in the author's clinical population. The maximal diameter of the VSD (4.40 ± 0.99 compared to 1.83 ± 0.83, $P < 0.01$) and the ratio of the VSD diameter to the aortic root (0.64 ± 0.06 compared to 0.31 ± 0.18, $P < 0.01$; see Figs. 15.5, 15.6) were significantly higher in horses presenting with congestive heart failure or exercise intolerance compared to those presenting with murmurs of VSD as an incidental finding (H. Whishart and C. M. Marr, unpublished data). Horses with muscular VSD, additional lesions such as severe aortic regurgitation (see Fig. 15.6) or in which the VSD is part of a more complex cardiac defect[4,6,35,42,43,45-49] and those that have concurrent severe valvular insufficiency[53] have a poor prognosis. Therefore, the echocardiogram should be evaluated carefully for additional lesions to provide accurate prognostic information.

Atrial septal defect

Atrial septal defects (ASD) are uncommon. A fossa ovalis defect has been reported as an isolated lesion in one foal with atrial fibrillation and progressive heart failure.[54] More often, ASD is part of more complex congenital cardiac defects.[6,46,48,55,56] A loud heart murmur is detected over the heart base and echocardiography demonstrates the defect, associated with enlargement of both atria and the right ventricle. Signs of right ventricular volume overload such as paradoxical septal motion and dilatation of the right ventricle are present. Care should be taken not to confuse the foramen ovale with an ASD. Flow within the foramen ovale can be seen in foals for several weeks after birth (see Fig. 15.1). Although anatomically and functionally closed, the foramen ovale may be visible as a circular anechoic area within the atrial septum in normal mature horses. Overall, the prognosis with ASD is poor, although the author has seen one horse with a small ASD and no signs of exercise intolerance.

Patent ductus arteriosus

As discussed above, the ductus arteriosus is a normal communication between the aorta and pulmonary artery during fetal life that closes during the neonatal adaptation period. The continuous murmur over the left heart base associated with flow in the ductus arteriosus disappears within the first week of life but colour flow Doppler echocardiography has demonstrated ductal flow in older pony foals.[26] Patent ductus arteriosus (PDA) is uncommon as an isolated defect[57-59] but is often part of complex congenital cardiac defects.[6,33,45,48,60] Isolated PDAs do not usually cause clinical signs during the first few months of life; however, if the defect is large, there is progressive left ventricular volume overload and ultimately left-sided congestive heart failure. Rupture of the pulmonary artery has also been reported to occur with PDA.[58] At the time of presentation, the classical continuous murmur of the PDA may be absent and replaced by a systolic murmur. This occurs as pulmonary hypertension that restricts the flow within the ductus during diastole. Alternatively, the loudest murmurs may be caused by atrioventricular valvular regurgitation that develops in response to the ventricular dilation. Occasionally with a small PDA, there are no clinical signs and it has been described as an incidental finding at post mortem.[59] In one horse, seen by the author, used throughout its life for light hacking, signs of congestive heart failure did not develop until the horse was in its twenties.

In young foals, the ductus arteriosus can be visualized echocardiographically in right or left parasternal images by angling the ultrasound beam dorsally and slightly caudally from a cranial location (see Fig. 15.2). However, because the ductus arises from the descending aorta and this area is difficult to image echocardiographically in older horses, it can be difficult to document the PDA itself. To confirm the diagnosis, continuous retrograde flow within the pulmonary artery should be documented with colour flow and spectral Doppler echocardiography. Signs of left ventricular volume overload, left ventricular dilatation, increased septal and free-wall movement, increased fractional shortening and globoid left ventricles should be assessed and, if present, warrant a poor prognosis. It is important to evaluate the pulmonary artery because rupture is associated with sudden death[58] (see Chapter 9).

Valvular dysplasia (VMD)

Valvular dysplasia, which is common in small animals, is an uncommon congenital defect in horses. Congestive

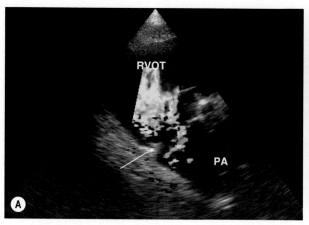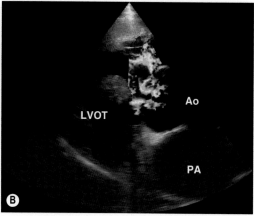

Figure 15.9 Right parasternal long-axis colour flow Doppler echocardiograms of the (**A**) right (RVOT) and (**B**) left (LVOT) ventricular outflow tracts from a 3-year-old pony with stunting, exercise intolerance and mild cyanosis. There is stenosis of the pulmonary artery (PA) at the level of the valve (arrow) and bidirectional flow in the VSD resulting in a complex arrangement of colours. The poststenotic portion of the PA is dilated when compared to the diameter of the aorta (Ao).

heart failure has been attributed to congenital aortic insufficiency in three horses[61-63] and echocardiograms from one horse with mitral valve dysplasia have been published.[64] Clinical findings are similar to other forms of valvular insufficiency (see Chapters 16 and 19). Valvular anomalies may also lead to stenosis and incomplete subaortic stenosis[65] and parachute mitral valve leading to both stenosis and regurgitation[66] are reported. The characteristics of stenotic murmurs are discussed in Chapter 8.

Pulmonic stenosis and atresia

Unlike small animals, stenosis of the semilunar valves is very uncommon in horses. Pulmonic stenosis has been described both as an isolated lesion[67] and in conjunction with other defects, whereas currently aortic stenosis has not. Pulmonic stenosis combined with VSD has also been reported sporadically.[33,68] This diagnosis is usually made early in life as affected foals are stunted and grow poorly. There are loud murmurs on both sides of the chest, but, unlike simple VSD, with combined VSD and pulmonic stenosis, the left-sided holosystolic crescendo–decrescendo murmur of pulmonic stenosis is louder than the right-sided murmur caused by the VSD. The stenotic area is visible on echocardiography with increased maximal velocity of the blood flow within a stenotic pulmonary artery and the VSD may have bidirectional shunting (Fig. 15.9). The prognosis is poor and it is extremely unlikely that affected animals can undertake any form of work; however, the author is aware of one case that was comfortable at pasture until it developed CHF at five years of age.

The term critical pulmonic stenosis refers to a severely stenotic lesion in which clinical signs are apparent from,

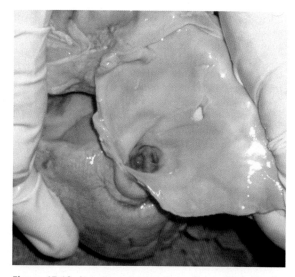

Figure 15.10 A post-mortem specimen from a Warmblood filly foal which died at around 15 hours of age with weakness, a loud systolic murmur, severe metabolic acidosis and hypoxia unresponsive to intranasal oxygen administration. The pulmonary artery has been opened and the valve area is viewed from above demonstrating critical pulmonic stenotis at the level of the valve.

or shortly after, birth.[33] The pulmonary artery is extremely stenotic (Fig. 15.10) and blood flows from the right atrium to the left atrium through the foramen ovale while the lungs are supplied by a left-to-right shunt through the ductus arteriosus. Affected foals have loud murmurs and severe hypoxaemia. There is no increase in arterial oxygen tension following the administration of intranasal oxygen. This presentation is similar to that of persistent fetal circulation[69] but the two conditions can be differentiated by echocardiographic or angiographic examination. A variation of this defect is atresia of the pulmonary artery.[35,70] In pulmonic atresia, the RV and PA do not communicate and this can also occur with[71] and without VSD.[70] Affected foals are likely to be extremely cyanotic with loud murmurs; they are able to survive in the short term due to a variety of alternative communications between the PA and the systemic circulation which may arise from the descending aorta.[71]

Tetralogy and pentalogy of Fallot (CCD)

Tetralogy of Fallot, which is a common congenital defect in ruminants, is seen occasionally in foals and it is the commonest form of right-to-left shunt.[16–22] The tetralogy consists of a large VSD, pulmonic stenosis, overriding of the aorta and right ventricular hypertrophy while the pentalogy has, in addition, an atrial septal defect.[6,56] The right-to-left shunt develops because due to the pulmonic stenosis, the pressures within the RV exceed those of the LV. This form of shunting creates systemic hypoxaemia, tissue hypoxia, cyanosis, exercise intolerance, polycythaemia, hyperviscosity of the blood and stunting of growth.[72] Foals typically have a loud systolic murmur with its point of maximal intensity over the pulmonary valve on the left side. Echocardiography illustrates the various components of the defect[22] (Fig. 15.11) The majority of cases die or are

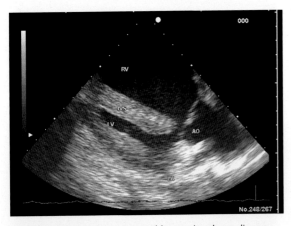

Figure 15.11 A right parasternal long-axis echocardiogram from a 9-day-old Welsh cob colt that presented with tetralogy of Fallot. Enlargement of the right ventricle (RV) and over-riding aorta (Ao) are visible. Image courtesy of Drs Jakub Plachy and Barbora Bezděková, Equine Clinic, Faculty of Veterinary Medicine, University of Veterinary and Pharmaceutical Sciences Brno, Czech Republic.

euthanased due to the severity of their clinical signs early in life; however, the degree of cardiac compromise is dependent on the degree of pulmonic stenosis and survival to 3[19] and 7 years of age[21] has been reported.

OTHER CONGENITAL CARDIAC DISEASE (CCD)

There are a range of other abnormalities that are attributed to abnormalities of the conotruncal development. The clinical and echocardiographic findings in atresia of the right atrioventricular (tricuspid) valve are well described[35,49,53,73–81] and are the result of abnormal truncoconal development. Foals present early in life with murmurs loudest over the right hemithorax, cyanosis and signs of severe cardiovascular compromise. On echocardiography, the right ventricle is extremely small, there is a muscular band in the area normally occupied by the tricuspid valve and there is a large VSD through which blood from the LV supplies the lungs. Persistent truncus arteriosus arises because the aorticopulmonary septum fails to form, leaving a single vessel from which the systemic, pulmonary and coronary arteries arise, and is accompanied by a VSD.[6,34,41,49,82–86] Other anomalies such as transposition of the great vessels,[87–89] aorticopulmonary septal defect,[90] hypoplastic left heart,[91] double outlet right ventricle[47,48] and anomalous origin of the left pulmonary artery[60] have all been described as individual case reports.

A variety of other forms of complex congenital defects are recognized in horses. AV canal defects are associated with abnormal development of the endocardial cushions. They have been reported sporadically in horses.[46,92–94] Young horses present with signs of congestive heart failure and systolic heart murmurs. However, because the defects are large, and pressures between the ventricles may be similar, the heart murmurs are not necessarily very loud.[93] More unusual defects arising from abnormal development of the aortic arches include absence of the aortic arch,[95] persistence of the right aortic arch[45] and coarctation of the aorta[96] while other embryological events can create a myriad of anatomical variation such as anomalous venous connections[97,98]) and atrial diverticulum.[99] These defects can all be detected echocardiographically. However, although these defects are interesting to differentiate using echocardiography, angiography or other diagnostic techniques, as a clinical problem they are rarely challenging because affected foals generally present with loud, widely radiating murmurs, and severe signs of cardiovascular compromise. As cardiac surgery is not a reasonable means of therapy, the prognosis for all of the major complex anomalies of the cardiac chambers and great vessels is hopeless.

REFERENCES

1. Collobert-Laugier C, Tariel G. Congenital abnormalities in foals: results of a seven year postmortem survey. Practique Veterinaire Equine 1993;25:105–110.

2. Puyalton-Moussu C, Collobert C, Tariel G, Foucher N. Study of congenital abnormalities in horses in Lower Normandy: incidence (1994–1998) and risk factors. Epidemiologie et Sante Animale 1999;35:87–96.

3. Crowe MW, Swerczek TW. Equine congenital defects. Am J Vet Res 1984;46:353–358.

4. Reef VB. Evaluation of ventricular septal defect in horses using two-dimensional and Doppler echocardiography. Equine Vet J Suppl 1995;19:86–95.

5. Buergelt D. Equine cardiovascular pathology: an overview. Animal Health Res Rev 2003;4(2).

6. Bayly WM, Reed SM, Leathers CW, et al. Multiple congenital heart anomalies in five Arabian foals. J Am Vet Med Assoc 1982;181(7): 684–689.

7. Palmers K, van Loon G, Jorissen M, et al. Situs inversus totalis and primary ciliary dyskinesia (Kartagener's syndrome) in a horse. J Vet Intern Med 2008;22(2): 491–494.

8. Turner SI, Jones RM. Complete situs inversus in a horse. Vet Rec 2004;155(3):96.

9. Angelini P. Embyrology and congenital heart disease. Texas Heart Institute Journal 1995;22(1): 1–12.

10. Larsen W. Human Embryology. New York: Churchill Livingstone, 1993.

11. Vitums A. The embryonic development of the equine heart. Anat Histol Embryol 1981;10(3): 193–211.

12. Glazier DB, Farrelly BT, O'Connor J. Ventricular septal defect in a 7-year-old gelding. J Am Vet Med Assoc 1975;167(1):49–50.

13. Lombard C, Scarratt WK, Buergelt CD. Ventricular septal defects in the horse. J Am Vet Med Assoc 1983;167:562–565.

14. Ueno Y, Tomioka Y, Kaneko M. Muscular ventricular septal defect in a horse. Bull Equine Res Instit 1992;29:15–19.

15. Deniau V, Delecroix A. A case of interventricular communication in a racehorse. Practique Veterinaire Equine 2004;36:25–31.

16. Prickett ME, Reeves JT, Zent WW. Tetralogy of fallot in a thoroughbred foal. J Am Vet Med Assoc 1973;162(7):552–555.

17. Reynolds DJ, Nicholl TK. Tetralogy of Fallot and cranial mesenteric arteritis in a foal. Equine Vet J 1978;10(3):185–187.

18. Keith J. Tetralogy of Fallot in a Quarter horse foal. Vet Med Small Animal Clin 1981;76(6):889–895.

19. Cargille J, Lombard C, Wilson JH, Buergelt CD. Tetralogy of Fallot and segmental uterine dysplasia in a three-year-old morgan filly. Cornell Vet 1991;81(4):411–418.

20. Houe H, Koch J, Bindseil E. Tetralogy of Fallot in horses. Dansk Veterinaertidsskrift 1996;79(2): 43–45.

21. Gesell S, Brandes K. Tetralogy of Fallot in a 7-year-old gelding. Pferdeheilkunde 2006;22:427–430.

22. Schmitz R, Klaus C, Grabner A. Detailed echocardiographic findings in a newborn foal with tetralogy of Fallot. Equine Vet Educ 2008;20(6):298–303.

23. MacDonald A, Fowden AL, Silver M, Ousey J, Rossdale PD. The foramen ovale of the foetal and neonatal foal. Equine Vet J 1988;20:255–260.

24. Machida N, Yasuda J, Too K, Kudo N, et al. A morphological study on the obliteration processes of the ductus arteriosus in the horse. Equine Vet J 1988;20(4):249–254.

25. Rossdale PD. Clinical studies on the newborn thoroughbred foal. II. Heart rate, auscultation and electrocardiogram. Br Vet J 1967;123(12):521–532.

26. Livesey L, Marr CM, Boswood A, Freeman S, Bowen IM, Corley KTT. Auscultation and two-dimensional, M mode, spectral and colour flow Doppler echocardiographic findings in pony foals from birth to seven weeks of age. J Vet Intern Med 1998;12:255.

27. Yamamoto K, Yasuda J, Too K. Arrhythmias in newborn Thoroughbred foals. Equine Vet J 1992;23:169–173.

28. Lombard C, Evans M, Martin L, Tehrani J. Blood pressure, electrocardiogram and echocardiogram measurements in the growing pony foal. Equine Vet J 1984;16:342–347.

29. Lamb C, O'Callaghan MW, Paradis MR. Thoracic radiography in the neonatal foal: a preliminary report. Vet Radiol Ultrasound 1990;31: 11–16.

30. Stewart J, Rose RJ, Barko A. Echocardiography in foals from birth to three months old. Equine Vet J 1984;16:332–341.

31. Reef VB. Echocardiographic findings in horses with congenital cardiac disease. Comp Contin Educ 1991;13:109–117.

32. Schwarzwald C. Sequential segmental analysis: a systematic approach to the diagnosis of congenital cardiac defects. Equine Vet Educ 2008;20:305–309.

33. Hinchcliff KW, Adams WM. Critical pulmonic stenosis in a newborn foal. Equine Vet J 1991;23: 318–320.

34. Steyn PF, Holland P, Hoffman J. The angiographic diagnosis of a persistent truncus arteriosus in a foal. J S Afr Vet Assoc 1989;60: 106–108.

35. Meurs KM, Miller MW, Hanson C, Honnas C, et al. Tricuspid valve atresia with main pulmonary artery atresia in an Arabian foal. Equine Vet J 1997;29(2):160–162.

36. Carlsten J, Kvart C, Jeffcott LB. Method for selective and non-selective angiocardiography in the horse. Equine Vet J 1984;16(1): 47–52.

37. Critchley KL. The importance of blood gas measurement in the diagnosis of an interventricular septal defect in a horse: a case report. Equine Vet J 1976;8: 120–129.

38. Koblik PD, Hornof WJ. Use of first pass nuclear angiocardiography to detect left-to-right cardiac shunts in the horse. Vet Radiol 1987;28(5):177–180.

39. Koblik PD, Hornof WJ. Diagnostic radiology and nuclear cardiology: their use in assessment of equine cardiovascular disease. Vet Clin North Am Equine Pract 1985;1(2):289–309.

40. Bonagura JD, Pipers FS. Diagnosis of cardiac lesions by contrast echocardiography. J Am Vet Med Assoc 1983;182(4):396–402.

41. Kvart C, Carlsten J, Jeffcott LB, Nilsfors L, et al. Diagnostic value of contrast echocardiography in the horse. Equine Vet J 1985;17(5):357–360.

42. Critchley KL. An interventricular septal defect, pulmonary stenosis and bicuspid pulmonary valve in a Welsh pony foal. Equine Vet J 1976;8(4):176–178.

43. Muylle E, De Roose P, Oyaert W, van den Hende C, et al. An interventricular septal defect and a tricuspid valve insufficiency in a trotter mare. Equine Vet J 1974;6(4):174–176.

44. Pipers FS, Reef VB, Wilson J. Echocardiographic detection of ventricular septal defects in large animals. J Am Vet Med Assoc 1985;187:810–816.

45. van der Linde-Sipman JS, Goedegebuure SA, Kroneman J. Persistent right aortic arch associated with a persistent left ductus arteriosus and an interventricular septal defect in a horse. Tijdschr Diergeneeskd 1979;104(20 suppl 4):189–194.

46. Reppas GP, Canfield PJ, Hartley WJ, et al. Multiple congenital cardiac anomalies and idiopathic thoracic aortitis in a horse. Vet Rec 1996;138(1):14–16.

47. Vitums A. Origin of the aorta and pulmonary trunk from the right ventricle in a horse. Pathol Vet 1970;7(6):482–491.

48. Chaffin MK, Miller MW, Morris EL. Double outlet right ventricle and other associated congenital cardiac anomalies in an American miniature horse foal. Equine Vet J 1992;24(5):402–406.

49. Rooney G, Franks WC. Congenital cardiac anomalies in horses. Pathol Vet 1964;1:454–464.

50. Reef VB, Spencer P. Echocardiographic evaluation of equine aortic insufficiency. Am J Vet Res 1987;48(6):904–909.

51. Menzel B, Kalmar P, Pokar H. Surgical correction of a ventricular septum defect in a mare with the help of extracorporeal circulation. Praktische Tierarzt 1995;76(12):1069–1072.

52. Bonagura JD, Blissitt KJ. Echocardiography. Equine Vet J Suppl 1995;19:5–17.

53. Davis JL, Gardner SY, Schwabenton B, Breuhaus BA, et al. Congestive heart failure in horses: 14 cases (1984–2001). J Am Vet Med Assoc 2002;220(10):1512–1515.

54. Taylor FG, Wotton PR, Hillyer MH, Barr FJ, Luce VM. Atrial septal defect and atrial fibrillation in a foal. Vet Rec 1991;128:80–81.

55. Physick-Sheard PW, Maxie MG, Palmer NC, Gaul C, et al. Atrial septal defect of the persistent ostium primum type with hypoplastic right ventricle in a Welsh pony foal. Can J Comp Med 1985;49(4):429–433.

56. Rahal C, Collatos C, Solano M, Bildfell R. Pentalogy of Fallot, renal infarction and renal abscess in a mare. J Equine Vet Sci 1997;17(11):604–607.

57. Guarda HI, Schifferlis RCA, Alvarez MLH, Probst A, Konig HE. A patent ductus arteriosus in a foal. Wiener Tieräztliche Monatsschrift 2005;92:233–237.

58. Buergelt C, Carmichael JA, Tashjian RJ, Das KM. Spontaneous rupture of the left pulmonary artery in a horse with patent ductus arteriosus. J Am Vet Med Assoc 1970;186:1210–1213.

59. Hare T. A patent ductus arteriosus in an aged horse. J Path Bact 1931;84:124.

60. Reimer JM, Marr CM, Reef VB, Saik JE. Aortic origin of the right pulmonary artery and patent ductus arteriosus in a pony foal with pulmonary hypertension and right sided heart failure. Equine Vet J 1993;25:466–470.

61. Gross DR, Clark DR, McDonald DR, McCrady JD, Allert JA. Congestive heart failure associated with congenital aortic valvular insufficiency in a horse. Southwestern Vet 1977;30:27–34.

62. Clark ES, Reef VB, Sweeny CR, Lichtensteiger C. Aortic valvular insufficiency in a one-year-old colt. J Am Vet Med Assoc 1987;191:841–844.

63. Taylor SE, Else RW, Keen JA. Congenital aortic valve dysplasia in a Clydesdale Foal. Equine Vet Educ 2007;19:463–468.

64. Reimer JM. Congenital defects and reversions to foetal circulation. In: Reimer JM, editor. Atlas of Equine Ultrasonography. St Louis: Mosby; 1998. p. 138–147.

65. King JM, Flint TJ, Anderson WI. Incomplete subaortic stenotic rings in domestic animals: a newly described congenital anomaly. Cornell Vet 1988;78:262–271.

66. McGurrin MK, Physick-Sheard PW, Southorn E. Parachute left atrioventricular valve causing stenosis and regurgitation in a Thoroughbred foal. J Vet Intern Med 2003;17(4):579–582.

67. Gehlen H, Bubeck K, Stadler P. Valvular pulmonic stenosis with normal aortic root and intact ventricular and atrial septa in an Arabian horse. Equine Vet Educ 2001;13(6):286–288.

68. Vitums A, Bayly WM. Pulmonary atresia with dextroposition of the aorta and ventricular septal defect in three Arabian foals. Vet Pathol 1982;19(2):160–168.

69. Cottrill C, O'Connor WN, Cudd T, Rantanen NW. Persistence of foetal circulatory pathways in a newborn foal. Equine Vet J 1987;19:252–255.

70. Young LE, Blunden AS, Bartram DH, Edgar A. Pulmonary atresia with an intact ventricular septum in a thoroughbred foal. Equine Vet Educ 1997;9:123–127.

71. Anderson R. The pathological spectrum of pulmonary atresia. Equine Vet Educ 1997;9(3):128–132.

72. Bonagura J, Reef VB. Disorders of the cardiovascular system. In: Reed S, Bayly WM, Sellon DC, editors. Equine Internal Medicine. Philadelphia: Saunders; 2004. p. 355–460.

73. Gumbrell RC. Atresia of the tricuspid valve in a foal. N Z Vet J 1970;18(11):253–256.

74. Button C, Gross DR, Allert JA, Kitzman JV, et al. Tricuspid atresia in a foal. J Am Vet Med Assoc 1978;172(7):825–830.

75. van Nie CJ, van der Kamp JS, [Congenital tricuspid atresia in a premature foal]. Tijdschr Diergeneeskd 1979;104(10):411–416.

76. van der Linde-Sipman JS, van den Ingh TS. Tricuspid atresia in a foal and a lamb. Zentralbl Veterinärmed A 1979;26A(3):239–242.

77. Hadlow W, Ward JK. Atresia of the right atrioventricular orifice in an Arabian foal. Vet Pathol 1980;17(5):622–626.

78. Honnas C, Puckett MJ, Schumacher J. Tricuspid atresia in a Quarter horse foal. Southwestern Vet 1987;38(1):17–20.

79. Wilson RB, Haffner JC. Right atrioventricular atresia and ventricular septal defect in a foal. Cornell Vet 1987;77(2):187–191.

80. Reef VB, Mann PC, Orsini PG. Echocardiographic detection of tricuspid atresia in two foals. J Am Vet Med Assoc 1987;191(2):225–228.

81. Zamora CS, Vitums A, Nyrop KA, Sande RD, et al. Atresia of the right atrioventricular orifice with complete transposition of the great arteries in a horse. Anat Histol Embryol 1989;18(2):177–182.

82. Rang H, Hurtienne H. [Persistent truncus arteriosus in a 2-year old horse]. Tierärztl Prax 1976;4(1):55–58.

83. Sojka JE. Persistent truncus arteriosus in a foal. Equine Pract 1987;9:24–26.

84. Stephen J, Abbott J, Middleton DM, Clarke C. Persistent truncus arteriosus in a Bashkir Curly foal. Equine Vet Educ 2000;12(5):251–255.

85. Jesty SA, Wilkins PA, Palmer JE, Reef VB. Persistent truncus arteriosus in two Standardbred foals. Equine Vet Educ 2007;19:307–311.

86. Greene H, Wray DD, Greenway JA. Two equine congenital cardiac anomalies. Irish Vet J 1975;29(7):115–117.

87. McClure JJ, Gaber CE, Watters JW, Qualls CW, et al. Complete transposition of the great arteries with ventricular septal defect and pulmonary stenosis in a Thoroughbred foal. Equine Vet J 1983;15(4):377–380.

88. Vitums A, Grant BD, Stone EC, Spencer GR, et al. Transposition of the aorta and atresia of the pulmonary trunk in a horse. Cornell Vet 1973;63(1):41–57.

89. Sleeper MM, Palmer JE. Echocardiographic diagnosis of transposition of the great arteries in a neonatal foal. Vet Radiol Ultrasound 2005;46(3):259–262.

90. Valdes-Martinez A, Easdes SC, Strickland KN, Roberts ED. Echocardiographic evidence of an aortic-pulmonary septal defect in a 4-day-old thoroughbred foal. Vet Radiol Ultrasound 2006;47:87–89.

91. Musselman EE, LoGuidice RJ. Hypoplastic left ventricular syndrome in a foal. J Am Vet Med Assoc 1984;185(5):542–543.

92. Ecke P, Malik R, Kannegieter NJ. Common atrioventricular canal in a foal. N Z Vet J 1991;39(3):97–98.

93. Kraus MS, Pariaut R, Alcaraz A, Gelzer ARM, Malik N, Renaud-Farrell S, et al. Complete atrioventricular canal defect in a foal: clinical and pathological features. J. Vet Cardiol 2005;7:59–64.

94. Kutasi O, Voros K, Biksi I, et al. Common atrioventricular canal in a newborn foal: case report and review of the literature. Acta Vet Hung 2007;55(1):51–65.

95. Scott E, Chaffee A, Eyster GE, Kneler SK. Interruption of the aortic arch in two foals. J Am Vet Med Assoc 1978;172:347–350.

96. Amend J, Ross JN, Garner HE, Rosborough JP, Hoff HE. Systolic time intervals in domestic ponies: alterations in a case of coarctation of the aorta. Can J Comp Med 1975;39:62–66.

97. Seco Diaz O, Desrochers A, Hoffmann V, Reef VB, et al. Total anomalous pulmonary venous connection in a foal. Vet Radiol Ultrasound 2005;46(1):83–85.

98. Machado G, Candioto CG, Carvalhal R, Vasconcelos R de O, Espirito-Sando EF, Oliveira DB. Congenital anomaly in the vessels at base of a foal heart. Brazilian J Vet Res Anim Sci 2006;43(3):408–411.

99. Patterson-Kane JC, Harrison LR. Giant right atrial diverticulum in a foal. J Vet Diagn Invest 2002;14(4):335–337.

Chapter | 16 |

Cardiac murmurs: valvular regurgitation and insufficiency

Celia M Marr

INTRODUCTION

One of the commonest cardiological dilemmas that faces the equine practitioner is the assessment of a horse, otherwise apparently healthy, in which a murmur is detected. This situation arises frequently in the context of examinations for suitability for purchase. Equally, in horses presented for investigation of poor performance, a murmur may have uncertain significance. The characteristic auscultatory features of equine cardiac murmurs are described in detail in Chapter 8. The investigation and management of horses with congenital cardiac disease (see Chapter 15), and infective endocarditis (see Chapter 17) and heart failure (see Chapter 19), are described elsewhere in this book. The purpose of this chapter is to discuss the investigation and management of cardiac murmurs in adult horses which are otherwise asymptomatic or have poor performance, the setting in which cardiac murmurs are most frequently encountered.

PATHOLOGICAL AND PHYSIOLOGICAL REGURGITATION

Valvular regurgitation is an important cause of murmurs in horses, second only to physiological flow murmurs in prevalence, and it occurs both in the presence and absence of valvular pathology.[1–6] Valvular lesions can be congenital, degenerative, inflammatory or idiopathic in nature[1,5,7–13] (see Chapter 4). The term valvular insufficiency can be defined as valvular regurgitation that is sufficiently severe to lead to some degree of haemodynamic changes and it is typically associated with some form of valvular pathology. However, it is important to recognize that valvular regurgitation can occur at structurally normal valves and in this setting it is described as physiological regurgitation. Furthermore, valvular regurgitation can be detected with Doppler echocardiography in many horses without murmurs.[2,4,6]

Valves are not inert structures; rather their tone and stiffness can be modified dynamically, under the influence of a variety of vasoactive mediators, just as is the case with blood vessels[14] (see Chapter 4). The factors that influence physiological regurgitation are not yet well understood and may involve not only neuroendocrine factors but also changes in the geometry of the ventricles that are part of cardiac adaptation to exercise and training. Physiological regurgitation is more common in human and canine athletes than sedentary individuals and it is well established that atrioventricular valvular regurgitation, both with and without murmurs, becomes more prevalent and more severe as Thoroughbred horses progress through training.[6,15] There is a higher prevalence of physiological regurgitation in racehorses trained for steeplechasing compared to flat races, suggesting that the cardiac adaptations that relate to the most intense, sustained exercise may be important in the development of physiological regurgitation[6] (see Chapter 3). There is no relationship between the presence and absence of physiological regurgitation and racing performance,[6,16] providing further evidence that this is a physiological rather than pathological phenomenon. The task of the clinician when called upon to examine a horse with a regurgitant murmur is first to distinguish between physiological and pathological regurgitation and then if pathological regurgitation is present, to determine whether it is of sufficient severity that it is likely to be affecting the horse's well-being and exercise capacity.

CLINICAL ASSESSMENT OF HORSES WITH MURMURS

Clinical assessment of a horse with a murmur due to valvular regurgitation involves:

- History taking, with an emphasis on identifying exercise intolerance, fatigue, weight loss and other features that might indicate cardiac disease or dysfunction.
- General physical examination.
- Auscultation to characterize and localize the valve involved.
- Echocardiography to confirm valvular regurgitation and estimate its severity.
- Electrocardiography to investigate concurrent dysrhythmias.

In horses with valvular regurgitation, M-mode, two-dimensional and Doppler echocardiography (see Chapter 9) are used to[3,5,17–26]:

- Identify specific forms of valvular pathology.
- Semiquantitate the severity of regurgitation.
- Document the size and shape of the cardiac chambers and great vessels.

The criteria recommended for the evaluation of severity of valvular regurgitation in horses include the presence and specific type of echocardiographically demonstrable valvular lesions, the degree of atrial and ventricular volume overload, and the timing of and area occupied by the regurgitant jet mapped by pulsed or colour flow Doppler echocardiography.[21] The chronicity of lesions can sometimes be inferred by the correlation of the jet size and the chamber enlargement and in acute, severe disease, a large jet may not necessarily be associated with chamber enlargement because this takes time to develop. The rate of progression can be assessed most accurately by repeated echocardiographic examinations.[21] Conventional, radiotelemetric and ambulatory electrocardiography can be useful to detect concurrent dysrhythmias (see Chapter 10). When the information generated with these techniques is considered in the light of the presenting signs and the owner's expectations for the horse, it is usually possible for the clinician to provide an accurate prognosis and advise the horse's owner on suitable management and the appropriate exercise level for the horse. Although in the following discussion, each valve is considered in turn, it is important for the clinician to remember that there may be valvular regurgitation in more than one valve and the clinical impact of multiple regurgitations may be additive.

AORTIC VALVULAR REGURGITATION AND INSUFFICIENCY (AR)

Prevalence

Estimates of the prevalence of aortic regurgitation (AR) have varied depending on the study populations and on the techniques used to define the diagnosis but AR appears to increase in prevalence with age and small riding breeds (i.e. Thoroughbred and Arab or crosses thereof) are at increased risk of having AR compared to small ponies.[27] The prevalence of audible murmurs of AR was 8.7% in cases at a referral hospital,[28] 2.2% in a mixed working population,[29] 5.5% in a mixed population with a median age of 14 years, many of whom were retired,[27] 7% in steeplechasers in the UK[6] but 0–1% in various categories of younger Thoroughbreds competing on the flat.[6] The true prevalence of AR is probably much greater, and with Doppler echocardiography, physiological AR can often be identified in horses with no murmurs.[2,4,6]

Pathogenesis

The aortic valve is the commonest site for valvular pathology, particularly in the middle-aged and older horse.[1,8] Degenerative lesions consisting of nodular or, less commonly, generalized fibrous thickenings are seen most often on the left coronary cusp, although any or all of the three cusps may be affected.[1,8,9,22] Valvular prolapse is a precursor to valvular disease in dogs[30] but this association has not been investigated in horses. The term aortic valvular prolapse refers to abnormal movement of the valve cusps during diastole such that they flop downwards into the ventricle. It is detected echocardiographically and must be visible in at least two perpendicular planes to confirm its presence. It can be seen in both the presence and absence of valvular pathology and in the presence or absence of AR.[4] It is a dynamic process that can be induced by application of a twitch and is extremely common in fit Thoroughbred racehorses compared to other breeds and those in lighter work.[31] It remains to be established whether aortic valvular prolapse is a risk factor for valvular disease later in life. (AR)

Infective endocarditis can affect the aortic valve[12,22,32,33] (see Chapter 17). All forms of congenital valvular lesions are extremely uncommon in isolation but congenital malformations have been reported in the aortic valve.[34,35] AR can accompany ventricular septal defects, when the presence of the defect immediately beneath the aortic root leads to instability and, in some cases, rupture of the aortic valve[22,36] (see Chapter 15). Fenestrations of the free edges of the cusps are a common feature of both the aortic and pulmonary valves in the horse and have been observed in both equine fetuses and mature animals.[7] Provided these are not extremely extensive, they are not thought to have any clinical significance, representing a normal variant rather than a pathological entity.[7]

Clinical findings

(AR, IE)

The murmur of AR is typically pan, holo- or early diastolic, decrescendo and has its point of maximal intensity over the aortic valve in the left fifth intercostal space and radiates variable distances ventrally towards the heart base (see Chapter 8). It may be musical in quality, and in some horses it has a bizarre "creaking" quality, which may be due to vibrations of cardiac structures, such as the mitral valve and the ventricular septum, rather than turbulent blood flow itself.[28]

The clinical findings that warrant further investigation in horses in which a murmur of AR is detected are summarized in Table 16.1. Horses with more severe AR are likely to have loud diastolic murmurs, multiple heart murmurs and hyperkinetic pulses.[37] The best clinical guide to severity of AR is the quality of the arterial pulses, rather than the grade of the murmur. It can also be useful to measure noninvasive arterial pressure, which provides a useful guide to severity: horses with severe AR have a diastolic arterial pressure below 50 mmHg and a pulse pressure (i.e. systolic – diastolic) of greater than 60 mmHg compared to horses with mild AR[37] (Fig. 16.1). As the insufficiency becomes more severe, increases in resting heart rate may also be observed.

Echocardiography

(ET, IE, VSD, AF)

Colour flow Doppler echocardiography can readily demonstrate the area occupied by the jet of AR (Fig. 16.2). Unfortunately, measurements of the maximum width, length and width at the base are not very repeatable or reproducible and changes over time must be in excess of 20% in order to document genuine progression of the AR. Doppler echocardiography can also be used to assess pressure gradients that arise as a result of AR. In human beings, the maximal velocity and pressure half-time of the regurgitant jet can be related to the severity of ventricular volume overload. In one study, horses with AR on Doppler echocardiography had significantly larger and faster regurgitant jets if a cardiac murmur was present, suggesting that these parameters do reflect severity to some extent.[26] However, critical prospective studies have not addressed the sensitivity, specificity and reliability of these variables in the horse.

The two-dimensional and M-mode echocardiographic features of AR and aortic insufficiency (AI) have been described extensively.[22,26,38] Prolapse of the noncoronary cusp is a common finding and is rarely associated with severe regurgitation. In the typical degenerative disease seen in older horses, echogenic foci, representing degenerative nodules, are commonly localized to the left coronary cusp. Generalized thickening of the aortic valve and flail cusp indicates more extensive pathology. Dilatation of the aortic root (>8 cm), diastolic vibrations of the mitral valve and septum, and premature closure of the mitral valve are seen with moderate to severe AI but are not necessarily related to severity.[22] The vibrations arise as a consequence of the turbulence created in the left ventricular outflow tract by the regurgitant jet.[22] Early closure of the mitral valve (closure of the valve before the onset of systole as indicated by the Q wave) is not present in horses with mild regurgitation.[22] Both two-dimensional and M-mode echocardiograms are useful in assessing the degree of left volume overload (see Chapter 9), which is diagnosed if the left ventricular diameter is increased, the apex of the ventricle takes on a globoid shape and the ventricle is hyperkinetic.

Electrocardiography

Horses with AR are more likely to have ventricular dysrhythmias compared to horses with other forms of valvular regurgitation (relative risk 1.87, 1.05–3.31, P = 0.035; C. M. Marr, unpublished data) and this appears to be independent of the severity of AR, while supraventricular premature depolarizations are more likely to be seen in horses with severe AR.[37] Therefore, ambulatory and exercising electrocardiography are recommended as part of the diagnostic work-up in cases of AR, particularly in horses with moderate to severe AI that are being used for riding purposes (Fig. 16.3). The pathogenesis of these dysrhythmias is not clear; in some cases, there may be valvular and myocardial disease of similar pathogenesis, for example, with infective endocarditis and myocarditis or endocardial and myocardial fibrosis (see Chapter 4). It is also possible that some of the dysrhythmias relate to neuroendocrine changes (i.e. increased circulating cathecholamines) or arise because coronary artery blood flow is disrupted.

Prognosis

When examined as a group, horses with murmurs of left-sided valvular regurgitation (i.e. aortic and/or mitral

Table 16.1 Guidelines for interpreting the clinical significance of valvular regurgitation in horses presented for investigation of murmurs

VALVE	INDICATIONS FOR FURTHER INVESTIGATIONS	ECHOCARDIOGRAPHIC FINDINGS USUALLY ASSOCIATED WITH A GOOD PROGNOSIS	ECHOCARDIOGRAPHIC FINDINGS USUALLY ASSOCIATED WITH A GUARDED PROGNOSIS	SPECIFICALLY ASSOCIATED ARRHYTHMIAS
Aortic	Hyperkinetic pulses Murmur grade ≥3/6 Young horse Older (>approx. 15 years) horse still used for ridden activities Concurrent murmurs of mitral regurgitation or ventricular septal defect Fever Poor performance Signs of congestive heart failure	Valvular prolapse or mild to moderate nodular changes No or moderate left ventricular dilation No or moderate increase in fractional shortening Small, low-velocity regurgitant jet with long pressure half-time	Flail cusp or severe thickening or nodular changes on valve Severe left ventricular dilation, marked globoid apex Marked increase in fractional shortening or normal to low fractional shortening with marked left ventricular dilation Large, high-velocity regurgitant jet with short pressure half-time Large regurgitant jet with minimal left ventricular dilation (suggests acute onset) Concurrent severe mitral regurgitation or ventricular septal defect Rapid progression on repeated examinations	Ventricular dysrhythmias
Mitral	Murmur grade ≥3/6 Loud third heart sound Fever Poor performance Signs of congestive heart failure	Valvular prolapse with no structural changes Normal left atrial diameter No left ventricular dilation Small regurgitant jet	Moderate to severe thickening or nodular changes on valve, flail cusp, ruptured chordae tendineae Left atrial enlargement Left ventricular volume overload; dilation, globoid apex Pulmonary artery dilation Large regurgitant jet with minimal left ventricular dilation (acute onset) Rapid progression on repeated examinations	Atrial fibrillation Other atrial dysrhythmias Ventricular dysrhythmias
Tricuspid	Murmur grade > 4/6 in Thoroughbreds or Standardbreds Murmur grade >3/6 in other breeds in which it is less common Increased jugular pulses Fever Poor performance Signs of congestive heart failure	Valvular prolapse with no structural changes No right atrial enlargement No right ventricular dilation Small to moderate low-velocity regurgitant jet	Severe thickening or nodular changes on valve, flail cusp, ruptured chordae tendineae Marked right atrial enlargement Right ventricular dilation, double-apex heart High-velocity regurgitant jet Paradoxical septal motion Rapid progression on repeated examinations	Atrial fibrillation (often coincidental)
Pulmonic	Murmur grade ≥1/6 Fever Poor performance Signs of congestive heart failure	No structural changes No right ventricular dilation Small to moderate low-velocity regurgitant jet	Severe thickening or nodular changes on valve, flail cups Right ventricular dilation, double-apex heart Paradoxical septal motion Rapid progression of repeated examinations	None

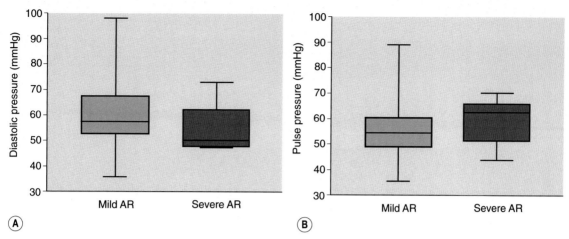

Figure 16.1 Diastolic (**A**) and pulse (**B**) pressures in horses with mild and severe aortic regurgitation (AR). Horses with severe AR were more likely to have diastolic pressure <50 mmHg (odds ratio = 5.34, 1.23–23.23, P = 0.017) and pulse pressure >60 mmHg (odds ratio 8.55, 1.84–39.62, P = 0.002). The box extends from the 25th to 75th percentile with a line at the median. The whiskers extend above and below the box to show the highest and lowest values. Reproduced with permission from Horn JNR (2002) Sympathetic nervous control of cardiac function and its role in equine heart disease, PhD thesis, University of London.

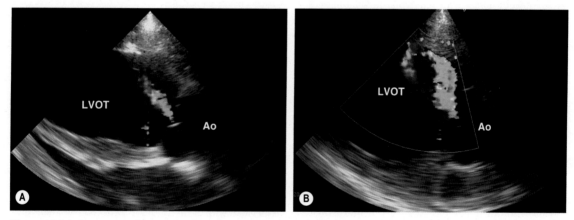

Figure 16.2 Left parasternal long-axis colour flow Doppler echocardiograms from: (**A**) a 9-year-old Thoroughbred gelding with mild aortic insufficiency; (**B**) a 14-year-old Arabian mare with degenerative valvular heart disease and moderate aortic insufficiency. Notice that the area occupied by the regurgitant jet (yellow and green) relates to its severity. RA, right atrium; RV, right ventricle; LVOT, left ventricular outflow tract; Ao, aorta; LA, left atrium.

regurgitation) have a similar life expectancy to those that do not have these murmurs.[27] Nevertheless, some individuals do develop cardiac failure as a result of aortic valve disease and the task of the clinician is to identify these specific individuals. In middle-aged horses, AR is usually well tolerated and horses with mild to moderate AI, which is slowly progressive and is not associated with ventricular dysrhythmias, can be used successfully as riding horses for several years after the diagnosis is made (see Table 16.1). Older horses should be investigated if they are to continue to be used for riding, and AR may be more clinically significant if it is detected in a young animal in which degenerative disease is unlikely to be present; thus the less common but more rapidly progressive forms of pathology must be considered (see Table 16.1). A poor prognosis is warranted with acute onset, severe AI and severe, advanced degenerative disease, particularly if the degree of left ventricular dilatation has caused dilatation of the mitral valve annulus and mitral regurgitation (MR) or if there is marked ventricular ectopy.

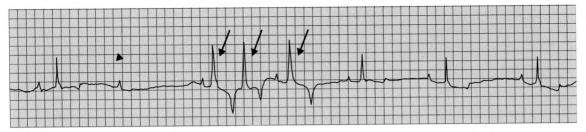

Figure 16.3 Ventricular premature depolarizations (arrows) and second-degree atrioventricular block (arrowhead) in an aged Thoroughbred gelding with severe aortic insufficiency.

In a group mainly comprising older, retired horses in the UK, a loud (>3/6) heart AR murmur, multiple heart murmurs, hyperkinetic pulses, systolic pressure ≥125 mmHg, diastolic pressure ≤50 mmHg, pulse pressure ≥60 mmHg, plasma noradrenaline concentration ≥130 pg/ml, plasma adrenaline ≥40 pg/ml and various indices of heart rate variability were all shown to have some value as predictors for progression of heart disease in horses with AI. However, the presence of ventricular dysrhythmias had much the highest likelihood ratio, suggesting that 30–50% of horses with ventricular premature depolarizations and AI are at risk of progression within 2 years.[37] Further studies are needed to validate this conclusion in other populations.

MITRAL REGURGITATION AND INSUFFICIENCY (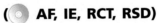 SFP, VMD)

Prevalence

Murmurs of MR are present in around 2.9–3.5% of the otherwise healthy, general horse population.[27,29] However, in racing Thoroughbreds the prevalence is much higher and it is at its highest in horses competing over jumps (19% of hurdlers and 23% of steeplechasers) compared to 7–18% of various groups of Thoroughbreds successfully engaged in flat racing.[6]

Pathogenesis

Physiological MR is common in equine athletes. The mitral valve is the second commonest location for valvular pathology, most often related to degenerative valvular disease.[1,13] Less often, the mitral valve may be affected by infective endocarditis, nonseptic valvulitis or congenital valvular dysplasia.[5,11,12] MR can arise secondary to dilation of the valve annulus in cardiomyopathy or as a result of severe AI or congenital malformations. Chordae tendineae

can rupture spontaneously or following inflammatory or degenerative disease (see Fig. 18.5) and this has an acute severe impact on left heart haemodynamics and therefore is poorly tolerated in comparison to the more slowly progressive lesions. (RCT) Occasionally, neoplasia, most notably lymphosarcoma, can affect the mitral valve. (CN) Mitral insufficiency (MI) is the most likely form of valvular insufficiency to lead to congestive heart failure or sudden death due to pulmonary rupture[5,10,13] (see Fig. 18.4) and both are the result of pulmonary hypertension, which ensues as MR leads first to increases in left atrial pressure, and ultimately to increased pressure within the pulmonary circulation. MI and increased left atrial size are also risk factors for the development of atrial fibrillation.[39]

Clinical findings

(AF, IE, RCT, RSD)

Horses with MR can present with murmurs found incidentally, with poor performance or occasionally in congestive heart failure (see Chapter 19). MR is the most frequent form of valvular regurgitation referred to specialist centres for cardiological investigation and is more likely to be associated with signs of poor performance than other forms of valvular regurgitation. In a study conducted between 1993 and 1998, 35% of horses presented to the author's clinic for investigation of valvular regurgitation had MR and in 50% of these there was a history of poor performance.

The MR murmur is holo- or pansystolic, typically band shaped and is loudest over the left fifth intercostal space, and radiates variable distances caudodorsally (see Chapter 8). A widely accepted and useful clinical guideline is that MR murmurs of grade 3/6 or greater warrant further investigation (Table 16.1), however, this "rule" serves as guide only and MR murmurs ≥grade 3/6 can be found in elite racehorses with no performance limitations.[6] The grade of the murmur does not necessarily relate to the severity of the disease, and it may reflect the direction of the regurgitant jet, frequently being louder if the jet is orientated towards the chest wall as opposed to the slightly more common caudodorsal direction. The degree of radiation of the murmur is an important guide to severity with more severe MR being audible over a wide area. Horses with MR and a loud third heart sound should also be investigated further: the third heart sound relates to early ventricular filling and increases in its volume raise the suspicion that there may be increased left ventricular diastolic filling and left ventricular volume overload. (*RCT*)

Echocardiography

(AF, ET, IE, RCT, RSD, VSD)

Severe degenerative disease of the mitral valve typically produces generalized or nodular thickening, although in milder cases there may be no echocardiographic evidence of structure changes in degenerative valve disease.[5,21] Mitral valve prolapse is a fairly common echocardiographic finding,[4] often associated with a mid-systolic murmur and it is usually non-progressive although as is the case with aortic valvular prolapse, the possibility of a link between mitral valve prolapse and subsequent valvular disease has not been investigated critically. Large, vibrating nodular lesions are suggestive of infective endocarditis. Portions of the chordae tendineae may flail into the left atrium with ruptured chordae tendinea.[5,40] These are usually found in left parasternal long-axis images and a careful search across the entire valve plane is required as they may be seen in only one image. (*RCT*)

Flow mapping can underestimate the severity of MR, because it is difficult to align the ultrasound beam parallel to the direction of regurgitant flow. (*RSD*) Therefore, care must be taken if a small jet is detected in a horse with other signs of severe MI, such as left atrial enlargement or left ventricular volume overload. Echocardiographic signs consistent with left ventricular volume overload include increases in the left atrial diameter and enlargement of the left ventricle with rounding of its apex such that the ventricle adopts a globular appearance. (*RCT*) The diameter of the pulmonary artery should be assessed as dilation is suggestive of pulmonary hypertension and may be a precursor to rupture, collapse and death.[5] Myocardial disease may accompany mitral valve disease.[5] If this has led to severe dilatation, the prognosis is poor, particularly if the fractional shortening is decreased. With mild ventricular dilatation and slight reduction in fractional shortening, the horse may experience reduced athletic performance but be able to perform light work provided that there are no concurrent exercise-associated dysrhythmias (Fig. 16.4).

Electrocardiography

(AF)

MR can lead to left atrial dilation and in turn atrial fibrillation. Chronic atrial fibrillation can also lead to or exacerbate MR. The MR rarely disappears, but can become less severe if the dysrhythmia is successfully treated. In the presence of moderate to severe MR, the AF is often

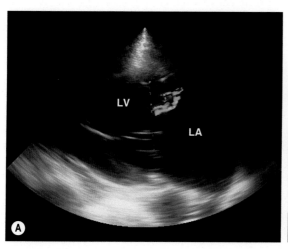

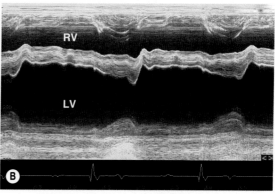

Figure 16.4 A left parasternal long-axis echocardiogram (**A**) of the left atrium (LA) and left ventricle (LV) and right parasternal M-mode echocardiogram (**B**) of the left and right ventricles (RV) from a 9-year-old event horse presented for lethargy with a grade 3/6 holosystolic murmur over the mitral valve. A small jet of mitral insufficiency is present and there is a mild reduction in the fractional shortening (27%) with poor left ventricular free-wall motility, suggesting myocardial dysfunction.

refractory to cardioversion, and in a performance horse, this may end a competitive career.[39] Horses with severe MI also have a high incidence of ventricular dysrhythmias, often associated with ventricular myocardial fibrosis.[5]

Prognosis

Physiological MR does not affect racing performance[6,16] and can also be assumed to have minimal impact on the majority of horses engaged in other, less arduous sports. In the general horse population, the presence of left-sided valvular regurgitation does not affect lifespan.[27] In attempting to formulate a prognosis in horses with MR, the jet should be semi-quantitated and the dimensions of the left ventricle, left atrium and pulmonary artery should be carefully evaluated. A good prognosis can be offered if the regurgitant jet is small, there are no valvular structural changes and no cardiac enlargement. Pulmonary artery dilatation is a particularly poor prognostic sign[5] (see Fig. 18.4), and care should be taken not to underestimate the importance of MR in horses with large regurgitant jets and minimal atrial enlargement, because this may indicate moderate or severe regurgitation of recent onset which may continue to progress; thus the echocardiographic examination should be repeated within 2–4 months to re-assess the degree of valvular insufficiency. In horses with degenerative valvular disease, progression does occur but this generally occurs slowly over months or years; repetition of the echocardiographic examination is recommended at 6 to 12 month intervals provided no further clinical signs are detected that might prompt an earlier re-assessment.

TRICUSPID REGURGITATION AND INSUFFICIENCY (VMD)

Prevalence

Murmurs of tricuspid regurgitation (TR) are frequently encountered, particularly in performance horses.[16,29] In one survey of 545 horses, the overall incidence was 9% but the incidence in Thoroughbred racehorses was 16.4%.[29] In another, TR murmurs were detected in around 20–25% of Thoroughbreds in flat racing and approximately 40–50% of Thoroughbreds in jump racing.[6] TR is even more common in surveys utilizing Doppler echocardiography.[2,4,6] Murmurs of TR are also often found in Standardbreds while TR is not found as frequently in non-athletic breeds: in a survey from the author's clinical population, 22% of Thoroughbreds presented for investigation of murmurs had TR, whereas there was an incidence of 8% in mixed pleasure horses and 5% in ponies.

Pathogenesis

The inciting mechanisms in physiological TR remain unclear and may relate to changes in the geometry of the ventricle or to haemodynamic or neuroendocrine changes associated with increased fitness. The tricuspid valve is rarely diseased[1] but ruptured chorda tendinea and dysplastic, inflammatory and degenerative diseases can occasionally occur. Infective endocarditis of the tricuspid valve tends to be associated with septic jugular thrombophlebitis (see Chapter 17).

Clinical findings (AF)

TR is rarely related to clinical signs such as exercise intolerance in performance animals, but if it is encountered in breeds in which it is less common, it may warrant further investigation (Table 16.1).

The murmur of TR is typically holo- or pansystolic and is loudest over the right heart base, in the right fourth intercostal space. It is usually blowing and crescendo–decrescendo in nature but can be harsh in some cases and tends to radiate concentrically from its point of maximal intensity (see Chapter 8). With severe tricuspid insufficiency (TI) signs of right heart compromise include distension and pulsation of the jugular veins, ventral oedema and pleural and peritoneal effusion. It is important to bear in mind that the main differential diagnosis for a right-sided murmur is a ventricular septal defect (see Chapter 8). It is also important to be aware that approximately 30% of horses with infective endocarditis of the tricuspid valve do not have murmurs.[41]

Echocardiography (AF, ET, IE, VSD)

Tricuspid valvular prolapse is seen commonly and, occasionally, lesions such as rupture of a chorda tendinea, infective endocarditis and severe degenerative valve disease are encountered. The severity of TR can be semiquantitated with Doppler echocardiography fairly easily and there is less difficulty in achieving alignment to regurgitant flow at the tricuspid valve. Signs of right ventricular volume overload include dilatation of the right ventricle, rounding of its apex so that the heart appears to have a double apex, and paradoxical septal motion.

Electrocardiography

TR was reported in 22% of horses presenting with atrial fibrillation, but in all but two of these this was secondary to severe MI.[39] Therefore, TR does not appear to predispose to the development of atrial fibrillation unless it is severe. Investigation of the association between TR and ventricular dysrhythmias in the author's clinical population produced insignificant results, with a tendency towards a reduced risk of development of dysrhythmias in horses with tricuspid regurgitation compared to other forms of valvular regurgitation.

Prognosis

TR is unlikely to affect athletic performance and loud TR murmurs and large TR jets have been documented in elite racehorses with no performance limitations.[6] Horses with normal valve structure or valvular prolapse, mild to moderate TR and no signs of right ventricular volume overload generally have a good prognosis for continued performance (see Table 16.1). Care must be taken to ensure that TR is the only cardiac abnormality, as where it occurs in association with other lesions such as MR or AR, or congenital defects, a more guarded prognosis is warranted.

PULMONIC REGURGITATION AND INSUFFICIENCY (AF, ET)

Isolated pulmonic valvular pathology is extremely rare;[1,42,43] although malformations of the pulmonary valve may be a component of congenital heart disease these usually lead to stenosis rather than regurgitation. On the other hand, physiological pulmonic regurgitation (PR) is common and horses will readily develop PR if there is pulmonary hypertension. Murmurs of PR are very unusual (Chapter 8). They are not readily auscultated because of the low pressures within the right side of the circulation. Therefore, if a murmur of PR is detected, particularly in a horse with other signs of right-sided heart failure or with fever that might suggest infective endocarditis, further investigation is justified. Echocardiography is the main diagnostic tool used to detect pulmonic valvular lesions, semiquantitate regurgitation and assess the status of the right ventricle (see Chapter 9).

REFERENCES

1. Else RW, Holmes JR. Cardiac pathology in the horse. 1. Gross pathology. Equine Vet J 1972;4(1): 1–8.

2. Blissitt KJ, Bonagura JD. Colour flow Doppler echocardiography in normal horses. Equine Vet J Suppl 1995;19: 47–55.

3. Blissitt KJ, Bonagura JD. Colour flow Doppler echocardiography in horses with cardiac murmurs. Equine Vet J Suppl 1995;19:82–85.

4. Marr CM, Reef VB. Physiological valvular regurgitation in clinically normal young racehorses: prevalence and two-dimensional colour flow Doppler echocardiographic characteristics. Equine Vet J Suppl 1995;19:56–62.

5. Reef VB, Bain FT, Spencer PA. Severe mitral regurgitation in horses: clinical, echocardiographic and pathological findings. Equine Vet J 1998;30(1):18–27.

6. Young LE, Rogers K, Wood JL. Heart murmurs and valvular regurgitation in thoroughbred racehorses: epidemiology and associations with athletic performance. J Vet Intern Med 2008;22(2):418–426.

7. Mahaffey L. Fenestration of the aortic and pulmonary semilunar valves in the horse. Vet Rec 1958;70:415–418.

8. Bishop S, Cole CR, Smetzer DL. Functional and morphologic pathology of equine aortic insufficiency. Path Vet 1966;3: 137–158.

9. Else R, Holmes JR. Cardiac pathology in the horse. 2. Microscopic pathology. Equine Vet J 1972;4:57–62.

10. Holmes J, Miller PJ. Three cases of ruptured mitral valve chordae in the horse. Equine Vet J 1984;16:125–135.

11. Buergelt CD. Equine cardiovascular pathology: an overview. Anim Health Res Rev 2003;4(2): 109–129.

12. Buergelt C, Cooley AJ, Hones SA, Pipers FS. Endocarditis in six horses. Vet Pathol 1985;22: 333–337.

13. Miller P, Holmes JR. Observations on seven cases of mitral insufficiency in the horse. Equine Vet J 1985;17:181–190.

14. Bowen IM, Marr CM, Chester AH, et al. In-vitro contraction of the equine aortic valve. J Heart Valve Dis 2004;13(4):593–599.

15. Young LE, Wood JL. Effect of age and training on murmurs of atrioventricular valvular regurgitation in young thoroughbreds. Equine Vet J 2000;32(3):195–199.

16. Kriz NG, Hodgson DR, Rose RJ. Prevalence and clinical importance of heart murmurs in racehorses. J Am Vet Med Assoc 2000;216(9): 1441–1445.

17. Reef VB. Heart murmurs in horses: determining their significance with echocardiography. Equine Vet J Suppl 1995;19:71–80.

18. Bonagura JD, Blissitt KJ. Echocardiography. Equine Vet J Suppl 1995;19:5–17.

19. Lombard CW, Evans M, Martin L, Tehrani J, et al. Blood pressure, electrocardiogram and echocardiogram measurements in the growing pony foal. Equine Vet J 1984;16(4):342–347.

20. Stewart JH, Rose RJ, Barko AM. Echocardiography in foals from birth to three months old. Equine Vet J 1984;16(4):332–341.

21. Reef VB. Advances in echocardiography. Vet Clin North Am Equine Pract 1991;7(2):435–450.

22. Reef VB, Spencer P. Echocardiographic evaluation of equine aortic insufficiency. Am J Vet Res 1987;48(6):904–909.

23. Reef V. Echocardiographic examination in the horse: the basics. Compend Contin Educ Pract Vet 1990;12:1312–1319.

24. Long K, Bonagura JD, Darke PGG. Standardised imaging technique for guided M mode and Doppler echocardiography in the horse. Equine Vet J 1992;24:226–235.

25. Reef VB, Lalezari K, De Boo J, et al. Pulsed-wave Doppler evaluation of intracardiac blood flow in 30 clinically normal Standardbred horses. Am J Vet Res 1989;50(1):75–83.

26. Stadler P, Hoch M, Fraunhaul B, Deegen E. Echocardiography in horses with and without heart murmurs in aortic regurgitation. Pferdeheilkunde 1995;11:373–383.

27. Stevens KB, Marr CM, Horn JN, et al. Effect of left-sided valvular regurgitation on mortality and causes of death among a population of middle-aged and older horses. Vet Rec 2009;164(1):6–10.

28. Holmes JR. Equine Cardiology, Vol 3. Langford, Bristol: JR Holmes; 1986.

29. Patteson MW, Cripps PJ. A survey of cardiac auscultatory findings in horses. Equine Vet J 1993;25(5):409–415.

30. Olsen LH, Fredholm M, Pedersen HD. Epidemiology and inheritance of mitral valve prolapse in Dachshunds. J Vet Intern Med 1999;13(5):448–456.

31. Hallowell G, Bowen IM. Aortic valve prolapse in the horse: epidemiology and the effects of training. J Vet Intern Med, in press.

32. Bonagura JD, Pipers FS. Echocardiographic features of aortic valve endocarditis in a dog, a cow, and a horse. J Am Vet Med Assoc 1983;182(6):595–599.

33. Maxson AD, Reef VB. Bacterial endocarditis in horses: ten cases (1984–1995). Equine Vet J 1997;29(5):394–399.

34. Rooney J, Franks WC. Congenital cardiac anomalies in horses. Vet Pathol 1964;1:454–464.

35. Clark ES, Reef VB, Sweeney CR, Lichtensteiger C, et al. Aortic valve insufficiency in a one-year-old colt. J Am Vet Med Assoc 1987;191(7):841–844.

36. Reef VB. Evaluation of ventricular septal defects in horses using two-dimensional and Doppler echocardiography. Equine Vet J Suppl, 1995(19):86–95.

37. Horn J. Sympathetic Nervous Control of Cardiac Function and its role in Equine Heart Disease. Royal Veterinary College University of London, 2002.

38. Patteson MW. Echocardiographic evaluation of horses with aortic regurgitation. Equine Vet Educ 1994;6:159–166.

39. Reef VB, Levitan CW, Spencer PA. Factors affecting prognosis and conversion in equine atrial fibrillation. J Vet Intern Med 1988;2(1):1–6.

40. Reef VB. Mitral valvular insufficiency associated with ruptured chordae tendineae in three foals. J Am Vet Med Assoc 1987;191(3):329–331.

41. Marr CM. Cardiovascular infections. In: Sellon E, Long MT, editors. Equine Infectious Diseases. Philadelphia: Saunders Elsevier; 2007. p. 21–38.

42. Reimer JM, Reef VB, Sommer M. Echocardiographic detection of pulmonic valve rupture in a horse with right-sided heart failure. J Am Vet Med Assoc 1991;198(5):880–882.

43. Nilsfors L, Lombard CW, Weckner D, Kvart C, et al. Diagnosis of pulmonary valve endocarditis in a horse. Equine Vet J 1991;23(6):479–482.

Chapter | 17 |

Fever: endocarditis and pericarditis

Abby Sage

INFECTIVE ENDOCARDITIS

Infective endocarditis is a microbial infection of the endothelial surface of the heart. In horses, infective endocarditis is characterized by bacterial or fungal invasion of the valves (valvular endocarditis) or wall of the endocardium (mural endocarditis) resulting in fibrinous clots or vegetations. Although infective endocarditis affects horses of all ages, the median age is 5 years with a range of reported cases from 2 months to 15 years.[1-20] Males are more likely to be affected than females. No breed predilection has been found.

Infective endocarditis predominantly affects the left side of the heart in the horse. The prognosis is poor in these cases because even with bacteriological cure, persistent regurgitation often leads to left ventricular volume overload, left heart failure and pulmonary hypertension.

Clinical signs

(IE)

The most frequently seen clinical signs are intermittent or continuous fever, cardiac murmur, tachycardia and tachypnoea.[1-20] Shifting leg lameness, intermittent joint distention, coughing, ventral oedema and depression are less commonly seen. Fever is present in almost all cases of infective endocarditis[1-22] and in many cases is the primary complaint.[5] Shifting leg lameness may be associated with effusion of one or more synovial structures. The lameness may be due to haematogenous synovial sepsis, emboli or immune complex deposition. Signs of congestive heart failure may be present in severely affected individuals. Clinical signs of left heart failure in the horse include tachypnoea, crackles and harsh lung sounds on thoracic auscultation. Signs of right heart failure are ventral oedema, venous distention and jugular vein pulsation.

The mitral valve is most often affected in the horse followed by the aortic, tricuspid and then the pulmonary valve.[5,18] The predominance of mitral valve endocarditis is also reported in some other species.[26] Cardiac murmurs associated with infective endocarditis in the horse are generally harsh holosystolic band-shaped grade 3/6 or louder if the atrioventricular valves are involved. If the semilunar valves are affected, the murmur is most often decrescendo holodiastolic grade 2/6 or louder. Cardiac murmurs are most often associated with regurgitation through the affected valve although murmurs of valvular stenosis can occur.[11] All horses with aortic or mitral valve involvement had a cardiac murmur.[1-3,6-20] Right-sided vegetative lesions may not produce a cardiac murmur as a result of a lower pressure difference between the right atrium and ventricle in comparison to left-sided pressures.[3-5] Mural and small valvular lesions also may not produce a cardiac murmur. If a cardiac murmur is not present and bacterial endocarditis is suspected, an echocardiogram should be performed to examine the valves for vegetative lesions.

Cardiac dysrhythmias in horses with bacterial endocarditis, although uncommon, may occur as a result of direct extension of the inflammatory lesion into the myocardium or thromboembolic myocardial ischaemia. Cardiac dysrhythmias reported in horses with bacterial endocarditis include atrial fibrillation, ventricular tachycardia and supraventricular and ventricular extrasystoles.[5,12,14,17,18]

© 2010 Elsevier Ltd.
DOI: 10.1016/B978-0-7020-2817-5.00022-5

Pathogenesis and microbiology

The source of infection is often not determined in the horse. Infective endocarditis has been associated with jugular vein thrombophlebitis[5,21,22] and with the presence of a transvenous pacing catheter[23] in the horse. Congenital heart disease is a frequent finding in human beings with infective endocarditis[24] but has not been reported in the horse. Many species of bacteria cause infective endocarditis in the horse. *Streptococcus* spp. and *Actinobacillus* spp. are the most common organisms cultured from horses with infective endocarditis although a wide range of pathogens has been reported.[1-20] Two reports of infective endocarditis were attributed to fungal infection with *Aspergillus* and *Candida* species.[7,18] *Borrelia burgdorferi* has also been implicated.[25]

Bacteraemia allows bacteria to reach the heart by haematogenous spread through blood in the chambers of the heart. Breaks in the endothelial surface may occur in three ways: (1) high-velocity jet impacting the endothelium; (2) flow from high to low pressure chamber; and (3) flow across a narrow orifice at high velocity.[24] The organism invades the valve through breaks in the endothelial surface. If the endothelium on the valve surface is damaged, platelets and fibrin are deposited. The platelet–fibrin complex is more receptive to bacterial colonization than intact endothelium and shields the bacteria from phagocytosis. Papilliferous masses of platelets, fibrin and bacteria supported by a bed of granulation tissue develop on the valve surface and are known as vegetations. Vegetations are found at the valve-closure line in the atrial surface of the atrioventricular valves and on the ventricular surface of the semilunar valves.

The clinical signs of infective endocarditis result from: (1) local destructive effects of intracardiac infection; (2) embolization of fragments of the vegetations to distant sites resulting in infection or infarction; (3) haematogenous seeding of remote sites during continuous bacteraemia and metastatic infection; and (4) deposition of immune complexes in tissues resulting in synovitis and glomerulonephritis.[24] The vegetations distort the valvular architecture, which leads to valvular incompetence and/or stenosis and cardiac murmur. If regurgitation through the affected valve is sufficient, congestive heart failure can develop. In addition, local destruction of tissues may lead to chordae tendineae rupture and perforation or fistulas between cardiac chambers or major blood vessels. Myocardial infection and myocardial microabscess may cause disruption of the conduction system, dysrhythmias and myocardial failure. Arterial emboli originating from the vegetation most commonly affect the coronary arteries, kidney, spleen, brain and lung, resulting in specific clinical signs.[24]

The haemodynamic consequences of infective endocarditis are dependent on the valve(s) affected, degree of regurgitation and severity of the infection. In cases of mitral valvular lesions and significant regurgitation, the excessive pressure in the left atrium may be transferred retrograde to the pulmonary vasculature and pulmonary oedema may develop. The high pressures may also be transferred to the pulmonary artery and right heart resulting in signs of right heart failure with the potential for pulmonary artery rupture. In general, aortic regurgitation is better tolerated in the horse. Moderate to severe aortic regurgitation may cause left ventricular volume overload, dilation and subsequent mitral regurgitation. Tricuspid regurgitation is less likely to have significant haemodynamic effects but the potential for right heart failure exists.

Clinical pathology

(IE)

Hyperfibrinogenaemia, leucocytosis with a mature neutrophilia, hyperproteinaemia and anaemia are the most common abnormal laboratory findings in horses with infective endocarditis.[1-19] Hyperproteinaemia reflects hypergammaglobulinaemia. The anaemia is nonregenerative and is typical of anaemia of chronic disease. Thrombocytopaenia occurs uncommonly. Prerenal azotaemia may accompany dehydration or shock. Azotaemia may also be found in patients with bacterial endocarditis if congestive heart failure, immune mediated glomerulonephritis or renal infarcts or emboli are present. Serum amyloid A and cardiac troponin I may also be useful in diagnosis and monitoring of treatment.

Bacteraemia associated with bacterial endocarditis is continuous but the number of bacteria at any one time may fluctuate.[27] Ideally, three blood cultures should be obtained at least 1 hour apart prior to the initiation of antimicrobial therapy. Blood should be cultured in aerobic and anaerobic media for at least 4 days before determining that the culture is negative. Obtaining blood for cultures during peak temperature elevation has not been shown to increase the number of positive cultures.[24] Previous antimicrobial administration has been shown to inhibit positive blood culture for 7–10 days in human beings.[24] Therefore, withholding antimicrobials to improve the success rate of a positive blood culture is not warranted in the acute case. Antimicrobial removal devices have been shown to be effective in increasing the likelihood of a positive blood culture in patients that are receiving antimicrobials.[28] Negative blood cultures should not rule out bacterial endocarditis especially in horses previously treated with antimicrobials.

Echocardiography

(IE)

Echocardiography provides an accurate diagnosis by identifying the location of the lesion(s) and determining its size. It should be performed in all patients suspected of infective endocarditis regardless of a negative blood culture. Echocardiography is also useful in formulating a prognosis by assessing degree of chamber enlargement, severity of regurgitation and extent of myocardial dysfunction. In humans transoesophageal echocardiography using biplane technology is the preferred approach. Due to size and financial limitations, this technology is not used in clinical practice in the horse. Vegetative lesions on the valves, chordae tendineae, mural endocardium or intimal surface of the great vessels appear as irregular shaggy hypoechoic to echogenic masses on the echocardiogram. Vegetative lesions that extend from the valve margins can result in a flailing motion with movement of the affected valve leaflet. The shaggy thickened appearance of the valve may also be detected on M-mode echocardiography. Ruptured chordae tendineae associated with vegetative lesions may also be detected with echocardiography as a flail valve leaflet. Extension of the infection beyond the valve leaflet worsens the prognosis. In less severe cases, the lesion may appear as an irregular thickening. These lesions may be difficult to distinguish from severe degenerative valvular disease. Clinical signs, clinical pathology data, age of the animal and response to therapy must all be taken into account in these cases. Appropriate antimicrobial therapy should be initiated until an alternative diagnosis is reached. (RCT)

Doppler interrogation of the affected valve should be performed to semiquantitate the severity of regurgitation or stenosis and spectral and colour flow Doppler are used to map the size and location of the regurgitant jet[29-33] (see Chapter 9). In significant mitral regurgitation, left atrial and ventricular enlargement are present.[33] The severity of the enlargement is dependent on the amount and duration of the regurgitation and may be relatively mild in the early stages of the disease even in the presence of severe regurgitation. Rounding of the left ventricular apex suggests left ventricular volume overload. The left parasternal 2-chamber view of the left atrium provides the best image to measure left atrial diameter.[29,33] Increases in left atrial pressures create a turgid round appearance of the left atrium and bulging of the interatrial septum to the right.[33]

Dilation of the pulmonary artery is an indicator of pulmonary hypertension.[33] The pulmonary artery diameter obtained in the two-dimensional right parasternal view of the right outflow tract should be less than or equal to the aortic diameter obtained in the right parasternal left outflow tract view.[33] If the pulmonary artery diameter exceeds the aortic diameter, pulmonary hypertension is present. Horses with pulmonary hypertension are at risk for sudden death secondary to rupture of the pulmonary artery.[33] A smaller than normal aortic diameter is compatible with low left ventricular output and left heart failure.[33]

Moderate to severe aortic regurgitation results in left ventricular volume overload[34] and in left ventricular dilation the interventricular septum and left ventricular free wall may become thin.[29,34] Fractional shortening is expected to be above normal in horses with volume overload and concurrent normal myocardial function. A normal or decreased fractional shortening is indicative of myocardial dysfunction.[29,34] The aortic root becomes dilated in moderate to severe aortic regurgitation most likely because of increased blood flow into the aorta.[29,34] Premature closure of the mitral valve may occur in cases of severe regurgitation due to the volume overload.[35] In addition, the septal leaflet of the mitral valve may have high-frequency diastolic flutter visible on M-mode echocardiography.[29,34,35]

Doppler echocardiography of the aortic valve can be performed from the right parasternal long-axis view of the left outflow tract, the right parasternal short-axis view of the aorta or the left parasternal long-axis view of the left outflow tract. The most parallel flow signal is from the left parasternal window.[29] Aortic regurgitation jets are either directed towards the left apex or travel laterally towards the left ventricular free wall.[32] A sharp decline (steep slope) in the continuous wave Doppler spectral tracing of the aortic regurgitation indicates a rapid increase in left ventricular diastolic pressure and severe aortic regurgitation.[32] The severity of regurgitation is determined by the distance the regurgitant jet travels into the left ventricular outflow tract and the width of the jet at its origin.[32] A regurgitant jet that extends into more than two-thirds of the left ventricular outflow tract beyond the septal leaflet of the mitral valve is considered severe.[32]

When tricuspid regurgitation is moderate to severe, right atrial enlargement will be present.[35] Volume overload of the right ventricle will present with right ventricle enlargement and possible dilation.[29] Paradoxical septal motion occurs when there is severe tricuspid regurgitation and right ventricular volume overload.[35] A regurgitant jet that occupies more than two-thirds of the atrium is considered severe.[29]

Serial echocardiography can be used to assess therapeutic success. A decrease in lesion size, increase in echogenicity of the lesion and smoothing of the vegetative lesion is consistent with resolution of the infection as a result of fibrous scar tissue formation and contracture. However, studies in human beings indicate that infective endocarditis that is ultimately successfully treated with antimicrobial therapy may not show any change in the appearance of the lesions.[24] Changes in vegetations must be interpreted in a clinical context and do not in themselves reflect the efficacy of therapy.[24]

Treatment and prognosis

Treatment of horses with bacterial endocarditis should be rapid, appropriate and prolonged. Bactericidal antimicrobial agents based on the sensitivity pattern of the organism should be chosen if possible. However, broad-spectrum antimicrobials should be initiated before blood culture results are available or if a negative blood culture is obtained. Delay in antimicrobial therapy may lead to progression of the associated cardiac disease. Penicillin and gentamicin are the most commonly selected choices.[2,3,5,7,8,10,12] Other antimicrobials including enrofloxacin, ampicillin,[8] trimethoprim sulphonamide,[3,7] metronidazole,[17] oxytetracycline,[6] ceftoxamine[11] and rifampicin[14] have also been described with none emerging as superior to the others.[2,54,5,7,12,13,17] Bactericidal drugs are preferable to bacteriostatic drugs in this life-threatening bacteraemia. Successful treatment of fungal infective endocarditis has not been described.[7] Although the appropriate duration of therapy is unknown, reports of successful outcome in the literature suggests a minimum of 5–6 weeks.[12–14] Resolution of clinical signs, a decrease in size, an increase in echogenicity and smoother appearance of the lesion on echocardiographic examination and reduction in leucocytosis and hyperfibrinogenaemia should be used to determine the duration of antimicrobial therapy.

A diagnosis of mitral and/or aortic valve infective endocarditis carries a grave prognosis. Only a few cases of successful treatment of bacterial endocarditis involving the mitral or aortic valve have been reported in the horse.[12,13] Although a bacteriological cure may be achieved, valvular endocarditis usually results in regurgitation through the affected valve. Because of the high left heart pressures regurgitation through the mitral or aortic valve often leads to left ventricular volume overload, ventricular dilatation and ventricular dysfunction resulting in congestive heart failure. Systemic arterial emboli originating from a left-sided vegetative lesion most commonly affects the coronary artery and kidneys.[5] Cardiac dysrhythmias may occur secondary to myocardial infarction. Renal failure may result from renal infarction or immune complex deposition.[24]

The prognosis for infective endocarditis involving the tricuspid and/or pulmonary valve is guarded. Although regurgitation through the tricuspid or pulmonary valve is persistent despite bacteriological cure, the lower right-sided pressures in the heart are less likely to lead to congestive heart failure. In human beings, death secondary to right-sided bacterial endocarditis is usually due to extracardiac manifestations.[24] Pneumonia and pulmonary embolism can occur due to dislodgement of part of a vegetative lesion.

PERICARDITIS

Pericarditis, an inflammatory condition of the pericardium, is classified as effusive, fibrinous or constrictive. Effusive pericarditis is characterized by fluid accumulation in the pericardial sac. Fibrinous pericarditis is typified by fibrin in the pericardium. Constrictive pericarditis occurs

when fibrous tissue of the pericardial or myocardial tissue results in compression of the heart. The right ventricle is more vulnerable to the increased pressure than the left and diastolic filling is impaired. Horses usually present with signs of right heart disease. With early recognition and appropriate aggressive treatment a successful outcome is possible.

Clinical signs

 PC)

There is no breed predilection. In two studies, younger horses seemed at increased risk.[36,37] Male intact horses were over-represented and geldings under-represented in one retrospective study.[36] It is more common in men than in women.[38] Reasons for presentation are equally as likely to be respiratory as cardiac and almost always include a history of fever and depression. Almost all horses have tachycardia.[36] Pericardial friction rubs are usually bi- or triphasic and most often occur when there is little to no effusion within the pericardial sac. The noise is generated by friction between the roughened visceral and epicardial surfaces. Muffled heart sounds were present in less than half of the horses examined in one retrospective study.[36] Other clinical signs include murmurs, venous distension, jugular pulses, weak arterial pulses and ventral oedema.[36,39,40] In one study, 75% of the cases also presented with respiratory signs, the most common of which was a dulling of the lung sounds ventrally suggestive of pleural effusion.[36] This frequent co-occurrence of pleuropneumonia/pleuritis and pericarditis highlights the necessity for careful cardiac evaluations in cases presenting for respiratory disease. Occasionally, horses may present with anorexia and signs of colic.[41,42]

Pathophysiology

 PC)

Three types of pericarditis have been distinguished: effusive, fibrinous and constrictive. Effusive pericarditis results in the accumulation of fluid in the pericardial sac.[41] A large amount of fluid in the pericardial sac interferes with diastolic filling of the heart and has the greatest impact on the more compressible lower pressure right heart. Venous return is impaired throughout the entire cardiac cycle. Impaired venous return results in decreased diastolic myocardial perfusion and myocardial hypoxia resulting in decreased myocardial contractility. This decreased myocardial contractility, in conjunction with the decreased stretching of the myocardium secondary to reduced diastolic ventricular filling, results in a decreased stroke volume and cardiac output. Clinical signs of right-sided heart failure become apparent with venous distention, jugular pulses, oedema and ascites developing. The severity of clinical signs increases proportionally with the absolute amount of fluid present and the rate of its accumulation. The state of haemodynamic compromise caused by excessive pericardial fluid and defeating cardiac compensatory mechanisms is termed cardiac tamponade.

With fibrinous pericarditis, fibrin is present within the pericardial sac. Fibrin in the pericardial sac, if plentiful enough, restricts cardiac function. If fibrin matures to fibrous tissue or pericardial or myocardial injury result in fibrosis, then ventricular compliance may be compromised and constrictive pericarditis may result. With constrictive pericarditis, initial diastolic filling is unimpeded but when a critical diastolic volume is reached filling ceases abruptly. The restricted filling decreases preload and therefore cardiac output is decreased. As the diastolic volume of the right side of the heart is greater than that of the left, signs of right-sided heart failure are apparent first.[43]

By far the most common form of pericarditis in the horse in a recent study was fibrino-effusive.[36] Both fibrin and fluid can theoretically muffle heart sounds although fluid is more characteristically associated with this phenomenon. Fluid and/or fibrin in the pericardial sac should be suspected if muffled heart sounds are present on auscultation but should not be ruled out if heart sounds are not muffled. Pericardial friction rubs are believed to be caused by the rubbing of the inflamed pericardial layers and sound like "a creaking leather saddle," "walking on dry snow" or a saw on wood.[38] They can be biphasic (systolic and diastolic) or triphasic (systolic, diastolic and presystolic). Infrequently they are monophasic and can be confused with cardiac murmurs. Their presence or absence appears also to be unrelated to the presence or absence of fluid or fibrin in the pericardial sac.

Aetiology

The most common causes of pericarditis in horses include immune-mediated diseases, bacterial infections and viral infections. Neoplasia is an infrequent cause of pericarditis and heart failure but trauma/vessel rupture are differentials for pericardial effusion. In most cases of pericarditis, the etiology is not determined, making idiopathic pericarditis the most frequent diagnosis.[36]

In human beings, the idiopathic form is a very common etiological diagnosis for pericarditis, second only to metastatic neoplasia.[44] Idiopathic pericarditis in human beings is believed to be viral in origin as it frequently occurs in patients with a history of viral respiratory illness and/or positive serum titres to respiratory viruses. Respiratory viruses have also been successfully isolated from the myocardium and pericardial fluid of human patients with pericarditis. Viruses may lead to the development of pericarditis

via numerous pathways.[45–47] They may play a primary role as they are capable of direct cytopathic activity. They may also be indirectly responsible for the development of pericarditis via the induction of immune-mediated processes. The presence of virus in tissues is associated with infiltration by cytotoxic lymphocytes. Viruses have also been demonstrated to encourage the formation of immune complexes that are secreted into serous effusions and induce inflammation by activating complement and attracting leucocytes.

In horses with pericarditis, as with human beings, there is often a history of respiratory disease or concurrent respiratory disease. The association of pericarditis with pleuritis or pleuropneumonia has been well documented.[36,48–50] In several cases, equine herpes virus has been implicated.[36,51] Sometimes, other clinical signs such as purpura haemorrhagica, vasculitis and haemolytic anemia also suggest an immune-mediated etiology.[36]

Bacteria infection is another major cause of pericarditis in the horse. *Streptococcus* and *Actinobacillus* species are the most common isolates from pericardial fluid in horses with bacterial pericarditis.[36,39,40,50–52] Other bacteria including *Escherichia coli*, *Enterococcus faecalis* and *Corynebacterium pseudobacterium* have been reported.[51,53] In the spring of 2001, an epidemic of equine pericarditis occurred in Kentucky in association with mare reproductive loss syndrome. *Actinobacillus* species was isolated from 11 of 34 cases from the pericardial fluid. Exposure to Eastern tent caterpillars was the greatest risk factor and temporal distribution suggested a point source infection.[54] Changes in immune system function may be responsible for facilitating infection with *Actinobacillus* species in these cases. (PC)

Other less common reported causes of equine pericarditis are *Mycoplasma felis*, trauma from an external thoracic injury, penetrating foreign bodies entering through the gastrointestinal tract and iatrogenic penetration during bone marrow aspiration.[55–57] The definitive identification of the etiology of pericarditis in horses is rare and the use of more sophisticated diagnostic tools such as virus isolation, immunohistochemical studies, and pericardial and myocardial biopsies will be necessary to decrease the number of cases labelled as idiopathic.

Clinical pathology
(PC)

No specific clinical laboratory findings are characteristically associated with pericarditis. Depending upon the etiology, one may see a leucocytosis or a hyperfibrinogenaemia. If the pericarditis is of longstanding duration, associated with another longstanding disease, or associated with immune-mediated processes, then anaemia may be evident. Pericarditis producing heart failure may result in prerenal or renal azotemia, hyponatraemia and hyperkalaemia.[36]

Although often unrewarding, diagnostic laboratory tests must include analyses of pericardial fluid. Normal pericardial fluid should contain <1500 × 10⁶ nucleated cells/L and have a protein content of <2.5 g/L.[58] The diagnosis of septic pericarditis is based on the presence of increased numbers of degenerative neutrophils in the pericardial fluid with or without the presence of bacteria. Cultures of pericardial fluid rarely yield positive results and if possible should be performed before antimicrobial therapy is instituted.[36,41,50,51] Idiopathic or immune-mediated pericarditis is characterized by increased protein and nondegenerate neutrophils in the pericardial fluid.[41,59] Other diagnostic tests that can be performed in an effort to determine the etiology include viral titres for equine herpes virus, equine viral arteritis and equine influenza. If respiratory disease is present, culture and sensitivity and cytology of pleural and transtracheal wash fluids are recommended.

Echocardiography

 PC)

Echocardiography is undoubtedly the most useful diagnostic tool in the diagnosis and treatment of pericarditis. The definitive characterization of the nature of the pericarditis is only possible with the aid of echocardiography. Pericardial fluid can be seen as an anechoic space separating the parietal pericardium from the epicardial surface of the heart. Fibrin is hypoechoic to hyperechoic, usually shaggy and variably distributed throughout the pericardial sac. Echocardiography is also invaluable for assessing the impact of the pericarditis on cardiac function. Echocardiographic findings consistent with cardiac tamponade include: overall decreases in cardiac chamber sizes, right atrial collapse, right ventricular early diastolic collapse, left atrial collapse, abnormal variations in ventricular dimensions and mitral and tricuspid valve flow with phases of respiration, decreased mitral valve anterior leaflet opening (DE) with a slowing of the closure (decreased EF slope), and decreased fractional shortenings of the left ventricle.[44] Appreciable echocardiographic changes occurring with constrictive pericarditis include the abrupt cessation of ventricular filling during early diastole, diastolic flattening of the left ventricular free wall and abnormal increases in tricuspid flow with abnormal decreases in mitral flow during inspiration.[49] Pericardial thickening is often not appreciable. Computed tomography and magnetic resonance imaging are the modalities of choice for demonstrating thickened pericardium in human beings. By permitting assessment of cardiac function, echocardiography plays an essential role in the determination of the necessity for pericardial drainage. In addition, it is useful for guidance of pericardiocentesis and monitoring for fluid reaccumulation and resolution of fibrin.

Electrocardiography

 PC)

Decreased amplitude of the QRS complex and electrical alternans are electrocardiographic findings traditionally associated with pericardial effusions.[44] Decreased QRS amplitude is due to fluid dampening and short circuiting the electrical signal. A decrease in QRS amplitude is not a specific finding, however, since it also occurs with chronic pleuritis, recurrent airway obstruction, obesity, diaphragmatic hernias, thoracic masses and chronic wasting disease. Electrical alternans is due to the swinging of the heart in the pericardial fluid and is a pathognomonic finding. ST segment and T wave abnormalities may also occur due to inflammation of subpericardial myocardium (superficial myocarditis) causing changes in the propagation of electrical signals.

Radiography

Thoracic radiographs are of questionable utility in the diagnostic work-up of pericarditis. No information about the heart can be obtained which is not more readily available using echocardiography. Radiographs may be useful in the work-up of concurrent respiratory disease especially in foals. Thoracic ultrasound is usually more useful in the work-up of concurrent respiratory disease in adults.

Cardiac catheterization

Cardiac catheterization and right ventricular pressure tracing can provide a definitive diagnosis in constrictive pericarditis.[43] There is equalization of the right atrial and ventricular pressures and dip-and-plateau configuration of the right ventricular pressure curve that reflects the abrupt termination of diastolic filling when the limit of compliance of the pericardium is reached.

Treatment and prognosis

 PC)

Treatment should include rest for all animals. Aggressive treatment with broad-spectrum antimicrobials is recommended if bacterial involvement is suspected. When viral- or immune-mediated etiologies are suspected, and signs of active bacterial infections are absent, corticosteroids can be administered. The use of corticosteroids in suspected virally mediated pericarditis is controversial in both human and equine medicine. The bulk of the evidence suggests that the benefit of decreasing the immune-mediated sequelae of viral infections outweighs the risk of viral recrudescence.[41,59,60]

When effusions are moderate to severe and compromising cardiac function, pericardiocentesis and lavage are the treatments of choice.[41,42,50,59] Drainage of the pericardial effusion usually results in immediate attenuation of the signs of cardiac compromise. An electrocardiogram should be performed during the procedure to monitor for dysrhythmias. Catheters can be left indwelling without complications until fluid production has decreased significantly which is usually between 24 and 48 hours. Lavage of the pericardial sac with 1–2 L of 0.9% saline is recommended. One litre of 0.9% saline spiked with antimicrobials such as sodium penicillin, gentomicin or ceftiofur has been found to be successful.[36,50] Twice daily lavage is recommended until the amount of fluid drained is less than the amount of fluid infused. The rationale underlying lavage is removal of fibrin, bacteria, immune complexes, inflammatory cells and their byproducts.[50,61] Although levels of intravenously administered antimicrobials have been demonstrated to be equivalent to or higher in pericardial fluid than in serum, intrapericardial administration of antimicrobials allows guaranteed high levels for aggressive treatment.[50,62]

Fortunately, in horses, constrictive pericarditis is rarely a sequela to other more common forms of pericarditis. There is only one report of an attempted pericardiectomy in a horse and the surgery proved unsuccessful.[43]

With prompt and aggressive treatment, the prognosis for horses with idiopathic pericarditis is favourable.[36,41] Septic pericarditis carries a guarded prognosis, but with drainage and lavage a positive outcome can be achieved.[36,63] Thus, current data demonstrate that when properly diagnosed and aggressively treated pericarditis need not be a fatal or even a future performance-limiting disease.

REFERENCES

1. Frohlich W, Wlaschitz S, Riedelberger K, Reifinger M, et al. Case report: aortic valve endocarditis in a horse. Dtsch Tierärztl Wochenschr 2004;111(9):370–373.

2. Sponseller BT, Ware WA. Successful treatment of staphlococcal endocarditis in a horse. Equine Vet Educ 2001;13(6):298–302.

3. Ramzan PHL. Vegetative bacterial endocarditis associated with septic tenosynovitis of the digital sheath in a Thoroughbred racehorse. Equine Vet Educ 2000;12(3):120–123.

4. Church S, Harrigan KE, Irving AE, Peel MM, et al. Endocarditis caused by *Pasteurella caballi* in a horse. Aust Vet J 1998;76(8):528–530.

5. Maxson AD, Reef VB. Bacterial endocarditis in horses: ten cases (1984–1995). Equine Vet J 1997;29(5):394–399.

6. Travers CW, van den Berg JS. *Pseudomonas* spp. associated vegetative endocarditis in two horses. J S Afr Vet Assoc 1995;66(3):172–176.

7. Pace LW, Wirth NR, Foss RR, Fales WH, et al. Endocarditis and pulmonary aspergillosis in a horse. J Vet Diagn Invest 1994;6(4):504–506.

8. Hines MT, Heidel JR, Barbee DR. Bacterial endocarditis with thrombus formation and abscessation in a horse. Vet Radiol Ultrasound 1993;34(1):47–51.

9. Ball MA, Weldon AD. Vegetative endocarditis in an Appaloosa gelding. Cornell Vet 1992;82(3):301–309.

10. Ewart S, Brown C, Derksen F, Kufuor-Mensa E, et al. Serratia marcescens endocarditis in a horse. J Am Vet Med Assoc 1992;200(7):961–963.

11. Nilsfors L, Lombard CW, Weckner D, Kvart C, et al. Diagnosis of pulmonary valve endocarditis in a horse. Equine Vet J 1991;23:479–482.

12. Collatos C, Clark ES, Reef VB, Morris DD, et al. Septicemia, atrial fibrillation, cardiomegaly, left atrial mass, and *Rhodococcus equi* septic osteoarthritis in a foal. J Am Vet Med Assoc 1990;197(8):1039–1042.

13. Hillyer MH, Mair TS, Holmes JR. Treatment of bacterial endocarditis in a Shire mare. Equine Vet Educ 1990;2(1):5–7.

14. Dedrick P, Reef VB, Sweeney RW, Morris DD, et al. Treatment of bacterial endocarditis in a horse. J Am Vet Med Assoc 1988;193(3):339–342.

15. Hatfield CE, Rebhun WC, Dietze AE, Carlisle MS, et al. Endocarditis and optic neuritis in a Quarter horse mare. Comp Contin Educ Pract Vet 1987;9(4):451–454.

16. Reef VB. Mitral valvular insufficiency associated with ruptured chordae tendineae in three foals. J Am Vet Med Assoc 1987;191(3):329–331.

17. Roby KAW, Reef VB. ECG of the month: myocardial infarction in a horse with bacterial endocarditis. J Am Vet Med Assoc 1986;188(6):570–571.

18. Buergelt CD, Cooley AJ, Hines SA, Pipers FS, et al. Endocarditis in six horses. Vet Pathol 1985;22(4):333–337.

19. McCormick KBS, Peet RL, Downes K. Erysipelothrix rhusiopathiae vegetative endocarditis in a horse. Aust Vet J 1985;62(11):392.

20. Bonagura JD, Pipers FS. Echocardiographic features of aortic valve endocarditis in a dog, a cow, and a horse. J Am Vet Med Assoc 1983;182(6):595–599.

21. Pipers FS, Hamlin RL, Reef V. Echocardiographic detection of cardiovascular lesions in the horse. J Eq Med Surg 1979;3:68–77.

22. Gardener SY, Reef VB, Spencer PA. Ultrasonographic evaluation of

horses with thrombophlebitis of the jugular vein: 46 cases (1985–1988). JAVMA 1991;199: 370–373.

23. Hamir AN, Reef VB. Complications of a permanent transvenous pacing catheter in a horse. J Comp Path 1989;101:317–326.

24. Karchmer AW. Infective endocarditis. In: Braunwald E, editor. Heart Disease. A Textbook of Cardiovascular Medicine. Philadelphia: WB Saunders; 1997. p. 1077–1104.

25. Liebisch G, Assmann G, Leibisch A. *Borrelia burgdorferi* and *Lyme borreliosis* in horses in Germany. Praktische Tierarzt 1999;80(6): 498–516.

26. Calvert CA. Valvular bacterial endocarditis in the dog. JAVMA 1982;180:1080–1084.

27. Pelletier LL, Petersdorf RG. Infective endocarditis: review of 125 cases from the University of Washington Hospital, 1963–1972. Medicine 1977;56:287–313.

28. Peterson LR, Shanholtzer CJ, Mohn ML, Gerding DN, et al. Improved recovery of microorganisms from patients receiving antibiotics with the antimicrobial removal device. Am J Clin Pathol. 1983;80(5): 692–696.

29. Reef VB. Heart murmurs in horses: determining their significance with echocardiography. Eq Vet J Suppl 1995;19:71.

30. Blissitt KJ, Bonagura JD. Colour flow Doppler echocardiography in normal horses. Eq Vet J Suppl 1995;19:47.

31. Blissitt KJ, Bonagura JD. Colour flow Doppler echocardiography in horses with cardiac murmurs. Eq Vet J Suppl 1995;19:82.

32. Marr CM, Reef VB. Physiological valvular regurgitation in clinically normal young racehorses: prevalence and two-dimensional colour flow Doppler echocardiographic characteristics. Eq Vet J Suppl 1995;19:56.

33. Reef VB, Bain FT, Spencer PA. Severe mitral regurgitation in horses: clinical, echocardiographic and pathological findings. Eq Vet J 1998;30:18.

34. Reef VB, Spencer P. Echocardiographic evaluation of equine aortic insufficiency. Am J Vet Res 1987;48:904.

35. Bonagura JD, Herring DS, Welker F. Echocardiography. Vet Clinics N Am: Eq Pract 1985;1:311.

36. Worth LT, Reef VB. Pericarditis in horses: 18 cases (1986–1995). J Am Vet Med Assoc 1998;212(2): 248–253.

37. Seahorn JL, Slovis NM, Reimer JM, Carey VJ, Donahue JG, Cohen ND, et al. Case-control study of factors associated with fibrinous pericarditis among horses in central Kentucky during spring 2001. J Am Vet Med Assoc 2003;223(6):832–838.

38. Lorell BH. Pericardial diseases. In: Braunwald E, editor. Heart Disease: A Textbook Of Cardiovascular Medicine. Philadelphia: WB Saunders; 1997. p. 1478–1534.

39. Buergelt CD, Wilson JH, Lombard CW. Pericarditis in horses. Comp Cont Ed 1990;12:872–876.

40. Dill SG, Simoncini DC, Bolton GR, Rendano VT, Crissman JW, King JM, Tennant BC, et al. Fibrinous pericarditis in the horse. J Am Vet Med Assoc 1982;180:266–271.

41. Freestone JF, Thomas, WP, Carlson GP, Brumbaugh GW, et al. Idiopathic effusive pericarditis with tamponade in the horse. Equine Vet J 1987;19:38–42.

42. Reef VB, Gentile DG, Freeman DE. Successful treatment of pericarditis in a horse. J Am Vet Med Assoc 1984;185:94–98.

43. Hardy J, Robertson JT, Reed, SM. Constrictive pericarditis in a mare: attempted treatment by partial pericardiectomy. Equine Vet J 1992;24:151–154.

44. Fowler NO. Pericardial disease. Heart Disease Stroke 1992;1:85–94.

45. Gold RG. Post-viral pericarditis. Eur Heart J 1988;9(Suppl G): 175–179.

46. Twardoski ZJ, Alpert MA, Gupta RC, Nolph KD, Madsen BT, et al. Circulating immune complexes: possible toxins responsible for serositis (pericarditis, pleuritis, and peritonitis) in renal failure. Nephron 1983;35:190–195.

47. Maisch B, Kochsiek K. Humoral immune reactions in uremic pericarditis. Am J Nephrol 1983;3:264–271.

48. Wagner PC, Miller RA, Merritt F, Pickering LA, Grant BD, et al. Constrictive pericarditis in the horse. J Equine Med Surg 1977;1:242–247.

49. Bernard W, Reef VB, Clark ES, Vaala W, Ehnen SJ, et al. Pericarditis in horses: six cases (1982–1986). J Am Vet Med Assoc 1990;196:468–471.

50. Bolin DC, Donahue JM, Vickers ML, Harrison L, Sells S, Giles RC, Hong CB, Poonacha KB, Roberts J, Sebastian MM, Swerczek TW, Tramontin R, Williams NM, et al. Microbiologic and pathologic findings in an epidemic of equine pericarditis. J Vet Diagn Invest 2005;17(1):38–44.

51. Davis JL, Gardner SY, Schwabenton B, Breuhaus BA, et al. Congestive heart failure in horses: 14 cases (1984–2001). J Am Vet Med Assoc 2002;220(10):1512–1515.

52. Perkins SL, Magdesian KG, Thomas WP, Spier SJ, et al. Pericarditis and pleuritis caused by *Corynebacterium pseudotuberculosis* in a horse. J Am Vet Med Assoc 2004;224(7): 1133–1138.

53. Seahorn JL, Slovis NM, Reimer JM, Carey VJ, Donahue JG, Cohen ND, et al. Case-control study of factors associated with fibrinous pericarditis among horses in central Kentucky during spring 2001. J Am Vet Med Assoc 2003;223(6):832–838.

54. Morley PS, Chirino-Trejo M, Petrie L, Krupka L, Schwab M, et al. Pericarditis and pleuritis caused by *Mycoplasma felis* in a horse. Equine Vet J 1996;28(3):237–240.

55. Voros K, Felkai C, Szilagyi Z, Papp A, et al. Two-dimensional echocardiographically guided pericardiocentesis in a horse with traumatic pericarditis. J Am Vet Med Assoc 1991;198(11): 1953–1956.

56. Bertone JJ, Dill SG. Traumatic gastropericarditis in a horse. J Am Vet Med Assoc 1985;187(7): 742–743.

57. Bernard W, Lamb J. Pericardial disease. In: Robinson NE, editor. Current Therapy in Equine

Medicine 3. Philadelphia: WB Saunders; 1992. p. 402–405.

58. Robinson JA, Marr CM, Reef VB, Sweeney RW, et al. Idiopathic, aseptic, effusive, fibrinous, nonconstrictive pericarditis with tamponade in a Standardbred filly. J Am Vet Med Assoc 1992;201: 1593–1598.

59. Spodick DH. The normal and diseased pericardium: current concepts of pericardial physiology, diagnosis and treatment. J Am Coll Cardiol 1983;1:240–251.

60. Tan JS, Holmes JC, Fowler NO, Manitsas GT, Phair JP, et al. Antibiotic levels in pericardial fluid. J Clin Invest 1974;53:7–12.

61. May KA, Cheramie HS, Howard RD, Duesterdieck K, Moll HD, Pleasant RS, Pyle RL, et al. Purulent pericarditis as a sequela to clostridial myositis in a horse. Equine Vet J 2002;34(6):636–640.

Chapter 18

Collapse and syncope

Richard J Piercy and Celia M Marr

DEFINITIONS

The term "collapse" is used to describe signs of varying severity and duration where animals fall and become recumbent with or without a loss of consciousness. The animal may recover, in which case it may suffer recurring episodes, or it may die. Collapse in the horse may be associated with disorders not only of cardiovascular origin, but also musculoskeletal, respiratory, neurological and metabolic disease. Note that many debilitating disease processes may cause recumbency secondary to weakness, but that in these cases no particular event initiating collapse can be identified: in these cases owners may describe their horse as having collapsed when it has lain down suddenly, for example, because of abdominal pain.

The term "syncope" describes a transient and abrupt loss of consciousness and postural tone associated with inadequate cerebral blood flow often due to a cardiovascular anomaly: either a sudden reduction in cardiac output or a loss of vasomotor tone resulting in peripheral vasodilatation. In both circumstances, the result is an abrupt fall in blood pressure. Therefore, horses with collapsing episodes of cardiovascular origin are often undergoing syncope. However, occasionally a disturbance of cerebral nutrient blood flow composition may be the cause of syncopal attacks (e.g. hypoxia, hypercapnia, hypoglycaemia).[1]

INTRODUCTION

Collapse in the adult horse poses a considerable challenge for the veterinary surgeon attempting to establish the diagnosis and any appropriate treatment. Not surprisingly, owners are often more concerned about prognosis than diagnosis and in horses with a history of collapse at exercise, human safety becomes a concern and an accurate prognosis is essential. This task is often made more difficult because the clinician may not have observed the episode and has to rely on descriptions from the owner, which may lack detail and clarity. Furthermore, the incident(s) may not have had any clear predisposing cause, may be sporadic and the animal may appear normal on clinical examination or by the time specific diagnostic procedures can be performed. In such cases, deliberately precipitating an attack may be impossible or may further alarm an already worried owner and potentially put the animal's life at risk. These constraints may tempt the clinician to offer an "on-the-spot" diagnosis by using lay terms such as "heart attack," "stroke" or "fit" without considering a logical and disciplined approach to the case. Indeed, a "heart attack" or "stroke" is often considered the most likely diagnosis by the owner because of the not unnatural extrapolation from the situation in humans.

The difficulty in establishing a diagnosis for many cases of nonfatal collapse is reflected by the lack of relevant studies and reports. For comparison, there are a number

DOI: 10.1016/B978-0-7020-2817-5.00023-7

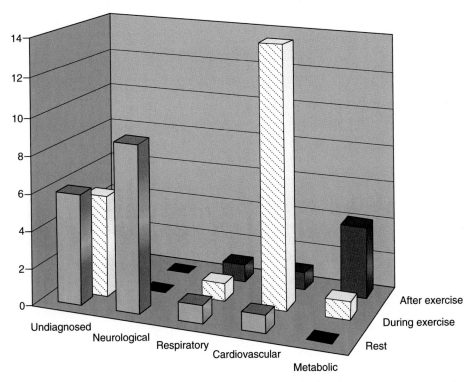

Figure 18.1 Diagnoses in 44 horses presented for cardiological investigation with a history of collapse. 18% were undiagnosed. Neurological conditions were most common in horses that collapsed at rest. Cardiological conditions were most common in horses that collapsed during exercise. Metabolic conditions, such as heat exhaustion, were most common in horses that collapsed after exercise. (R. Piercy, V. B. Reef and C. M. Marr, unpublished data.)

of reports of studies associated with investigating sudden death in the horse,[2–16] which is due in part to the relative ease in establishing a diagnosis at necropsy. Nevertheless, even with extensive post-mortem examination, the cause of death is not determined in approximately 30% of horses that die suddenly. However, it is important to consider that the cause of collapse in one horse may be the cause of sudden death in another, or that a number of collapsing episodes may occur in an individual before a fatal attack, or that a collapsed horse may subsequently die. In a review of 69 cases of sudden and unexpected death, in 24 of the cases, collapse and subsequently death were observed; in 6 of those 24 horses, death was due to trauma. Cardiovascular reasons were implicated as the cause of death in nine horses: six died from internal haemorrhage, one had aortic valvular disease, one had ruptured chordae tendineae of the mitral valve and one had a verminous granuloma in the coronary artery. In the remaining nine, seven of which had died at exercise, a post-mortem examination failed to reveal pathological changes and a functional cardiac disorder was postulated.[15]

Circulatory causes of nonfatal collapse in the horse occur commonly: 8.5% of horses referred for a second opinion for evaluation of the cardiovascular system at a referral centre had actually collapsed, and a further 11% had a history of inco-ordination, stumbling or unsteadiness and/or recumbency.[17] Figure 18.1 details the final diagnosis for 44 horses presented with a history of collapse after referral for cardiac investigation at a veterinary hospital. The cardiovascular causes of collapse in this group are illustrated in Figure 18.2.

CARDIOVASCULAR AND CIRCULATORY CAUSES OF COLLAPSE

Syncope

Horses that have suffered one or more episodes of acute, nonfatal collapse may be suspected of suffering from syncope. Usually there is little or no warning of collapse and, because of cerebral hypoxia, a temporary, quiet, comatose state ensues.[18] The animal may go on to recover or progress to die, in which case other signs of cardiac failure usually become evident.

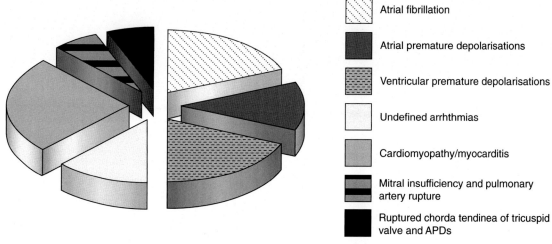

Atrial fibrillation

Atrial premature depolarisations

Ventricular premature depolarisations

Undefined arrhthmias

Cardiomyopathy/myocarditis

Mitral insufficiency and pulmonary artery rupture

Ruptured chorda tendinea of tricuspid valve and APDs

Figure 18.2 Specific cardiological conditions in 16 horses presented for investigation of collapse. Undefined dysrhythmias were diagnosed if a dysrhythmia had been auscultated at or around the time of the collapse episodes but was not documented electrocardiographically. Myocardial disease and dysrhythmias were much more frequent than valvular disease. In both horses that collapsed because of valvular insufficiency, the valvular regurgitation was severe and there were additional cardiovascular problems. APDs, atrial premature depolarizations. (R. Piercy, V. B. Reef and C. M. Marr, unpublished data.)

An alert state is maintained through multiple sensory inputs to the reticular activating system in the rostral brain stem and subsequently to the thalamus and cerebral cortex where consciousness is maintained[18]: in human beings it has been estimated that cerebral oxygen delivery of approximately 3.5 mL oxygen/100 g tissue each minute is required for consciousness.[19,20] A reduction of cerebral oxygen delivery below this level for periods of 10 seconds or more is associated with loss of consciousness and postural tone.[21] Cerebral blood flow is usually carefully maintained at a relatively constant level of 50–60 mL/100 g of tissue/minute by autoregulation: a drop to half this level may precipitate a syncopal attack. Cerebral blood flow is influenced by $PaCO_2$, PaO_2 and pH; however, autonomic control mechanisms (that profoundly affect blood flow in the rest of the body) appear to be capable of only fairly small changes in brain blood flow because of relatively sparse innervation.[22]

An abrupt fall in systemic arterial blood pressure may result from acute haemorrhage, pump failure, the sudden onset of a dysrhythmia, autonomic effects following carotid sinus stimulation or changes in vagal tone. It may also occur following the sudden failure of a mechanism that has previously compensated for a pre-existing cardiovascular problem. If the mechanisms discussed above for the regulation of cerebral blood flow cannot compensate for the fall in blood pressure, then syncope will result. If short lived, the attack is only transient; however, prolonged lack of oxygen and other nutrients to the brain lead to severe global cerebral dysfunction, irreversible damage and eventually death.

Acute haemorrhage

Acute haemorrhage leading to collapse occurs with the rupture of major vessels such as the aorta[23,24] (Fig. 18.3), the pulmonary artery[24] (Fig. 18.4), the anterior mesenteric artery and the uterine arteries.[25] Shock and rapid death can follow profuse haemorrhage into the pleural or abdominal cavities. Collapse and haemorrhagic shock may also occur following rupture of vessels associated with the guttural pouch in disorders such as empyema and mycosis or with severe exercise-induced pulmonary haemorrhage.[11]

While rupture of any major vessel is possible, if the horse survives the episode, the specific site may not be identified. However, certain vessels appear to be ruptured more commonly because of pre-existing disease. Rupture of the pulmonary artery leading to syncope or sudden death has been reported in association with pulmonary hypertension caused by patent ductus arteriosus[26] and severe mitral insufficiency[27] (see Fig. 18.4).

Aorto-cardiac fistula is a particularly well-documented cause of vessel rupture, occurring most commonly in stallions: in one report, four of the eight cases collapsed and died within minutes of covering.[28] On post-mortem examination, tears of the aortic ring were identified extending from the right coronary sinus into the right ventricle similar to that shown in Figure 18.3. Some cases die suddenly[29] but horses can survive formation of an aorto-cardiac fistula for periods varying up to 12 months.[30–33] A characteristic low-pitched continuous murmur may be auscultated over the right thorax and monomorphic

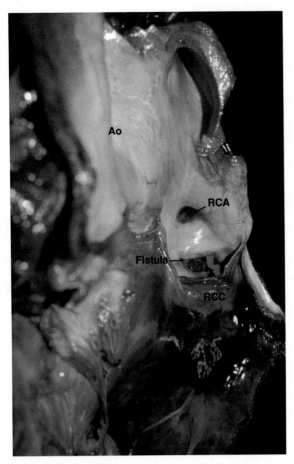

Figure 18.3 A post-mortem specimen from a 7-year-old Thoroughbred gelding that collapsed while galloping and subsequently died. There is a ruptured aneurysm forming a fistula between the right sinus of Valsalva and the right atrium. Ao, aorta; RCA, right coronary artery; RCC, right coronary cusp of the aortic valve.

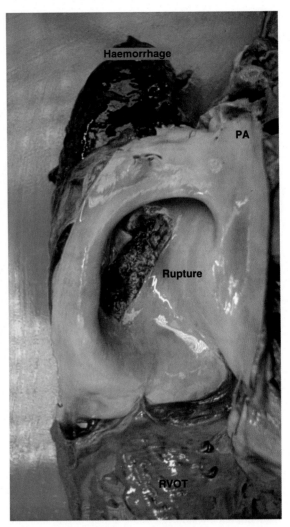

Figure 18.4 A post-mortem specimen from an aged mixed breed gelding that collapsed several times over the weeks preceding euthanasia due to pulmonary artery (PA) rupture secondary to severe mitral insufficiency and congestive heart failure. RVOT, right ventricular outflow tract.

ventricular tachycardia is often present due to disruption of the conduction tissue by a dissecting haematoma[33] that can be visualized by echocardiography. Some horses appear to have abdominal pain but this may in fact be thoracic pain that can be difficult to distinguish from that arising from the abdomen.[30,33] The pathogenesis remains unclear: aortic root rupture may be due to congenital abnormalities, cardiac degenerative changes, associated with chronic aortic insufficiency or occur because of pre-existing sinus of Valsalva aneurysm.[30–34] (ACF)

Collapse and death may occur as a result of the rupture of arteries at or near parturition: the utero-ovarian, middle uterine and external iliac arteries are most commonly affected. This is also a common cause of abdominal pain and haemoperitoneum in the periparturient brood mare. Pre-existing degenerative changes are thought to be responsible, in combination with the stresses associated with late gestation and parturition.[25]

Neoplasia should be considered as a possible underlying cause of pleural or abdominal haemorrhage. The rupture of a thoracic haemangiosarcoma with corresponding collapse and death from haemorrhagic shock has been reported[35] as has sudden death, caused by thoracic lymphosarcoma.[2] Collapse and sudden death in a Thoroughbred stallion during breeding have been associated with intraseptal haemorrhage and atrioventricular node disruption caused by a malignant melanoma.[14]

Acute cardiac failure

Inadequacy of the pumping mechanism of the heart can have profound effects on arterial blood pressure and hence cerebral blood flow. The most notable spontaneous example is probably mitral valve chorda tendinea rupture leading to severe valve incompetence, regurgitation into the left atrium during systole, pulmonary congestion and oedema[7] (Fig. 18.5, see Chapter 19). (RCT) These horses may collapse with severe dyspnoea and cyanosis.[36] A loud pansystolic murmur is audible over the left thorax with often a palpable thrill. If the horse survives, clinical signs may improve; however, generally the murmur remains, loudest over the mitral value, and a loud third heart sound may be audible and there may be caudal extension of the cardiac area of auscultation associated with left atrial dilatation. This may be followed by the progression to cardiac failure, possibly with further episodes of collapse, often exacerbated by exercise.[7,27,37]

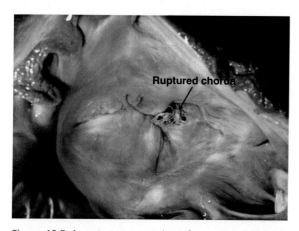

Figure 18.5 A post-mortem specimen from a 6-year-old Irish Draught gelding with rupture of a chorda tendinea of the mitral valve. The ventricle has been filled with water which causes the valve to close and the ruptured chorda is visible within the atrium.

Dysrhythmias

Cardiac rhythm disturbances are amongst the more common causes of collapse, particularly in horses that collapse during exercise (Fig. 18.6). Collapsing episodes occur as a result of failure to maintain cardiac output, caused by the inability to regulate either heart rate or stroke volume in periods of either brady- or tachyarrhythmia.[38] A normal horse will increase cardiac output at submaximal rates (less than 210 bpm) primarily by tachycardia; at maximum heart rates of between 210 and about 240 bpm increasing cardiac output is achieved with increased stroke volume[39] (see Chapter 3). With tachyarrythmias such as atrial fibrillation[40,41] and ventricular tachycardia, heart rates in excess of 240 bpm may be reached. In these circumstances there may be limited perfusion of the myocardium during diastole, leading to poor contractility and compromised cardiac output as a result of inadequate ventricular filling. Disease processes that alter myocardial contractility (e.g. focal ischaemia) will compound this effect, which may become apparent even at submaximal heart rates. (AF, RCT)

Bradydysrhythmias

Many normal horses at rest, particularly if fit, show varying degrees of first- and second-degree atrioventricular (AV) block: sinus rhythm is re-established when heart rate rises in response to exercise or excitement. Horses may also drop isolated beats immediately following a period of exercise as the heart rate slows; again sinus rhythm quickly returns. Second-degree AV block is generally of Mobitz type 1 classification: i.e. variation in conduction time between the atria and ventricles often with the progressive lengthening of the R–R interval up to the missed beat. Mobitz type 2 AV block with pathology and disruption of conduction in the bundle of His is associated with severe bradycardia and syncope in humans, but is rare in horses. It may, however, be a precursor of complete (third-degree) AV block.[42] Physiological first- and second-degree AV

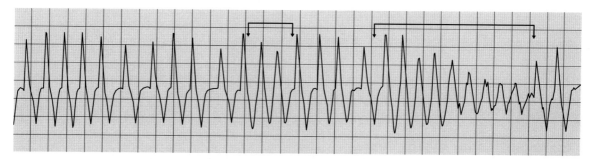

Figure 18.6 An exercising ECG from a middle-aged riding horse with a history of collapse at exercise. Sustained atrial fibrillation was present at rest. During exercise, atrial fibrillation was present and there were runs of rapid ventricular tachycardia (under arrows). Recorded at paper speed of 25 mm/second, sensitivity of 5 mm = 1 mV.

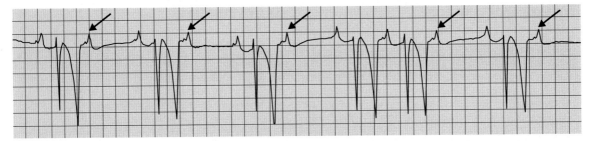

Figure 18.7 An ECG recorded following light exercise from a middle-aged riding horse with a history of collapse. Advanced second-degree AV block is present and there are numerous unconducted P waves (arrows). The significance of this dysrhythmia was uncertain, because normal sinus rhythm was present during exercise. Recorded at paper speed of 25 mm/ second, sensitivity of 5 mm = 1 mV.

block, which disappear with exercise and excitement, are very unlikely to be the cause of collapsing episodes and other causes should be considered.

Second-degree AV block should be regarded with suspicion though, if there is a history of collapse and it is very frequent, it cannot be abolished by exercise or excitement or is accompanied by ventricular premature depolarizations (Fig. 18.7). In one horse with a history of collapse at exercise: sinus bradycardia and second-degree AV block were detected on 24-hour ambulatory ECG and the horse had a maximal heart rate of only 183 beats per minute at exercise and an exaggerated bradycardic response following exercise. Sick sinus syndrome and chronotropic incompetence were diagnosed.[43]

Third-degree AV block, where there is no conduction between atria and ventricles, often precipitates syncope, in which case the term Adams–Stokes syndrome is used[44,45] (see Chapter 13). In one such horse that was observed for 6 months, collapse occurred towards the beginning of the illness, in the first month and in the last days of life; however, during the intervening period, attacks did not occur spontaneously and could not be precipitated. Adams–Stokes attacks appeared to occur when the ventricular pause was measured between 15 and 18 seconds; however, intervals of complete heart block were recorded lasting up to 65 seconds and another horse survived for 9 months with up to 100 attacks per day, before dying suddenly during an attack.[44,45] Haemodynamic measurements demonstrated a drop in systolic blood pressure of 100 mmHg or more during such episodes, with a return to normality following each attack. Cases of complete AV block (and certain other rhythm disturbances) may show resolution of clinical signs following the implantation of a pacemaker[42,43,46] (see Chapter 14).

Supraventricular dysrhythmias

Exercise-induced supraventricular tachycardia or frequent supraventricular premature depolarizations (see Figs. 18.2, 18.8) has been detected in horses presented with histories of collapse, however, this appears to be generally an uncommon presentation with supraventricular dysrhythmias, and the severity of signs may be dependent on the underlying cause rather than the dysrhythmia itself (see Chapter 13). Frequent supraventricular premature depolarizations may however predispose the horse to paroxysmal or sustained atrial fibrillation. Atrial fibrillation may occur spontaneously in an apparently normal horse or in horses with a previous good track record, during maximal exertion.[47,48] There is an abrupt cessation of the normal co-ordinated atrial contraction, which terminates ventricular filling. This, combined with the disordered rhythm, may cause a sudden reduction in cardiac output and hence systolic blood pressure with a corresponding drop in peripheral perfusion, most notably to the skeletal musculature. However, atrial fibrillation is a relatively rare cause of collapse: it was detected in only 6 out of 94 horses with this presenting history.[48] Similarly, most horses with atrial fibrillation are observed to stop or slow dramatically in a race (and are therefore exercise intolerant). Collapse itself is rare in horses with atrial fibrillation: of 106 horses with atrial fibrillation only two had a history of collapse whereas 64 demonstrated exercise intolerance.[49] (AF)

In conscious, resting horses, atrial fibrillation is often not associated with poor haemodynamic function, particularly if there is no underlying cardiac disease.[50,51] Although there are no reports documenting measurements of blood pressure before and after the spontaneous development of atrial fibrillation during exercise, it appears that atrial fibrillation is most likely to result in collapse if it occurs suddenly during exercise, causing an acute change in haemodynamics, or if there is concurrent ventricular ectopy (see Fig. 18.6). In horses with sustained atrial fibrillation without ventricular ectopy and normal exercising heart rates, collapse is unlikely.

Ventricular dysrhythmias

The identification of ventricular premature depolarizations in a horse presented with collapse should be regarded

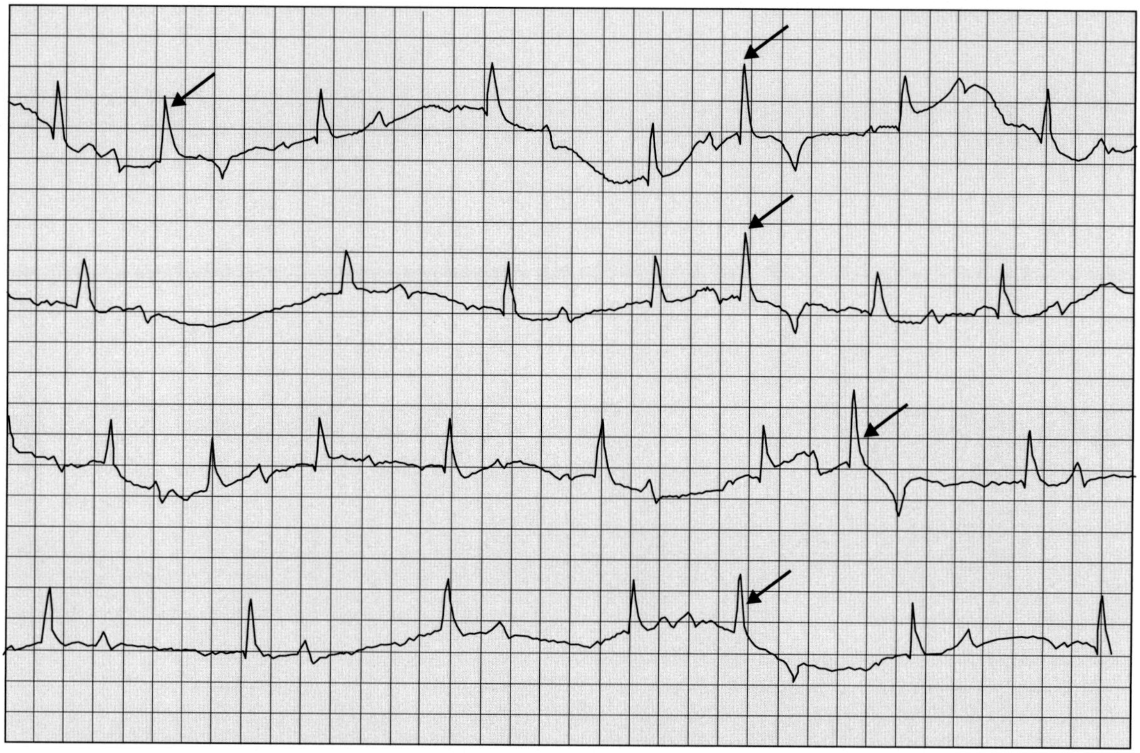

Figure 18.8 Samples of a 24-hour ambulatory electrocardiogram from a 10-year-old event horse with a history of collapse. Frequent supraventricular premature depolarizations (arrows), occurring at a frequency of more than 100 per hour, were detected. This suggests that the collapsing episodes may be related to paroxysmal atrial fibrillation or rapid supraventricular tachycardia. Recorded at a paper speed of 25 mm/second, sensitivity of 5 mm = 1 mV.

with suspicion (see Fig. 18.1) even though they are commonly encountered in apparently normal racehorses during exercise[52] (see Chapter 11). However, although the occasional ventricular premature depolarization is probably insignificant, in some circumstances it may progress to ventricular tachycardia. A horse with a history of collapse at exercise in which dysrhythmia is identified therefore warrants further investigation with the use of ambulatory and exercising electrocardiography. Ventricular dysrhythmias are less common than supraventricular dysrhythmias in horses and are more likely to cause a reduction in cardiac output sufficient to induce collapse. Therefore, if frequent ventricular premature depolarizations or ventricular tachycardia are present then these are likely to be significant (Figs. 18.6, 18.9, 18.10, see Chapters 11 and 13). (⬤ AF, RCT)

Ventricular tachycardia has been associated with collapse in a horse that also demonstrated intermittent complete AV dissociation.[42] Syncope was associated with prolonged diastolic pauses, immediately followed by paroxysms of ventricular tachycardia. The horse demonstrated stupor followed by staggering and collapse. The reported causes of ventricular tachycardia include electrolyte distur-bances, myocarditis, endocarditis (see Fig. 18.10) and cardiotoxins[53,54] (see Chapter 13). In a survey of sudden death in race horses, in 17 of the 25 cases no clear pathological lesion was identified and it was speculated that death was attributed to exercise-induced acute myocardial failure. It was suggested that small foci of myocardial degeneration within the Purkinje fibres may have led to focal hypoxia, ventricular tachycardia and fatal ventricular fibrillation.[10]

Vagal stimulation

In comparison with other animals and human beings, the horse has a slow resting heart rate, associated with high vagal tone. Partial AV block, common at rest in the horse (see above), is probably a means of regulating blood pressure. It has been suggested however that abrupt bradycardia and a precipitous fall in systolic blood pressure may be a sequel to sudden vagal stimulation and cause transient weakness, inco-ordination and collapse. Collapsing episodes associated with lifting the head, stretching the neck, tacking up, tightening the girth and hosing down after exercise are not uncommon.[17,55] In 17% of 94 horses

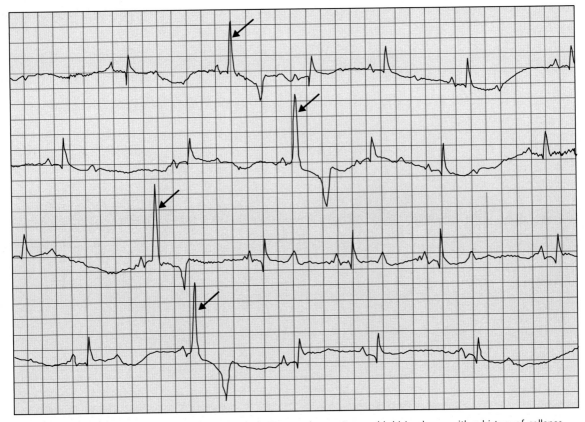

Figure 18.9 Samples of a 24-hour ambulatory electrocardiogram from a 9-year-old driving horse with a history of collapse. Ventricular premature depolarizations (arrows) were detected at a rate of up to 60/hour. Recorded at paper speed of 25 mm/ second, sensitivity of 5 mm = 1 mV.

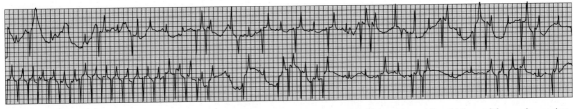

Figure 18.10 Paroxysmal monomorphic ventricular tachycardia in a 13-year-old riding mare with a history of fever, depression and syncope and a loud diastolic murmur. Bacterial endocarditis and myocarditis were diagnosed.

presented with a history of collapse, the episode appeared to be associated with some form of restraint.[17] A baroreceptor mechanism associated with the carotid sinus may be involved. The horse or pony may stagger, slump backwards and fall. Recovery generally occurs within a few seconds and no abnormalities can be identified.

This collapsing syndrome seen in horses and ponies may be compared with the so-called vasovagal faint (cardioneurogenic syncope) that has been extensively studied in humans. Many individual causes have been identified; however, they all appear to be associated with the stimula-

tion of the medullary vasodepressor region in the brain stem. Efferent signals cause increased parasympathetic tone via the vagus nerve and vasodilatation. Diminished cardiac filling and bradycardia follow, leading to syncope.[56] In human beings, it is thought that vasodilatation is more important than the bradycardia in producing symptoms; however, whether this is the case in horses, which have a very slow resting heart rate, remains to be determined. Stimulation of the medullary vasodepressor region occurs after receiving afferents (cardiac C fibres) from mechanocardiac receptors within the ventricular myocardium when a volume-depleted ventricle contracts vigorously. It is tempting to suggest that this stimulus may be occurring as a result of the various forms of restraint that precede collapse in horses and ponies (described above). In certain susceptible human beings,[56] increasing sympathetic tone is not combined with increasing heart rate and peripheral vascular resistance, hence venous return progressively decreases to the point where eventually the contraction of the relatively empty ventricles causes firing of the C fibres; sudden sympathetic withdrawal ensues with corresponding vagal stimulation, vasodilatation, bradycardia and syncope. In human beings, cardioneurogenic syncope has been treated effectively by the administration of β-blockers,[57] which at first appears paradoxical; however, the eradication of the triggering hypersympathetic tone may explain their efficacy. Their use in the treatment of horses that repeatedly suffer bouts of this syndrome has not been evaluated.

It has also been suggested that the collapse response seen in horses and ponies after tacking up or raising the head or neck may be related to the carotid-sinus syndrome seen particularly in older people.[58] In the original classical case, a syncopal attack was precipitated by pressure from a stiff collar, presumably on an oversensitive carotid sinus. Overactive baroreceptors causing sudden reflex vagal stimulation may be associated with altered structure of the head and neck blood vessels as a result of atherosclerotic disease or in human patients who have undergone neck surgery or radiation.[22] It is also described in patients with local neoplastic disease in the neck, or aneurysmal dilatation of the sinus. The usual precipitant for a syncopal attack is a sudden turn of the head, inducing dizziness and fainting similar to that reported in ponies that appeared to collapse following stretching of the neck.[55]

Sleep disorders and narcolepsy/cataplexy

(RSD)

One of the commoner noncardiac causes of episodic collapse in horses is sleep disorder (Fig. 18.1). Narcolepsy/cataplexy syndrome is a familial condition in Miniature horse foals,[59] but similar signs also occur in a variety of breeds as an acquired adult-onset condition.[18] Some clinicians now favour chronic sleep deprivation[60] rather than a primary neurological abnormality as the more likely cause in most acquired cases, particularly as episodes may become more frequent during an unrelated systemic illness or painful condition, in particular musculoskeletal disorders. In some circumstances an episode may be incited by a particular, repeatable event (e.g. tacking up, grooming). Generally, narcoleptic/sleep-deprived horses appear sleepy immediately prior to an attack and often fall forwards onto their carpi.[61] In comparison with the syncopal attacks

described above, these horses may be roused from sleep and often correct themselves before falling to the ground completely. Attacks do not usually occur while an animal is exercising vigorously.[18]

CLINICAL INVESTIGATION OF THE COLLAPSING HORSE

History

A general history may reveal relevant details and a specific history should include a description of the collapsing episode in an attempt to determine if the horse lost consciousness, the duration of the episode and the horse's behaviour immediately before and afterwards. In particular, the circumstances leading to the episode of collapse should be determined because the common differential diagnoses differ, depending on whether the collapse occurred at rest or during exercise (see Fig. 18.1).

Clinical examination

When presented with a horse that has collapsed a thorough investigation is warranted. If the horse is still recumbent then the safety of the owner should be taken into consideration as well as the immediate safety of the horse. Primary objectives of first aid may well apply in an acutely collapsed horse and the veterinary surgeon should determine that a patent airway is present, that the horse is breathing and that any external haemorrhage is adequately controlled.

Particular attention should be paid to examination of the cardiovascular system, to detect pallor and tachycardia associated with haemorrhage, dysrhythmias or cardiac murmurs, and to the neurological system (see Fig. 18.1). However, because many horses seem clinically normal by the time of veterinary examination, further diagnostic tests are often required. In episodic collapse, it is particularly helpful to obtain video footage of the event and in particular this may allow the clinician to distinguish events such as sleep deprivation from seizures. This can be achieved by housing the horse in a stable fitted with CCTV; however, owners should also be encouraged to capture the event on their mobile phones if possible. In specific cases, further evaluation of the musculoskeletal or respiratory systems may be necessary and the reader should refer to more specific texts for further details. The remainder of this discussion will focus on the differential diagnoses described above.

Acute haemorrhage

Haemorrhage is suspected if there are clinical signs of pallor, sinus tachycardia or haematological evidence of blood loss. With severe epistaxis, endoscopy is used to determine the source of blood and, in the case of severe pulmonary haemorrhage, thoracic radiographs may be helpful. Haemoperitoneum and haemothorax can be documented by abdominocentesis and thoracocentesis respectively. Abdominal or thoracic ultrasonography is useful to document the presence of large volumes of free fluid in body cavities and may demonstrate neoplastic lesions or other sources of haemorrhage.

Acute cardiac failure and dysrhythmias

Echocardiography is the technique of choice for investigating many cardiac diseases that can be associated with collapse, such as chorda tendinea rupture,[7,37] dilated cardiomyopathy or aorto-cardiac fistula[33] (see Chapters 9, 16 and 19). However, in horses with dysrhythmias caused by focal myocardial lesions or by hypoxia or electrolyte disturbances, the echocardiogram is often normal. Equally, horses with intermittent dysrhythmias frequently have normal ECGs if these are recorded for a short period at rest. Ambulatory electrocardiography can provide a much more accurate assessment of intermittent dysrhythmias (see Figs. 18.8. 18.9, 18.10) (see Chapter 10). In horses that have collapsed during exercise, an exercising ECG is extremely helpful (see Figs. 18.6, 18.7) (see Chapter 11). Some horses with exercise-induced upper airway obstruction[62] develop ventricular dysrhythmias in association with hypoxia, in which case, concurrent exercising endoscopy is helpful in evaluating upper airway obstruction. The appropriate management of dysrhythmias is dependent on determining its precise nature and underlying cause (see Chapters 13 and 14).

Vagal stimulation and vasovagal syncope

At this time, no specific diagnostic tests for these syndromes exist. It may be helpful and often reassuring for the client if the signs can be recreated by observing the horse while subjected to the specific stimulus though the animal's safety should be taken into account. In horses that collapse (or lie down) while being tacked up, investigations for possible causes of back or rib pain are often undertaken, but are rarely productive; however, occasionally, the rare exception rewards the clinician's efforts.

Sleep disorders and narcolepsy/cataplexy (RSD)

Narcolepsy/cataplexy is diagnosed in other species by provocative testing. The administration of physostigmine (0.05–0.1 mg/kg intravenously), a parasympathomimetic that can cross the blood–brain barrier, induces narcoleptic attacks in some horses.[61] However, in five of nine cases with adult-onset sleep disorders, physostigmine did not produce clinical signs (C. M. Marr and S. W. J. Reid, unpublished data). The most effective means of diagnosing sleep disorders is to record the episodes by surveillance video monitoring. Prodromal signs include drooping of the lips, head and shoulders and knuckling at the knees. Affected individuals often have a history of multiple lacerations and traumatic injuries that they sustain while suffering unobserved episodes. Frequently, once the owner is made aware of the implications of the disease and its triggering factors in their particular horse, they can manage the problem by avoiding those factors. Also, by careful observation it is often possible to detect the onset of signs and wake the horse up. Successful treatment with imipramine, a tricyclic antidepressant (0.5 mg/kg orally, s.i.d.), has been described.[61] However this drug must be used with care; variable efficacy and adverse effects of muscle fasciculations, tachycardia, hyper-resonsiveness to sound and haemolysis have been reported.[63] Clinicians should also consider a diagnosis of sleep deprivation, particularly in those that may be reluctant to lie down because of chronic pain and those that show the signs following a change in their stabling or alteration in herdmates (either loss of a companion or addition of an animal that is perceived as threatening). In these animals, analgesic medication and/or a change in their environment may be beneficial.

REFERENCES

1. Hay WP, Baskett A, Abdy MJ. Complete upper airway obstruction and syncope caused by a subepiglottic cyst in a horse. Equine Vet J 1997;29(1):75–76.
2. Lawn K. Sudden death due to thoracic lymphoma in a standardbred racing horse. Can Vet J 2005;46:528–529.
3. Boden LC, Slocombe JA, Sandy RF, et al. Sudden death in racing Thoroughbreds in Victoria, Australia. Equine Vet J 2005;37(3): 269–271.
4. Kiryu K, Nakamura T, Kaneko M, et al. Pathologic and electrocardiographic findings in sudden cardiac death in racehorses.

J Vet Med Sci 1999;61(8):921– 928.
5 Johnson BJ, Stover SM, Daft BM, et al. Causes of death in racehorses over a 2 year period. Equine Vet J 1994;26(4):327–330.
6. Johnson PJ, Moore LA, Mrad DR, et al. Sudden death of two horses associated with pulmonary

aspergillosis. Vet Rec 1999;145(1):
16–20.

7. Reef VB. Mitral valvular
insufficiency associated with
ruptured chordae tendineae in
three foals. J Am Vet Med Assoc
1987;191(3):329–331.

8. Reppas GP, Harper CG. Sudden
unexpected death in a horse due
to a cerebral oligodendroglioma.
Equine Vet J 1996;28(2):163–
165.

9. Brown CM, Kaneene JB, Taylor RF.
Sudden and unexpected death in
horses and ponies: an analysis of
200 cases. Equine Vet J 1988;20(2):
99–103.

10. Gelberg HB, Zachary JF, Everitt JI,
et al. Sudden death in training and
racing Thoroughbred horses. J Am
Vet Med Assoc 1985;187(12):
1354–1356.

11. Gunson DE, Sweeney CR, Soma
LR. Sudden death attributable to
exercise-induced pulmonary
hemorrhage in racehorses: nine
cases (1981–1983). J Am Vet Med
Assoc 1988;193(1):102–106.

12. Hughes P, Howard EB. Endocardial
fibroelastosis as a cause of sudden
death in the horse. Equine Pract
1984;6:23–26.

13. Lucke VM. Sudden death. Equine
Vet J 1987;19(2):85–86.

14. Pascoe RR, O'Sullivan BM. Sudden
death in a Thoroughbred stallion.
Equine Vet J 1980;12(4):211–212.

15. Platt H. Sudden and unexpected
deaths in horses: a review of 69
cases. Br Vet J 1982;138(5):417–
429.

16. Schiff P, Knottenbelt DC. Sudden
death in an 11 year old
thoroughbred stallion. Equine Vet
Educ 1990;2:8–10.

17. Holmes J. Equine Cardiology, Vol
1. Langford, Bristol: JR Holmes;
1987.

18. Mayhew I. Large Animal
Neurology: A Handbook for
Veterinary Clinicians. Philadelphia:
Lea and Febiger; 1989.

19. Gibson GE, Pulsinelli W, Blass JP,
Duffy TE, et al. Brain dysfunction
in mild to moderate hypoxia. Am J
Med 1981;70(6):1247–1254.

20. McHenry L, Fazekas JF, Sullivan JF.
Cerebral haemodynamics of
syncope. Am J Med Sci 1961;241:
173.

21. Wood E. Hydrostatic homeostatic
effects during changing force
environments. Aviat Space
Environment Med 1990;61:366.

22. Benditt D. Syncope. In: Willerson J,
Cohn P, editors. Cardiovascular
Medicine. Edinburgh: Churchill
Livingstone: Edinburgh; 1995.

23. Holmes JR, Rezakhani A, Else RW.
Rupture of a dissecting aortic
aneurysm into the left pulmonary
artery in a horse. Equine Vet J
1973;5(2):65–70.

24. van der Linde-Sipman JS,
Kroneman J, Meulenaar H, Vos JH,
et al. Necrosis and rupture of the
aorta and pulmonary trunk in four
horses. Vet Pathol 1985;22(1):
51–53.

25. Rooney JR. Internal hemorrhage
related to gestation in the mare.
Cornell Vet 1964;54:11–17.

26. Buergelt C, Carmichael JA, Tashjian
RJ, Das KM. Spontaneous rupture
of the left pulmonary artery in a
horse with patent ductus arteriosus.
J Am Vet Med Assoc 1970;186:
1210–1213.

27. Reef VB, Bain FT, Spencer PA.
Severe mitral regurgitation in
horses: clinical, echocardiographic
and pathological findings. Equine
Vet J 1998;30(1):18–27.

28. Rooney JR, Prickett, ME, Crowe
MW. Aortic ring rupture in
stallions. Path Vet 1967;4:
268–274.

29. Shirai W, Momotani E, Sato T,
et al. Dissecting aortic aneurysm in
a horse. J Comp Pathol 1999;
120(3):307–311.

30. Sleeper MM, Durando MM, Miller
M, et al. Aortic root disease in four
horses. J Am Vet Med Assoc
2001;219(4):491–496, 459.

31. Roby KA, Reef VB, Shaw DP,
Sweeney CR, et al. Rupture of an
aortic sinus aneurysm in a
15-year-old broodmare. J Am Vet
Med Assoc 1986;189(3):305–308.

32. Lester G, Lombard CW, Ackerman
N. Echocardiographic detection of
a dissecting aortic root aneurysm
in a Thoroughbred stallion. Vet
Radiol Ultrasound 1992;33:
202–205.

33. Marr CM, Reef VB, Brazil TJ, et al.
Aorto-cardiac fistulas in seven
horses. Vet Radiol Ultrasound
1998;39(1):22–31.

34. Reef VB, Klumpp S, Maxson AD,
Sweeney RW, et al.
Echocardiographic detection of an
intact aneurysm in a horse. J Am
Vet Med Assoc 1990;197(6):
752–755.

35. Freestone J, Williams MM,
Norwood G. Thoracic
haemangiosarcoma in a 3 year old
horse. Aust Vet J 1990;67(7):
269–270.

36. Holmes J, Miller PJ. Three cases of
ruptured mitral valve chordae in
the horse. Equine Vet J 1984;16:
125–135.

37. Marr CM, Love S, Pirie HM,
Northridge DB, et al. Confirmation
by Doppler echocardiography of
valvular regurgitation in a horse
with a ruptured chorda tendinea of
the mitral valve. Vet Rec 1990;
127(15):376–379.

38. Miller R, Holmes JR. Effect of
cardiac arrhythmias on left
ventricular and aortic blood
pressure parameters in the horse.
Res Vet Sci 1983;35:190–199.

39. Evans D. Cardiovascular
adaptations to exercise and
training. Vet Clin North Am
Equine Pract 1985;1(3):513–531.

40. Buntenkotter S, Deegen E.
Behaviour of the heart rate of
horses with auricular fibrillation
during exercise and after treatment.
Equine Vet J 1976;8(1):26–29.

41. Amada A, Senta T, Katsuyoski K.
Atrial fibrillation in the horse:
clinical and histopathological
studies of two cases. Exp Rep
Equine Health Lab 1974;11:51–69.

42. Reef VB, Clark ES, Oliver JA,
Donawick WJ, et al. Implantation
of a permanent transvenous pacing
catheter in a horse with complete
heart block and syncope. J Am
Vet Med Assoc 1986;189(4):
449–452.

43. van Loon G, Fonteyne W,
Rottiers H, et al. Implantation of
a dual-chamber, rate-adaptive
pacemaker in a horse with
suspected sick sinus syndrome.
Vet Rec 2002;151(18):541–545.

44. Bosnic L, Rapic S. The Adams-
Stokes syndrome in partial heart
block in a horse. Vet Archiv
1941;11:1–17.

45. Bosnic L, Rapic S. Two further
cases of Adams-Stokes disease in

horses. Vet Archiv 1941;11: 166–179.

46. Taylor D, Mero MA. The use of an internal pacemaker in a horse with Adams-Stokes syndrome. J Am Vet Med Assoc 1967;151(9):1172–1176.

47. Ohmura H, Hiraga A, Takahashi T, et al. Risk factors for atrial fibrillation during racing in slow-finishing horses. J Am Vet Med Assoc 2003;223(1):84–88.

48. Holmes JR, Henigan M, Williams RB, et al. Paroxysmal atrial fibrillation in racehorses. Equine Vet J 1986;18(1):37–42.

49. Deem DA, Fregin GF. Atrial fibrillation in horses: a review of 106 clinical cases, with consideration of prevalence, clinical signs, and prognosis. J Am Vet Med Assoc 1982;180(3): 261–265.

50. Muir WW, McGuirk SM. Hemodynamics before and after conversion of atrial fibrillation to normal sinus rhythm in horses. J Am Vet Med Assoc 1984;184(8): 965–970.

51. Gehlen H, Stadler P. Comparison of systolic cardiac function before and after treatment of atrial fibrillation in horses with and without additional cardiac valve insufficiencies. Vet Res Commun 2004;28(4):317–329.

52. Ryan N, Marr CM, McGladdery AJ. Survey of cardiac arrhythmias during submaximal and maximal exercise in Thoroughbred racehorses. Equine Vet J 2005; 37(3):265–268.

53. Reef V. A monensin outbreak in horses in the eastern United States. Paper presented at Eighth Annual Vet Med Forum. Washington, 1990.

54. Reimer JM, Reef VB, Sweeney RW. Ventricular arrhythmias in horses: 21 cases (1984–1989). J Am Vet Med Assoc 1992;201(8): 1237–1243.

55. Cross E. Equine syncope. Vet Rec 1988;122(15):215.

56. Fogoros R. Cardiac arrhythmias, syncope and stroke. Neurol Clin 1993;11(2):375–390.

57. Akhatar M, Jazayeri M, Sra J. Cardiovascular causes of syncope. Postgrad Med 1991;90:87.

58. Kerr S. Carotid sinus hypersensitivity in asymptomatic older persons: implications for diagnosis of syncope and falls. Arch Intern Med 2006;166(5):87.

59. Lunn DP, Cuddon PA, Shaftoe S, Archer RM, et al. Familial occurrence of narcolepsy in miniature horses. Equine Vet J 1993;25(6):483–487.

60. Bertone JJ. Excessive drowsiness secondary to recumbent sleep deprivation in two horses. Vet Clin North Am Equine Pract 2006; 22(1):157–162.

61. Sweeney CR, Hendricks JC, Beech J, Morrison AR, et al. Narcolepsy in a horse. J Am Vet Med Assoc 1983;183(1):126–128.

62. Maxson-Sage A, Parente EJ, Beech J, et al. Effect of high-intensity exercise on arterial blood gas tensions and upper airway and cardiac function in clinically normal quarter horses and horses heterozygous and homozygous for hyperkalemic periodic paralysis. Am J Vet Res 1998;59(5):615–618.

63. Peck K, Hines MT, Mealey KL, Mealey RH. Pharmacokinetics of imipramine in narcoleptic horses. Am J Vet Res 2001;62(5):783–786.

Chapter 19

Heart failure

Celia M Marr

CHAPTER CONTENTS

INTRODUCTION

Heart failure is the pathophysiological state in which an abnormality of cardiac function is responsible for failure of the heart to fill with or eject blood sufficient to meet the metabolic requirements of the tissues[1,2] (see Chapter 5). Failure of the myocardium is usually present, however the initiating pathology may be elsewhere within the heart, for example, involving the endocardium, pericardium or great vessels (see Chapter 4). Historically, medical and veterinary students were taught to consider heart failure as having two forms: forward and backward failure. These theories focused on cardiovascular haemodynamics and postulated that clinical signs of heart failure could be attributed to either failure of the cardiac pump (forward failure) or damming up of blood behind one or both ventricles (backward failure).[2] These concepts are now outmoded and it is clear that heart failure is a complex process involving not only structural abnormalities and haemodynamic mechanisms but also neuroendocrine, biochemical and genetic pathways through which either an increased haemodynamic burden or a reduction in myocardial oxygen delivery leads to abnormal myocardial

structure and function.[1,2] Although not yet fully investigated the autonomic nervous system is activated in horses with heart failure[3] and there is also some evidence supporting activation of the renin–angiotensin activating system, and plasma aldosterone concentrations rise as the severity of valvular disease increases.[4] Initially, these neuroendocrine adaptations have beneficial effects in maintaining cardiac output, but ultimately they create deleterious effects on the heart, and also on the vasculature and organs such as the kidney[1,2,5] (see Chapters 2 and 4).

CLINICAL SIGNS OF HEART FAILURE

The clinical signs of heart failure can be attributed to a combination of reduced cardiac output and increased ventricular filling pressures. Increased ventricular filling pressures can lead to signs of congestion affecting one or both sides of the heart. These processes occur in combination to varying degrees in most of the cardiac conditions that lead to heart failure, and provided that oversimplification is avoided, it can be helpful for the clinician to differentiate the signs of reduced cardiac output from congestion of each side of the circulation as this may lead to the formation of the most accurate list of differential diagnoses. The term congestive heart failure (CHF) should be reserved for those cases showing left, right or biventricular venous congestion and it is important to recognize that the term heart failure not only encompasses CHF but also includes cases in which the ventricle fails and cardiac output drops without development of congestion. The clinical consequences of reduced cardiac output include tachycardia, weight loss, weakness, exercise intolerance, pale mucous membranes, weak arterial pulses, ataxia and syncope. Reduced renal output is common and increases in serum

DOI: 10.1016/B978-0-7020-2817-5.00024-9

creatinine concentration arise through both prerenal and direct renal mechanisms.[6] (PC, VMD)

Increased ventricular filling pressure leads to congestion of the systemic, the pulmonic or both sides of the circulation and the clinical signs of CHF. The exact range of signs will depend on the specific causative lesion and its location. Lesions that cause the left heart to fail, such as severe mitral insufficiency (MI) and large ventricular septal defects, lead to congestion of the pulmonary circulation.[6,7] The distribution of fluid between the interstitium and the plasma is dependent on the balance between oncotic pressure and hydrostatic forces. The hydrostatic forces rise in response to increased ventricular filling pressure and pulmonary venous engorgement in heart failure, forcing fluid from the pulmonary capillaries into the pulmonary interstitium faster than the lymphatics can remove it, to create pulmonary oedema. Oedema fluid is relatively low in protein and as it moves from the pulmonary capillaries into the interstitium, the protein is returned to the blood, raising the plasma oncotic pressure and lowering the interstitial oncotic pressure and thereby counteracting the tendency for fluid to leave the circulation under hydrostatic forces. Therefore, pulmonary oedema can be self-limiting for a considerable period of time.[8] In slowly progressive lesions, early or mild heart failure, raised respiratory rates, particularly after exercise, and crackles and moist bronchovesicular sounds may be the only clinical signs of pulmonary oedema.[8] Thoracic radiographs demonstrate an interstitial pattern and pulmonary venous congestion. If pulmonary capillary pressure rises acutely, the oncotic pressure within the interstitium rises rapidly to produce alveolar flooding.[8] With a more acute onset or in advanced heart failure, there may be dyspnoea, coughing and profuse nasal discharge which is typically white or pink-tinged and frothy (Fig. 19.1) and thoracic radiographs demonstrate a fluffy alveolar pattern (Fig. 19.2). Pulmonary hypertension can also lead to dilatation and eventually rupture of the pulmonary artery[6,9,10] (see Fig. 18.4). Rupture of the pulmonary artery is not necessarily immediately fatal and there may be a history of episodes of syncope and distress on several occasions before the horse dies (see Chapter 18). (AF, IE)

Right ventricular volume overload is less common as an isolated state. However, clinical signs of left heart failure may frequently go unnoticed, with slowly progressive disease until the right heart fails in response to pulmonary hypertension.[6] Clinical signs of right-sided CHF include jugular distension, pulsations of the jugular veins extending beyond the normal distal one-third of the neck, distension of other peripheral veins such as the lateral thoracic veins, and ventral, muzzle, preputial and limb oedema. Ascites is difficult to appreciate on physical examination in horses, but ultrasonography may reveal increased volumes of fluid in the abdominal cavity and congestion of the hepatic vessels. Horses also frequently develop pleural effusions with heart failure which can be demon-

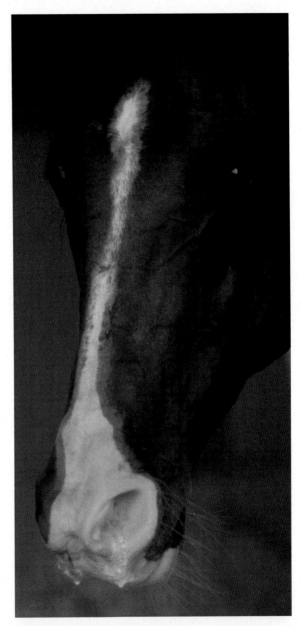

Figure 19.1 A frothy nasal discharge in an 11-year-old Arabian mare with congestive heart failure caused by acute myocarditis.

strated by absence of respiratory sounds over the ventral lung field and percussion of ventral thoracic dullness, and which can be visualized radiographically or ultrasonographically. (ACF, PC, VMD)

Many of the lesions associated with heart failure lead to enlargement of either the left or right atrium. This predisposes the horse to the development of atrial fibrillation, an extremely common finding in CHF[11] (Fig. 19.3). It is

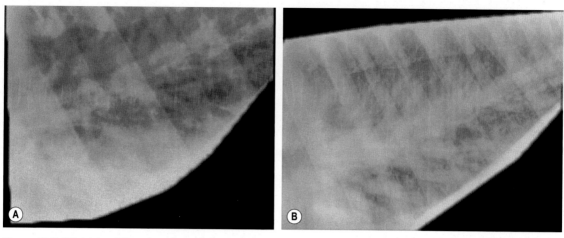

Figure 19.2 (**A**) A lateral thoracic radiograph from an 18-year-old Irish Draught gelding with chronic heart failure due to a ventricular septal defect and mitral insufficiency. There is an interstitial pattern characterized by generalized increase in opacity and loss of detail of the lung field. (**B**) A lateral thoracic radiograph from a 5-year-old warmblood mare with acute heart failure due to infective endocarditis of the aortic and mitral valves. There is an interstitial-alveolar pattern resulting in fluffy opacities and a generalized increase in opacity of the lung field.

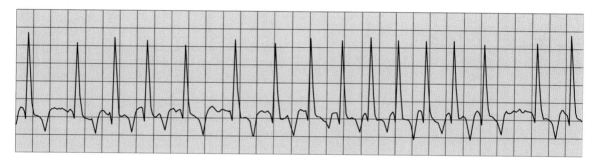

Figure 19.3 An ECG recorded on lead Y demonstrating atrial fibrillation with a ventricular rate of around 90/minute in an aged gelding with congestive heart failure associated with degenerative valvular heart disease and rupture of a chorda tendinea of the mitral valve. Paper speed 25 mm/second, sensitivity of 5 mm = 1 mV.

important to differentiate horses in which atrial fibrillation is a consequence of heart failure rather than a primary condition, because as discussed in Chapter 13, quinidine sulphate is indicated in lone (uncomplicated) atrial fibrillation and contraindicated in CHF.[11] A heart rate of greater than 60 bpm, loud cardiac murmurs and echocardiographic evidence of valvular or other cardiac lesions suggest CHF is present in horses with atrial fibrillation (see Fig. 19.3). (AF)

DIFFERENTIAL DIAGNOSIS OF HEART FAILURE

The prevalence of CHF in horses is unknown and is likely to vary considerably between different horse populations. In one study examining causes of death among a group of

1153 horses the majority of which were middle-aged or older, there were no cardiac-related deaths in horses less than 17 years of age, and 5% of deaths in the 15–23 years age group and 8.5% of deaths in the >24 years age group were considered to relate to cardiac disease.[12] In the author's cardiological practice serving a wide range of racing, sports, pleasure and breeding horses of all ages, approximately 2% of cardiac admissions have CHF.

Disorders affecting a variety of body systems can present in a similar manner to CHF. In addition to CHF, the main differential diagnoses for horses presenting with peripheral oedema can be broadly classified: as (1) conditions associated with protein loss, such as protein-losing enteropathy; (2) conditions associated with obstruction to lymphatic drainage, such as lymphoma or lymphadenopathy; and (3) peripheral vasculitis such as purpura haemorrhagica. In horses presenting with mild to moderate respiratory disease, there are numerous possible conditions that must be considered while with acute severe pulmonary disease, in addition to left-sided heart failure, conditions such as interstitial pneumonia and acute lung injury must be included in the list of differential diagnoses. The clinical signs associated with low cardiac output are nonspecific and myocardial failure must be differentiated from other conditions associated with circulatory failure (i.e. shock) such as abdominal catastrophes and haemorrhage (see Chapter 21).

Causes of heart failure in the horse are listed in Table 19.1. The majority of these diseases can also present at less advanced stages and are described in more general terms elsewhere in this book. The reader is advised to consult specific chapters for additional details (see Chapters 13–18). The aim of this section is to assist the clinician in devising an appropriate diagnostic and therapeutic plan when presented with a horse showing signs of heart failure.

Biventricular CHF is most commonly seen in association with severe, acquired disease of the aortic and/or mitral valves.[6,13-18] However, occasionally horses with large ventricular septal defects and other congenital cardiac defects can present with left-sided or bilateral CHF.[7,19] Primary right-sided CHF is less common but occasionally occurs with severe tricuspid (TI) or pulmonic insufficiency, congenital disease and cor pulmonale.[20,21] Pericarditis causes heart failure because cardiac tamponade due to effusion within the pericardial sac or loss of elasticity in restrictive pericarditis increases the intrapericardial pressure and prevents diastolic filling. This process affects both sides of the heart, but typically signs associated with the systemic circulation predominate because the lower pressures within the right side of the circulation can more readily be overwhelmed.[22-25] Rapid tachycardia can also impede diastolic function sufficiently to induce signs of heart failure by decreasing the time available for the heart to fill in diastole.[1] In this situation, signs of left-sided congestion predominate.

DIAGNOSTIC APPROACH IN HEART FAILURE

Echocardiography is an extremely valuable diagnostic aid when cardiac failure is suspected as both cardiac structure and function can be assessed with this imaging modality.[26-29] Echocardiography can be useful, in particular in identifying chamber dilation and compromised myocardial function. In compensated left ventricular volume overload, the fractional shortening and ejection fraction should be increased and where normal or decreased fractional shortening and ejection fraction are detected in the presence of volume overload, ventricular remodelling and loss of myocardial function should be suspected (see Chapter 9). Regardless of cause, typical echocardiographic features of generalized myocardial dysfunction include ventricular dilatation, hypomotility, increased septal–mitral E-point separation, reduced fractional shortening and reduction in the movement of the aortic root on M-mode echocardiography. (AF, PC, VMD) There is often mitral insufficiency secondary to valve annulus dilatation. Where the myocardial dysfunction has arisen as a consequence of valvular insufficiency and volume overload, the left ventricular free wall is often more obviously affected than interventricular septum. (VMD)

Direct measurement of pulmonary artery and capillary wedge pressure is the most reliable method for documenting pulmonary hypertension. (PH) Radiology can be limited in its ability to demonstrate milder forms of oedema and clinical signs do not necessarily relate closely to the degree of oedema visible radiographically. Nevertheless, radiography is frequently the most practical means of identifying pulmonary oedema and evaluating the response to therapy (see Fig. 19.2). Severe pulmonary oedema can be visualized with diagnostic ultrasonography as multifocal areas of hypoechoic, nonaerated lung at

Table 19.1 Conditions that commonly cause heart failure in the horse
Predominantly left-sided or biventricular failure
Mitral insufficiency
Rupture of a chorda tendinea
Severe degenerative lesions
Infective endocarditis
Secondary to dilation of the valve annulus
Aortic insufficiency
Severe degenerative lesions with dilation of the left ventricle and consequent mitral insufficiency
Infective endocarditis
Rupture of an aortic valve leaflet
Myocardial disease
Myocarditis
Myocardial fibrosis
Myocardial ischaemia
Dilated cardiomyopathy
Congenital cardiac disease
Ventricular septal defect
Patent ductus arteriosus
Aortocardiac fistula
Predominantly right-sided failure
Pericarditis
Effusive
Constrictive
Tricuspid insufficiency
Rupture of a chorda tendinea
Infective endocarditis
Congenital cardiac disease
Right atrioventricular valvular atresia
Tetralogy of Fallot
Atrial septal defect
Great vessel anomalies
Others

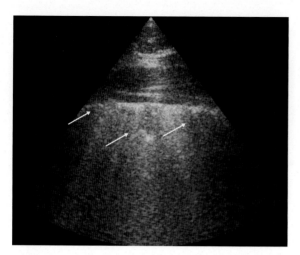

Figure 19.4 A thoracic ultrasonogram in an 11-year-old Arabian mare with acute myocarditis and pulmonary oedema (see Fig 19.1). The periphery of the lung is irregular with hypoechoic nonaerated areas representing oedema (arrows) and the lung has lost the horizontal reverberation pattern that is seen in normal aerated lung.

the periphery (Fig. 19.4). However, pulmonary oedema is most severe at the hilar area and often does not always extend to the periphery of the lung where it can be visualized with ultrasonography. Diagnostic ultrasonography is more useful in documenting the presence of pleural effusion, hepatic congestion and ascites. (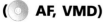 *PC*)

The identification of myocardial disease and dysfunction is an important component of assessment of horses with heart failure. Electrocardiography is required to demonstrate arrhythmias that may accompany heart failure, such as atrial tachycardia, atrial fibrillation, supraventricular or ventricular premature depolarizations, ventricular tachycardia or pre-excitation syndrome. Ambulatory ECG techniques are particularly useful in demonstrating paroxysmal arrhythmias and documenting their frequency over prolonged periods (see Chapters 6 and 10). Novel biomarkers are currently being assessed in horses and these are discussed in more detail in Chapter 12. Cardiac troponin may be increased in some cases[6,30] but it is important to recognize that a normal cardiac troponin concentration does not rule out the presence of myocardial pathology, particularly myocardial fibrosis.

SPECIFIC FORMS OF HEART FAILURE

Left-sided valvular insufficiency (AF, VMD)

Degenerative valvular disease of the aortic valve is extremely common in horses[12,31,32] (see Chapter 16). In the majority of horses with aortic insufficiency (AI), the lesion is well tolerated and the proportion of affected individuals that progress to develop CHF is unknown: in one study, 86% of horses with AI showed no signs of heart disease at rest while 13.2% had signs of CHF at rest, however, this population was drawn from an elderly population and horses that develop CHF with AI are typically in their late teens or older. Clinical signs of hyperkinetic pulses and a widely radiating diastolic murmur are consistent with severe AI.[13] With echocardiography, nodular lesions of the aortic valve and large regurgitant jets are visualized.[13,14,28,33] The onset of myocardial failure often appears to herald the onset of clinical signs of CHF; in horses with well-compensated but severe AI, the left ventricle is usually dilated but hyperkinetic[13,14] (Fig. 19.5). Left ventricular volume overload increases end-diastolic left ventricular diameter and causes the ventricle to adopt a globoid shape with a rounded apex.[13] In the hyperkinetic ventricle, septal and left ventricular free-wall movement is exaggerated and the fractional shortening is increased.[13] As the ventricle begins to fail, myocardial contractility is often depressed. Fractional shortening, which is influenced by a variety of factors including myocardial contractility, will decrease and subjectively the ventricle may appear to be hypomotile (see Fig. 19.5). Most horses that develop overt CHF with degenerative AI have ventricular dilatation to a degree that can disrupt the mitral valve annulus and cause MI (Fig. 19.6). In fact, it is the onset of MI that may be the event that has ultimately caused the cardiac decompensation and horses with multiple murmurs are more likely to go into CHF than those with AI alone.[3] Therefore, the development of a murmur of MI in a horse with previously well-compensated AI should alert the clinician to the possibility of progression of the disease. These horses typically have end-diastolic left ventricular diameters in excess of 16 cm (see Fig. 19.5).

Severe MI can be caused by valvular degeneration or inflammation[6,15,31] and may also arise secondary due to ventricular dilation as a result of myocardial, congenital or aortic disease. In one study of horses with severe MI, almost 50% of affected horses had evidence of concurrent myocardial disease.[6] Severe MI is seen in a wider range of age groups than AI. Auscultation reveals a loud pan- or holosystolic murmur radiating over a wide area with severe MI and the third heart sound is often loud because there is increased ventricular filling in diastole.[6] In chronic degenerative cases, nodular thickening of the valve may be visible echocardiographically and subsequently on post-mortem examination. Severe mitral regurgitation occupies the majority of the left atrium, has a wide base, may originate from more than one source at the valve leaflets and may demonstrate proximal flow convergence[29] (Fig. 19.7). Severe MI is poorly tolerated and consequences include atrial enlargement (see Fig. 19.6), atrial fibrillation (see Fig. 19.5), ventricular tachyarrhythmias, pulmonary

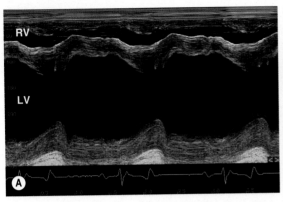
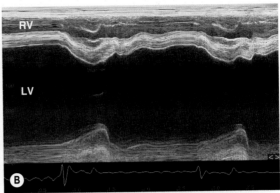

Figure 19.5 M-mode echocardiograms of the right (RV) and left ventricle (LV) in horses with severe aortic and mitral insufficiency. (**A**) This horse has a left ventricular end-diastolic diameter of 16.6 cm, a fractional shortening of 43% and a hyperkinetic ventricle and is currently in compensated heart failure. (**B**) This horse has a hyperkinetic septum but the left ventricular end-diastolic diameter is 18.9 cm, the fractional shortening is 33% and the left ventricular free-wall is hypokinetic, suggesting myocardial dysfunction, and consequently the horse is showing more severe clinical signs. Note the ECG also demonstrates that the horse has atrial fibrillation.

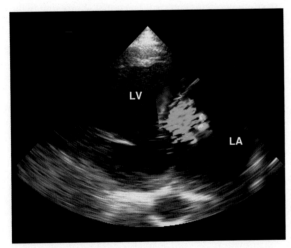

Figure 19.6 A left parasternal long-axis echocardiogram of the left atrium (LA) and ventricle (LV) from the horse illustrated in Fig. 19.5B. The mitral valve annulus is dilated and there is a large jet of mitral regurgitation (green). The LA has an increased diameter of 18.9 cm (normal <13.5 cm).

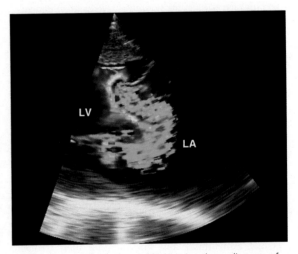

Figure 19.7 A left parasternal long-axis echocardiogram of the left atrium (LA) and ventricle (LV) from a 7-year-old Thoroughbred with severe mitral insufficiency and myocardial disease. Two jets of mitral regurgitation (green) coalesce to occupy the majority of the LA. In the left ventricular inflow tract, regurgitant flow accelerating towards the regurgitant orifice depicted by bands of colour from blue to yellow to red represents proximal flow convergence.

oedema (see Fig. 19.4) and, occasionally, pulmonary artery dilatation and rupture[6,15–18] (see Fig. 18.4). Dilatation of the left atrium can be appreciated most readily from two-chamber left parasternal images (see Fig. 19.6), and in mature horses with severe MI, left atrial diameters of 16.2–23 cm have been reported, normal being less than 13.5 cm.[6,29] The normal ratio of the pulmonary artery measured in long-axis to the aortic root diameter measured in long-axis is around 0.8. Dilatation of the pulmonary artery is diagnosed if its diameter is greater than that of the aorta (Fig. 19.8).[6,9] In many horses with pulmonary artery dilatation, pulmonic valvular insufficiency is present (see Fig. 19.8), again probably the result of pulmonary hypertension.[6] Horses with severe MI also often have reduction in the aortic root diameter due to reduced cardiac output (see Fig. 19.8). In one report describing horses with severe mitral valve disease, 64% of horses had pulmonary artery diameters which exceeded that of the aorta by greater than 1 cm.[6]

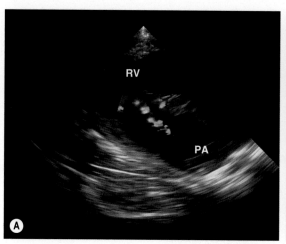
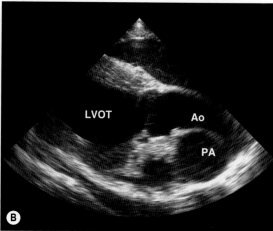

Figure 19.8 A right ventricular inflow–outflow (**A**) and a right parasternal long-axis echocardiogram of the left ventricular outflow tract (LVOT) (**B**) from the horse illustrated in Fig 19.7. There is pulmonic regurgitation and the pulmonary artery (PA) is dilated because of pulmonary hypertension: its diameter in the right ventricular inflow-outflow image is 7.8 cm and the diameter of the aorta (Ao) in long-axis is reduced (6.1 cm) because of reduced cardiac output. Dilation of the PA can also be appreciated in the LVOT image. On post-mortem examination, a partial rupture of the PA was observed. RV, right ventricle.

Rupture of a chorda tendinea of the mitral valve is the most common form of acute, severe mitral valve disease described in the horse.[6,15–18,34] This can occur spontaneously or secondary to degenerative or inflammatory valve disease. Frequently, it is one of the accessory cusps that is affected and, while acute onset CHF is the most common presentation, occasionally the clinical signs are less severe.[6,15–18,34] Echocardiography can accurately demonstrate rupture of a chorda tendinea, and portions of the valve are seen everting into the left atrium or a flail leaflet is visualized. Usually, there is a large regurgitant jet but the atrium and ventricle may not necessarily be markedly dilated because, with the onset of acute severe regurgitation, there is little time for changes in atrial compliance or volume. The heart cannot compensate for acute volume overload rapidly, which explains the severity of the typical clinical signs.[6] (RCT)

Infective endocarditis typically causes vegetative lesions which are visible echocardiographically[9,35–41] (see Chapter 17). Aortic and mitral valves are affected most commonly, but mural portions of the endocardium and the pulmonic and tricuspid valves can be affected, particularly if the endocarditis arises secondary to septic jugular thrombophlebitis.[9,35–41] The clinical signs are dependent on the specific location of the lesions. Because the onset of regurgitation is rapid, there may be large regurgitant jets with little or no ventricular or atrial dilatation. Clinical signs such as fever and depression, and laboratory evidence of infection such as leukocytosis and hyperfibrinogenaemia, support the diagnosis of infective endocarditis.[35,40,41] (IE)

Right-sided valvular insufficiency and cor pulmonale

(PH, VMD)

Tricuspid and pulmonic regurgitation very rarely lead to CHF. Exceptions include rupture of a chorda tendinea of the tricuspid valve or leaflet of the pulmonary valve.[42] (ACF) The echocardiographic appearances of these valvular lesions are similar to those described above for the corresponding valves of the left heart. Although uncommon, right-sided CHF does occasionally occur in horses or ponies with long-standing respiratory disease. This syndrome, cor pulmonale, is much more common in cattle. In response to hypoxia, pulmonary vasoconstriction and pulmonary hypertension can develop.[21,43,44] This can lead to increased pulmonary artery diameter, abnormal septal motion, decreased left ventricular diameter and decreased stroke volume. These changes are reversible[21] but with chronic hypoxia, ultimately right heart failure can ensue.[20,27] Generally, there are not only signs consistent with right heart failure such as jugular distension and pulsation but also severe respiratory compromise, reflecting the underlying cause. The prognosis is poor. Regardless of the cause, care must be taken to accurately measure the dimensions of the right ventricle because of the crescent shape of the ventricle[45] (see Chapter 9 and Fig. 9.3). With severe right ventricular volume overload, the heart adopts a double-apex appearance and paradoxical septal motion is present.[26,28,29,42]

Congenital cardiac disease

(VSD)

Congenital cardiac disease is usually suspected in foals, weanlings or yearlings presenting with CHF, particularly if loud cardiac murmurs are present. A segmental approach to the echocardiographic examination is used to document the size, shape and relative location of each cardiac structure[7,46,47] (see Chapter 15).

Aorto-cardiac fistula

(ACF)

Aorto-cardiac fistula occurs when there is disruption of the aortic wall, usually in the right sinus of Valsalva, occasionally the non-coronary sinus, and a dissecting tract extends from the aorta to the right atrium, the right ventricle and/or the interventricular septum (see Chapter 18, Fig. 18.3). The aetiology is unknown: there may be congenital or acquired degeneration of the media of the aorta[48,49] and intact aneurysms may be present prior to the rupture.[50] Some reports have associated the condition with chronic aortic insufficiency although this may be coincidental rather than causative.[51] Males are more prone to this condition than mares and typically affected animals are middle-aged or older.[52] Presenting signs range from sudden death, often during breeding or exercise, acute thoracic pain, often mistaken for colic by observers, and CHF.[51–54] There is typically a low-pitched, continuous murmur with its point of maximal intensity over the right hemithorax. There is frequently a rapid ventricular tachycardia, most likely due to disruption of the conducting tissue by a tract extending into the interventricular septum.[52] Emergency treatment includes stabilization of the ventricular dysrhythmia and management of CHF. Horses can survive the initial episode for periods of up to 2 years but generally the condition is eventually fatal.[51,52,54,55]

Myocardial disease

With underlying structural disease such as valvular pathology or congenital heart disease, over time, neuroendocrine, haemodynamic and genetic factors can lead to ventricular remodelling (see Chapter 4 and Fig. 15.7). Eventually, cardiac fibrosis may develop and the subsequent myocardial dysfunction may precipitate the development of clinical signs of cardiac failure and the progression from compensated to decompensated heart failure. Other forms of primary myocardial disease are relatively uncommon in horses, particularly when compared with human beings in whom coronary artery disease and myocardial ischaemia is such an important cause of

Table 19.2 Potential causes of myocardial failure and disease in horses

Viruses
    Equine herpes virus 1
    Equine influenza
    Mobillivirus
    African horse sickness
Bacteria
    Streptoccal toxic shock
    Piroplasmosis
Nutritional
    Vitamin E and selenium deficiency
    Cooper deficiency
    Excessive molybdenum
    Excessive sulphates
Toxins
    Rattlesnake venom
    Ionophores
    Digitalis species
    Taxus (yew)
    Pimelea species
    Oleander
    Cantharidin (blister beetle)
    Sodium fluoroactetate rodenticides
Neoplasia
    Haemangiosarcoma
    Lymphosarcoma
    Melanoma
    Mesothelioma
Genetic
    Glycogen branching enzyme deficiency in Quarter horse foals
Idiopathic
    Dilated cardiomyopathy
    Amyloidosis

morbidity and mortality worldwide. Nevertheless, primary myocardial disease does lead to heart failure in horses and potential infectious,[56–61] toxic,[62–74] nutritional,[75–77] neoplastic,[78–80] genetic[81] and idiopathic[82] causes are listed in Table 19.2. (CN)

Dilated cardiomyopathy

(VMD)

Cardiomyopathy is a subacute or chronic disease of the ventricular myocardium that occurs in the absence of pulmonary disease, congenital defects or structural disease of the valves, although cardiomyopathy can lead to valvular dysfunction. In horses, only dilated cardiomyopathies occur and these are rare and sporadic and the idiopathic forms are of unknown causes but in some cases they may represent a sequel to myocarditis.[75]

Glycogen branching enzyme deficiency

Recently, a glycogen branching enzyme (GBE) deficiency has been reported in Quarter horse foals that died by 7 weeks of age.[81] The condition has an autosomal recessive mode of inheritance. Glycogen is important for glucose homeostasis in foals and is composed of straight and branched chains of linked glucose molecules. GBE is responsible for the formation of the α1,6 branch points that are essential to rapid mobilization of glucose in a range of tissues. In human beings, deficiency is associated with a range of age-dependent presentations, including cardiomyopathy. Affected foals show a range of nonspecific signs and in addition to cardiac arrest these include still birth, respiratory arrest, seizures and progressive muscle weakness. Because the signs are nonspecific it is possible that this disease has gone unrecognized in the past.[81] Clinicopathological findings include increased serum activity of aspartate transaminase and creatine kinase and hypoglycaemia but there are no specific findings on gross post-mortem examination, requiring the demonstration of lack of GBE activity for confirmation of diagnosis.[81]

Nutritional myodegeneration (white muscle disease)

Vitamin E and/or selenium deficiency is associated with a variety of disorders including nutritional myodegeneration or white muscle disease that is usually seen in foals of less than 2 months of age and has been reported in the fetus.[76] The condition affects skeletal and smooth muscle, including the heart, the diaphragm and muscles of mastication. The presenting signs include sudden death, cardiac and respiratory failure, cardiac dysrhythmias, pulmonary oedema and in less acute cases, weakness, stiffness, lethargy and dysphagia. There may be painful subcutaneous swellings. Clinicopathological findings include increased serum activity of aspartate transaminase and creatine kinase, decreased serum activity of glutathione peroxidase and concentrations of vitamin E and myoglobinuria may be present. Some foals may recover with supportive treatment and vitamin E administered orally on a daily basis coupled with intermittent intramuscular injections of vitamin E/selenium preparations that can be repeated in 3–7 days if necessary.[77]

Ionophore toxicity

Ionophores are used as growth promoters in cattle and as coccidiostats for poultry (monensin, salinomycin and lasalocid).[67,69,70,83–85] The horse is exquisitely sensitive to the toxic effects of ionophores and interspecies differences in sensitivity are related to differences in oxidative meta-

bolism of ionophores by cytochrome P450 in hepatic microsomes. Ionophores enhance cell membrane permeability, affecting both ion influx and efflux, and this is detrimental in excitable cells such as those in nervous tissue, and cardiac and skeletal muscle. The mechanism of toxicity of ionophores varies slightly between different products: Monensin has a higher affinity for sodium ions than potassium ions whereas salinomycin has higher affinity for potassium than sodium and lasalocid binds to both calcium and magnesium ions. Loss of intracellular potassium suppresses ATP production and decreases cell energy production, increase in intracellular sodium leads to cellular water influx and mitochondrial swelling, ionophores potentiate intracellular calcium influx, and all of these effects contribute to cell death. Clinical effects and mortality rates are likely to be influenced by the amount of ionophore ingested.[83] With large amounts, the progression can be extremely rapid with death ensuing within 1–15 hours. Structural skeletal and cardiac lesions are not necessarily found in horses that die very acutely.[68,84] With lesser amounts, signs and pathological abnormalities related to skeletal and cardiac myopathy are observed. Some more mildly affected horses develop a delayed form of cardiomyopathy,[73] which depending on its severity, may lead to variable degrees of cardiac compromise evident weeks or months after initial exposure.

Horses of any age, breed or sex can be exposed to ionophore-contaminated feed. The contamination may come from feed accidentally contaminated at the feed mill or from accidental feeding of or exposure to ionophore-containing cattle or poultry feed. Feed samples should be obtained for toxicological analysis if ionophore exposure is suspected. Gastrointestinal samples should be similarly analysed in any horses that experienced sudden death. Sudden death is often the first indication of exposure of horses to high doses of ionophores.[68,83,84] Fever, depression, lethargy, restlessness, exercise intolerance and profuse sweating are some of the signs first noticed by the owners and/or trainers of affected horses. Anorexia, poor appetite and feed refusal are common because ionophore-contaminated feed is less palatable. Muscle weakness, trembling and ataxia often occur. Horses may be polyuric and become oliguric or anuric. Diarrhoea, colic and/or ileus have frequently been reported. Muddy or injected mucous membranes with thready arterial pulses may be detected initially. Cardiac dysrhythmias may develop at any time following ionophore exposure but are most likely in the first few days to weeks following exposure. Generalized venous distention, jugular pulses, ventral oedema and murmurs of mitral and/or tricuspid regurgitation may develop weeks to months following ionophore exposure.[68,83,84]

Electrocardiographic abnormalities may be detected in horses recently exposed to ionophores but are not good prognostic indicators of the severity of the myocardial injury. Axis shifts, ST segment depression, T wave changes,

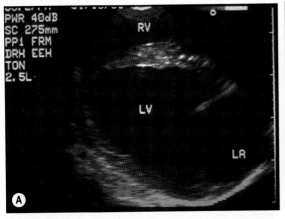 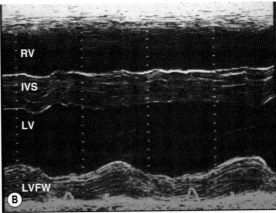

Figure 19.9 (A) A right parasternal long-axis echocardiogram of the left (LV) and right (RV) ventricles and left atrium (LA) and **(B)** a ventricular M-mode echocardiogram from a 6-year-old Standardbred gelding with dilated cardiomyopathy due to monensin toxicosis. The cardiac chambers are dilated and globular in shape and the movement of the interventricular septum (IVS) and left ventricular free wall (LVFW) is markedly depressed.

atrial and ventricular premature depolarizations, atrial fibrillation, ventricular tachycardia and a variety of brady-dysrhythmias have been reported in horses exposed to ionophores. The majority of horses exposed to ionophores in the field situation, however, do not have cardiac dysrhythmias. Increases in serum cardiac troponin I concentrations and activities of the cardiac isoenzymes of creatine kinase (CK) and lactate dehydrogenase (LDH) have been reported in some outbreaks of ionophore toxicity, but were only slight or not detected in other field outbreaks. Echocardiographic signs are typical of dilated cardiomyopathy and include dilation and rounding of the ventricles and reduction in fractional shortening (Fig. 19.9) together with other signs of reduced cardiac output (see Chapter 9).

If ionophore exposure is suspected the possibly contaminated feed should be removed. Activated charcoal or mineral oil should be administered to decrease further absorption of the ionophore from recently ingested feed. Large doses of vitamin E to attempt to stabilize cell membranes and control peroxidation-mediated cell injury may be helpful if administered as soon as possible after exposure. Supportive care should be provided as needed. Exposed horses should receive stall rest for a minimum of 2 months. Digoxin is contraindicated in acute monensin exposure because monensin and digoxin also affect the transmembrane transport of electrolyes and have an additive effect causing calcium to flood into the myocardial cell. The use of digoxin in horses recently exposed to monensin may result in the intracellular calcium sequestration mechanisms being further overloaded, increasing the amount and severity of myocardial cell injury and cell death.

Ionophore toxicity may have significant medicolegal implications. The client should be advised to make detailed records of events leading up to the onset of signs and to have these corroborated by third parties where possible. Where a group of horses has been exposed to ionophores, it can be impossible to determine which individual horses may have ingested the toxin and how much they have consumed. Horses that do not show clinical signs in the acute stages may be at risk of developing cardiac compromise later. Clients should be advised not to use the horses for ridden activities for 2–3 months and after this time, an echocardiogram and exercising ECG should be performed in order to identify signs of chronic cardiomyopathy before returning the horse to ridden work.

TREATMENT AND MANAGEMENT OF CONGESTIVE HEART FAILURE

Given that in most forms of CHF associated with structural heart disease the prognosis may ultimately be hopeless, once the severity of the disease has been established, euthanasia is often the appropriate course of action. Therefore, the equine clinician may frequently serve his/her patient and client most appropriately by providing an accurate assessment of the causes and severity of the CHF with the methods described above. Management of CHF in the short and medium term can be effective; however, in the long term, it is rarely successful: nine of 14 horses presenting in CHF were euthanazed and the remainder died or were euthanazed within 1 year.[27] Notable exceptions include pericarditis that can be managed effectively with pericardial drainage and medical therapy (see Chapter 17). Specific therapy should be directed towards the causative lesion, such as relieving cardiac tamponade in pericarditis and antimicrobial therapy in infective endocarditis (see Chapter 17). The general goals of therapy in CHF are to reduce congestion and improve cardiac output. The involvement of the renin–angiotensin–aldosterone system, endothelin and β-adrenoceptors activation in the progression of myocardial enlargement suggests that these pathways may provide sites for pharmacological intervention. In human patients and animal models, β-adrenergic blockers have been shown to reverse cardiac remodelling in aortic valve regurgitation[86,87] while angiotensin-converting enzyme inhibitors, mineralocorticoid receptor antagonists and endothelin receptor antagonists have all shown benefits in reversing cardiac remodelling in humans and animal models with pressure-induced cardiac hypertrophy as well as improvements in cardiac function in those with valvular pathology. There is currently no species-specific evidence to support the use of β-blocking agents in equine valvular or myocardial disease, although, based on studies of cardiac disease in human patients, these may represent a potential area for pharmacological intervention in horses with chronic cardiac enlargement brought about by valvular regurgitation. Some horses may benefit from digoxin that is used to control the ventricular rate in supraventricular tachycardia. Further details of the pharmacology and appropriate use of these drugs can be found in Chapter 7 and the discussion below focuses on the clinical use of these drugs.

Vasodilators

 AF, IE)

There is anecdotal evidence that ACE inhibitors such as enalapril may be beneficial in horses. However, pharmacokinetic studies have shown poor oral bioavailability.[88,89] The ACE inhibitor quinapril, given orally at a dose of 120 mg/horse/day, lead to increased stroke volume and cardiac output, a reduction in the amount of valvular regurgitation, but no clinically significant changes in cardiac size after 8 weeks of therapy in horses with mitral insufficiency but no CHF. This corresponded with an owner-reported improvement in exercise tolerance.[90] Further studies are required before specific recommendations can be made on the clinical use of ACE inhibitors in CHF.

Acepromazine has been suggested as a more economical alternative to conventional vasodilators. However, there is neither retrospective nor prospective data to support its use. Hydralazine is an arteriolar dilator that acts directly on vascular smooth muscle, decreases total peripheral resistance and increases cardiac output in normal horses.[91] In other species, it is indicated in low-output failure and acute mitral valvular insufficiency. Its efficacy in horses with CHF has not been established but it can be used at 0.5–1.5 mg/kg every 12 hours orally. Hydralazine can induce severe hypotension and therefore must be used with care, ideally titrating the dose against blood pressure

measurements. The venedilator nitroglycerine ointment is useful in the short-term management of pulmonary oedema in other species. Its mechanism of action is dependent on its ability to dilate the veins. Intravenous infusions of nitroglycerin in normal horses cause a dose-related decrease in right atrial, pulmonary artery, pulmonary artery wedge and pulmonary capillary pressure but have a more potent effect on pulmonary veins than arteries. The efficacy of nitroglycerin ointment in the treatment of pulmonary oedema in the horse has not been critically evaluated.

Diuretics

Furosemide is the most effective and popular diuretic used in horses. It inhibits chloride transport in the ascending loop of Henle, increasing the excretion of sodium, chloride, potassium, hydrogen ions and water. This produces a decrease in plasma volume, extracellular fluid volume, left ventricular end-diastolic pressure and pulmonary capillary wedge pressure, resulting in a reduction in pulmonary hydrostatic pressure, pulmonary fluid volume and the work of ventilation.[92] Furosemide is usually administered at 1–2 mg/kg two to three times per day intravenously or intramuscularly. In many horses it is effective orally; however, occasionally, beneficial effects abate when the route of administration is changed from intravenous to oral. Long-term administration may produce hyponatraemia, hypokalaemia, hypomagnesaemia and metabolic alkalosis.[93] Therefore, periodic monitoring of serum electrolyte concentrations is advisable during furosemide therapy.

Digoxin

 AF)

The role of digoxin in CHF is controversial and, like the other digitalis glycosides, it has a variety of effects including positive inotropic actions mediated by inhibition of the myocardial cell sodium–potassium pump and a negative chronotropic effect. This arises both directly by prolonging the refractory period of the atrioventricular node and indirectly by increasing parasympathetic and decreasing sympathetic tone. Digoxin also suppresses plasma renin and aldosterone activity and promotes diuresis, thereby reducing venous pressure and congestion (see Chapter 7). The main indication for the use of digoxin in horses with heart failure is to control tachycardia in atrial fibrillation (see Fig. 19.3).

The recommended maintenance dosage is 0.011 mg/kg orally daily and 0.0022 mg/kg intravenously twice daily.[94,95] There is considerable variation in plasma half-life of digoxin in the horse.[94] Adverse side effects are common and serum digoxin concentrations should be monitored to maintain therapeutic concentrations (see Chapter 7). Adverse side effects include anorexia, depression, abdominal pain and ventricular arrhythmias.[55] Antiarrhythmic drugs that are used in human beings with digoxin-induced arrhythmias include phenytoin, lignocaine and propanolol. Regimens involving loading doses increase the likelihood of toxicity and particular care

should be taken in horses with renal dysfunction in which excretion may be affected. Abnormalities in serum potassium, magnesium, calcium and sodium concentrations and acid–base status may alter the individual's sensitivity to digoxin, and drug interaction increases the steady-state serum concentration of digoxin if quinidine is administered concurrently.[96]

REFERENCES

1. Colucci W, Braunwald E. Pathophysiology of heart failure. In: Zipes DP, Bonow RO, Braunwald E, editors. Braunwald's Heart Disease: A Textbook of Cardiovascular Medicine. Philadelphia: Elsevier Saunders; 2005. p. 509–538.

2. Givertz M, Colucci WS, Braunwald E. Clinical aspects of heart failure. In: Zipes DP, Bonow RO, Braunwald E, editors. Braunwald's Heart Disease: A Textbook of Cardiovascular Medicine. Philadelphia: Elsevier Saunders; 2005. p. 539–602.

3. Horn J. Sympathetic nervous control of cardiac function and its role in equine heart disease. Royal Veterinary College, University of London; 2002.

4. Gehlen H, Sundermann T, Rohn K, Stadler P, et al. Aldosterone plasma concentration in horses with heart valve insufficiencies. Res Vet Sci 2008;85(2):340–344.

5. Richards AM. The renin-angiotensin-aldosterone system and the cardiac natriuretic peptides. Heart 1996;76(Suppl 3):36–44.

6. Reef VB, Bain FT, Spencer PA. Severe mitral regurgitation in horses: clinical, echocardiographic and pathological findings. Equine Vet J 1998;30(1):18–27.

7. Reef VB. Evaluation of ventricular septal defects in horses using two-dimensional and Doppler echocardiography. Equine Vet J Suppl 1995;19:86–95.

8. Ware W, Bonagura JD. Pulmonary oedema. In: Fox P, editor. Canine and Feline Cardiology. New York: Churchill Livingstone; 1988. p. 205–217.

9. Dedrick P, Reef VB, Sweeney RW, Morris DD, et al. Treatment of bacterial endocarditis in a horse. J Am Vet Med Assoc 1988;193(3):339–342.

10. Buergelt C, Carmichael JA, Tashjian RJ, Das KM. Spontaneous rupture of the left pulmonary artery in a horse with patent ductus arteriosus. J Am Vet Med Assoc 1970;186:1210–1213.

11. Reef VB, Levitan CW, Spencer PA. Factors affecting prognosis and conversion in equine atrial fibrillation. J Vet Intern Med 1988;2(1):1–6.

12. Stevens KB, Marr CM, Horn JN, et al. Effect of left-sided valvular regurgitation on mortality and causes of death among a population of middle-aged and older horses. Vet Rec 2009;164(1):6–10.

13. Reef VB, Spencer P. Echocardiographic evaluation of equine aortic insufficiency. Am J Vet Res 1987;48(6):904–909.

14. Patteson MW. Echocardiographic evaluation of horses with aortic regurgitation. Equine Vet Educ 1994;6:159–166.

15. Miller P, Holmes JR. Observations on seven cases of mitral insufficiency in the horse. Equine Vet J 1985;17:181–190.

16. Marr CM, Love S, Pirie HM, Northridge DB, et al. Confirmation by Doppler echocardiography of valvular regurgitation in a horse with a ruptured chorda tendinea of the mitral valve. Vet Rec 1990;127(15):376–379.

17. Brown C, Bell TG, Paradis MR, Breeze RG. Rupture of the mitral chordae tendineae in two horses.

J Am Vet Med Assoc 1987;182:281–331.

18. Reef VB. Mitral valvular insufficiency associated with ruptured chordae tendineae in three foals. J Am Vet Med Assoc 1987;191(3):329–331.

19. Reef VB. Echocardiographic findings in horses with congenital cardiac disease. Comp Contin Educ 1991;13:109–117.

20. Sage AM, Valberg S, Hayden DW, Firshman AM, Jacob K, et al. Echocardiography in a horse with cor pulmonale from recurrent airway obstruction. J Vet Intern Med 2006;20(3):694–696.

21. Johansson AM, Gardner SY, Atkins CE, LaFevers DH, Breuhaus BA, et al. Cardiovascular effects of acute pulmonary obstruction in horses with recurrent airway obstruction. J Vet Intern Med 2007;21(2):302–307.

22. Robinson JA, Marr CM, Reef VB, Sweeney RW, et al. Idiopathic, aseptic, effusive, fibrinous, nonconstrictive pericarditis with tamponade in a standardbred filly. J Am Vet Med Assoc 1992;201(10):1593–1598.

23. Bernard W, Reef VB, Clark ES, Vaala W, Ehnen SJ, et al. Pericarditis in horses: six cases (1982–1986). J Am Vet Med Assoc 1990;196(3):468–471.

24. Dill S, Simoncini DC, Bolton GR, Rendano VT, Crissman JW, King JM, et al. Fibrinous pericarditis in the horse. J Am Vet Med Assoc 1982;180:266–271.

25. Freestone J, Thomas WP, Carlson GP, Brumbaugh GW. Idiopathic effusive pericarditis with tamponade in the horse. Equine Vet J 1987;19:38–42.

26. Bonagura JD, Blissitt KJ. Echocardiography. Equine Vet J Suppl 1995;19:5–17.

27. Davis JL, Gardner SY, Schwabenton B, Breuhaus BA, et al. Congestive heart failure in horses: 14 cases (1984–2001). J Am Vet Med Assoc 2002;220(10):1512–1515.

28. Marr CM. Equine echocardiography: sound advice at the heart of the matter. Br Vet J 1994;150(6): 527–545.

29. Reef VB. Heart murmurs in horses: determining their significance with echocardiography. Equine Vet J Suppl 1995;19:71–80.

30. Cornelisse CJ, Schott HC, 2nd, Olivier NB, et al. Concentration of cardiac troponin I in a horse with a ruptured aortic regurgitation jet lesion and ventricular tachycardia. J Am Vet Med Assoc 2000;217(2): 231–235.

31. Else RW, Holmes JR. Cardiac pathology in the horse. 1. Gross pathology. Equine Vet J 1972;4(1): 1–8.

32. Patteson MW, Cripps PJ. A survey of cardiac auscultatory findings in horses. Equine Vet J 1993;25(5): 409–415.

33. Stadler P, Hoch M, Fraunhaul B, Deegen E. Echocardiography in horses with and without heart murmurs in aortic regurgitation. Pferdeheilkunde 1995;11:373–383.

34. Holmes J, Miller PJ. Three cases of ruptured mitral valve chordae in the horse. Equine Vet J 1984;16: 125–135.

35. Maxson AD, Reef VB. Bacterial endocarditis in horses: ten cases (1984–1995). Equine Vet J 1997;29(5):394–399.

36. Bonagura JD, Pipers FS. Echocardiographic features of aortic valve endocarditis in a dog, a cow, and a horse. J Am Vet Med Assoc 1983;182(6):595–599.

37. Nilsfors L, Lombard CW, Weckner D, Kvart C, et al. Diagnosis of pulmonary valve endocarditis in a horse. Equine Vet J 1991;23(6): 479–482.

38. Collatos C, Clark ES, Reef VB, Morris DD, et al. Septicemia, atrial fibrillation, cardiomegaly, left atrial mass, and *Rhodococcus equi* septic osteoarthritis in a foal. J Am Vet Med Assoc 1990;197(8): 1039–1042.

39. Buergelt CD, Cooley AJ, Hines SA, Pipers FS, et al. Endocarditis in six horses. Vet Pathol 1985;22(4): 333–337.

40. Marr CM. Cardiovascular infections. In: Sellon D, Long MT, editors. Equine Infectious Diseases. Philadelphia: Saunders Elsevier; 2007. p. 21–38.

41. Porter SR, Saegerman C, van Galen G, et al. Vegetative endocarditis in equids (1994–2006). J Vet Intern Med 2008;22(6):1411–1146.

42. Reimer JM, Reef VB, Sommer M. Echocardiographic detection of pulmonic valve rupture in a horse with right-sided heart failure. J Am Vet Med Assoc 1991;198(5): 880–882.

43. Slack J, Durando MM, Ainsworth DM, Reef VB, Jesty SA, Smith G, et al. Non-invasive estimation of pulmonary arterial pressure in horses with recurrent airway obstruction. J Vet Intern Med 2006;20:757.

44. Durando M, Collins N, Slack J, Marr CM, Ousey J, Palmer L, et al. Echocardiographic estimation of pulmonary arterial pressures in hypoxemic foals. J Vet Emerg Crit Care 2008;18:422.

45. Helwegen MM, Young LE, Rogers K, Wood JL, et al. Measurements of right ventricular internal dimensions and their relationships to severity of tricuspid valve regurgitation in national hunt thoroughbreds. Equine Vet J Suppl 2006;36:171–177.

46. Reef V. Echocardiographic findings in horses with congenital heart disease. Compend Contin Educ Pract Vet 1991;13:109–117.

47. Schwarzwald C. Sequential segmental analysis: a systematic approach to the diagnosis of congenital cardiac defects. Equine Vet Educ 2008;20:305–309.

48. Rooney JR, Prickett ME, Crowe MW. Aortic ring rupture in stallions. Path Vet 1967;4:268–274.

49. Rooney JR. Rupture of the aorta. Mod Vet Pract 1979;60(5):391–392.

50. Reef VB, Klumpp S, Maxson AD, Sweeney RW, et al. Echocardiographic detection of an intact aneurysm in a horse. J Am Vet Med Assoc 1990;197(6): 752–755.

51. Sleeper MM, Durando MM, Miller M, et al. Aortic root disease in four horses. J Am Vet Med Assoc 2001;219(4):491–496, 459.

52. Marr CM, Reef VB, Brazil TJ, et al. Aorto-cardiac fistulas in seven horses. Vet Radiol Ultrasound 1998;39(1):22–31.

53. Shirai W, Momotani E, Sato T, et al. Dissecting aortic aneurysm in a horse. J Comp Pathol 1999; 120(3):307–311.

54. Lester G, Lombard CW, Ackerman N. Echocardiographic detection of a dissecting aortic root aneurysm in a Thoroughbred stallion. Vet Radiol Ultrasound 1992;33: 202–205.

55. Roby KA, Reef VB, Shaw DP, Sweeney CR, et al. Rupture of an aortic sinus aneurysm in a 15-year-old broodmare. J Am Vet Med Assoc 1986;189(3):305–308.

56. Hooper PT, Ketterer PJ, Hyatt AD, Russell GM, et al. Lesions of experimental equine morbillivirus pneumonia in horses. Vet Pathol 1997;34(4):312–322.

57. Machida N, Tanguchi T, Nakamura T, Kiryu K. Cardiohistopathological observations on aborted equine fetuses infected with equid herpesvirus 1 (EHV-1). J Comp Pathol 1997;116(4):379–385.

58. Dolente BA, Seco OM, Lewis ML. Streptococcal toxic shock in a horse. J Am Vet Med Assoc 2000;217(1):64–67, 30.

59. Peet RL, McDermott J, Williams JM, Maclean AA, et al. Fungal myocarditis and nephritis in a horse. Aust Vet J 1981;57(9): 439–440.

60. Diana A, Guglielmini C, Candini D, Pietra M, Cipone M. Cardiac arrhythmias associated with piroplasmosis in the horse: a case report. Vet J 2007;174:193–194.

61. Marr CM. Cardiovascular infections. In: Sellon D, Long MT, editors. Equine Infectious Diseases. Philadelphia: Saunders Elsevier; 2007. p. 21–38.

62. Tiwary AK, Puschner B, Kinde H, Tor ER, et al. Diagnosis of Taxus (yew) poisoning in a horse. J Vet Diagn Invest 2005;17(3):252–255.

63. Wilson SJ, Taylor JD, Gibson JA, McKenzie RA, et al. Pimelea trichostachya poisoning (St George disease) in horses. Aust Vet J 2007;85(5):201–205.

64. Hoffman A, Levi O, Orgad U, Nyska A, et al. Myocarditis following envenoming with Vipera palaestinae in two horses. Toxicon 1993;31(12):1623–1628.

65. Dickinson C, Traub-Dargatz JL, Dargatz DA, Bennett DG, Knight AP. Rattlesnake venom poisoning in horses; 32 cases (1973–1993). J Am Vet Med Assoc 1996;208(11):1866–1871.

66. Schmitz D. Toxicological problems. In: Reed S, Bayly WM, Sellon DC, editors. Equine Internal Medicine. Philadelphia: Saunders; 2004. p. 1441–1512.

67. Aleman M, Magdesian KG, Peterson TS, Galey FD, et al. Salinomycin toxicosis in horses. J Am Vet Med Assoc 2007;230(12):1822–1826.

68. Peek SF, Marques FD, Morgan J, et al. Atypical acute monensin toxicosis and delayed cardiomyopathy in Belgian draft horses. J Vet Intern Med 2004;18(5):761–764.

69. Bezerra PS, Driemeier D, Loretti AP, Riet-Correa F, et al. Monensin poisoning in Brazilian horses. Vet Hum Toxicol 1999;41(6):383–385.

70. Doonan GR, Brown CM, Mullaney TP, Brooks DB, et al. Monensin poisoning in horses: an international incident. Can Vet J 1989;30(2):165–169.

71. Ordidge RM, Schubert FK, Stoker JW. Death of horses after accidental feeding of monensin. Vet Rec 1979;104(16):375.

72. Matsuoka T. Evaluation of monensin toxicity in the horse. J Am Vet Med Assoc 1976;169(10):1098–1100.

73. Muylle E, Vandenhende C, Oyaert W, et al. Delayed monensin sodium toxicity in horses. Equine Vet J 1981;13(2):107–108.

74. Rollinson J, Taylor FG, Chesney J. Salinomycin poisoning in horses. Vet Rec 1987;121(6):126–128.

75. Reef V, McGuirk SM. Diseases of the cardiovascular system. In: Smith B, editor. Large Animal Internal Medicine. St Louis: Mosby; 1996. p. 507–549.

76. Dill S, Rebhun W. White muscle disease in foals. Comp Cont Educ Pract Vet 1996;7:627.

77. MacLeay JM. Diseases of the musculoskeletal system. In: Reed SM, Bayly, WM, Sellon ED, editors. Equine Internal Medicine. Philadelphia: Saunders; 2004. p. 461–531.

78. Delesalle C, van Loon G, Nollet H, Deprez P, et al. Tumor-induced ventricular arrhythmia in a horse. J Vet Intern Med 2002;16(5):612–617.

79. Southwood LL, Schott HC, 2nd, Henry CJ, et al. Disseminated hemangiosarcoma in the horse: 35 cases. J Vet Intern Med 2000;14(1):105–109.

80. Sugiyama A, Takeuchi T, Morita T, et al. Mediastinal lymphoma with complete atrioventricular block in a horse. J Vet Med Sci 2008;70(10):1101–1105.

81. Valberg SJ, Ward TL, Rush B, et al. Glycogen branching enzyme deficiency in quarter horse foals. J Vet Intern Med 2001;15(6):572–580.

82. Bonagura J, Reef VB. Disorders of the cardiovascular system. In: Reed S, Bayly WM, Sellon DC, editors. Equine Internal Medicine. Philadelphia: Saunders; 2004. p. 355–460.

83. Reef V. A monensin outbreak in horses in the eastern United States. Paper presented at the Eighth Annual Vet Med Forum, Washington, 1990.

84. Reef V. Pericardial and myocardial diseases. In: Koblick C, Ames TR, Geor RJ, Trent AM, editors. The Horse: Diseases and Clinical Management. Edinburgh: Churchill Livingstone; 1993. p. 185–197.

85. Bila CG, Perreira CL, Gruys E. Accidental monensin toxicosis in horses in Mozambique. J S Afr Vet Assoc 2001;72(3):163–164.

86. Plante E, Lachance D, Champetier S, et al. Benefits of long-term beta-blockade in experimental chronic aortic regurgitation. Am J Physiol Heart Circ Physiol 2008;294(4):H1888–1895.

87. Dell'Italia LJ. The renin-angiotensin system in mitral regurgitation: a typical example of tissue activation. Curr Cardiol Rep 2002;4(2):97–103.

88. Gardner SY, Atkins CE, Sams RA, et al. Characterization of the pharmacokinetic and pharmacodynamic properties of the angiotensin-converting enzyme inhibitor, enalapril, in horses. J Vet Intern Med 2004;18(2):231–237.

89. Sleeper MM, McDonnell SM, Ely JJ, Reef VB, et al. Chronic oral therapy with enalapril in normal ponies. J Vet Cardiol 2008;10(2):111–115.

90. Gehlen H, Vieht JC, Stadler P. Effects of the ACE inhibitor quinapril on echocardiographic variables in horses with mitral valve insufficiency. J Vet Med A Physiol Pathol Clin Med 2003;50(9):460–465.

91. Bertone J. Cardiovascular effects of hydralazine HCl administration in horses. Am J Vet Res 1998;49:618–621.

92. Muir W, Milne DW, Skarda RT. Acute haemodynamic effects of furosemide administered intravenously in the horse. Am J Vet Res 1976;37:1177–1180.

93. Freestone J, Carlson GP, Harrold DR, Church H. Influence of furosemide treatment on fluid and electrolyte balance in the horse. Am J Vet Res 1988;49:1899–1902.

94. Pedersoli W, Belmonte AA, Purohit RC, Nachreiner RF. Pharmacokinetics of digoxin in the horse. J Equine Med Surg 1978;2:384–388.

95. Sweeney RW, Reef VB, Reimer JM. Pharmacokinetics of digoxin administered to horses with congestive heart failure. Am J Vet Res 1993;54(7):1108–1111.

96. Parraga M, Kittleson MD, Drake CM. Quinidine administration increases steady state serum digoxin concentrations in horses. Equine Vet J Suppl 1995;19:114–119.

Chapter | **20** |

Cardiovascular emergencies associated with anaesthesia

Sheilah A Robertson

INTRODUCTION

Despite the utilization of new anaesthetic drugs, techniques and equipment and improved patient monitoring, the risk associated with general anaesthesia in horses has not significantly decreased over the past 10 years. The Confidential Enquiry into Perioperative Equine Fatalities (CEPEF), a prospective epidemiological multi-centre study, has furnished accurate perioperative mortality rates after extensive analysis of over 50 000 anaesthetic records.[1-5] The overall perioperative mortality rate is 1.6–1.9% and if anticipated "high-risk" horses that underwent emergency abdominal surgery ("colics" and dystocias) are excluded from the analysis, the anaesthetic-related death rate is still alarmingly high at 0.9%.[3-5] This is 4 to 5 times higher than the mortality rate recently established for dogs

and cats using a similar data collection technique[6]. Further analysis of the unanticipated deaths in healthy horses undergoing elective procedures reveals that the commonest cause of death (32–33%) is due to cardiac arrest or irreversible cardiovascular collapse, with fractures and myopathies being the second and third reasons.[4,5] Cardiac arrest represents one extreme end of the spectrum of cardiac emergencies that can occur in horses. Other common anaesthetic-related complications include cardiac dysrhythmias, hypotension and hypertension. The causes, recognition, prevention and treatment of these problems will be discussed.

RISK FACTORS

The CEPEF identified several risk factors that should influence the anaesthetic management of horses. These factors include the choice of premedicant agent and the maintenance technique[4]; these will be discussed in greater detail later in this chapter. Risk of dying increased with duration of anaesthesia;[3] therefore, speed is of the essence and all procedures should be well planned and all stages expedited efficiently. Other risk factors included age; young foals and older horses were at higher risk.[4]

PREOPERATIVE EVALUATION AND PREMEDICATION

Most horses scheduled for surgery, whether for an elective or emergency procedure, do not have cardiac disease and these patients are the focus of this discussion. Horses with cardiac disease are not good candidates for surgery.

DOI: 10.1016/B978-0-7020-2817-5.00025-0

However, any patient with heart disease should be stabilized as much as possible prior to anaesthesia (these conditions including atrial fibrillation are discussed comprehensively elsewhere in this book, see Chapters 13 and 14). Standing sedation and local anaesthetic techniques should always be considered in these animals and the advent of laparoscopic surgery has expanded the scope of procedures that can be performed in conscious horses.

Before anaesthetizing any equine patient a thorough clinical examination with an emphasis on the respiratory and cardiovascular system is mandatory. Bradydysrhythmias may be detected in as many as 25% of horses at rest but most are categorized as physiological and considered benign. The resting adult horse has high vagal tone with normal heart rates ranging from 25 to 45 bpm. At low heart rates, first- or second-degree atrioventricular (AV) block, sinoatrial (SA) block, wandering atrial pacemaker, sinus bradycardia and sinus arrhythmia are often present (see Chapters 6 and 13). In a pre-anaesthetic work-up, one should confirm that exercise or excitement increases the heart rate and abolishes these dysrhythmias; careful auscultation and palpation of a peripheral pulse is usually sufficient. If they are not easily overridden, an electrocardiogram (ECG) and further investigation is warranted. The administration of atropine is not recommended as a first step to counteract vagal tone because of the CNS excitement and gastrointestinal stasis that may result from its use.[7] If surgery is elective, it should be postponed until a definitive diagnosis is reached. In an emergency situation there is no option but to proceed with caution. If an anticholinergic is used, glycopyrrolate would be preferable as it has fewer undesirable side effects.

Horses, including foals, should be adequately sedated prior to induction of anaesthesia. Omitting premedication is associated with a striking increase in the risk of death.[4] The benefits of sedation include a more manageable patient and increased safety for personnel, decreased excitement and release of endogenous catecholamines that may produce dysrhythmias, a reduction in requirements of induction and maintenance agents that have potent cardiopulmonary depressive effects, smoother maintenance of anaesthesia and a calmer recovery. Does the choice of premedicant agent matter? The most commonly used premedicants are the phenothiazine acepromazine and the α_2-adrenergic agents xylazine, detomidine and romifidine. More recently medetomidine has been used in horses although it has no market authorization in this species.[8,9] These drugs have cardiovascular actions that are important to consider in the equine patient.

The use of acepromazine alone or in combination with α_2-agonists was correlated with a lower anaesthetic risk compared to other commonly used drugs.[3,4] Acepromazine has antiarrhythmic properties and may offer some myocardial protection. In dogs[10] it reduces the sensitivity of the myocardium to catecholamines. Acepromazine can cause a decrease in arterial blood pressure as a result of CNS depression, α-adrenergic blockade and decrease in total peripheral resistance. A decrease in after-load may decrease the workload of the myocardium thereby improving blood flow and oxygen delivery to peripheral tissues, which would be beneficial during the maintenance phase of anaesthesia. Steffey demonstrated a significant fall in arterial blood pressure but an increase in cardiac output in halothane anaesthetized horses given acepromazine.[11] Acepromazine has marked anaesthetic sparing effects; 0.05 mg/kg reduced the minimum alveolar concentration of halothane in ponies by approximately 37%[12] and this is likely to contribute to its beneficial cardiovascular effects. Recently acepromazine was shown to improve the haemodynamic variables associated with romifidine, butorphanol and tiletamine-zolazepam anaesthesia in horses.[13] In addition acepromazine decreased the shunt fraction and ventilation-perfusion mismatch with resultant improvement in PaO_2 during recumbency.[13] There is unequivocal evidence that acepromazine exerts a positive benefit on horses that are anaesthetized.

Acepromazine is unlikely to produce satisfactory tranquillization in an excited animal and may cause a profound fall in blood pressure in these animals because α-blockade is superimposed on pre-existing β-mediated vasodilatation from endogenous catecholamines;[14] the same could happen in horses that have very recently been exercised. Acepromazine is likely to cause an exaggerated cardiovascular response in the face of hypovolaemia so should be reserved for healthy, hydrated elective surgery candidates.

The α-adrenergic agonist agents produce reliable sedation,[15] predictable, dose-related cardiovascular effects[16] and a decrease in the requirements for inhalant agents.[17] Bradycardia and first- or second-degree AV blocks are common. Initially, total peripheral resistance and arterial blood pressure rise, but this is followed by a period of hypotension secondary to a significant decrease in cardiac output. The cardiovascular effects of the α_2-adrenergic agents are most obvious when given intravenously. In a fit racehorse with a low resting heart rate and pre-existing AV block, high doses of intravenous α_2-adrenergic drugs can cause syncope. Under these circumstances, intramuscular administration would be preferable. Slow intravenous administration of lower doses of xylazine (<0.03 mg/kg) combined with the opioid analgesic butorphanol (0.02 mg/kg) will often provide excellent sedation with fewer cardiovascular problems. If syncope does occur, atropine or glycopyrrolate will usually, but not always, increase the heart rate. Fortunately the acute bradycardia and AV block are short lived (<5 minutes).

Collapse following injection of premedicant agents can result from inadvertent intra-carotid injection; this is easily differentiated from syncope by the violent nature in which the horse collapses to the ground. If it is possible to safely approach the animal, intravenous access should be confirmed, and diazepam, acepromazine or xylazine administered in an attempt to sedate the animal. Additional therapy includes fluids and respiratory support. The final outcome depends on how much CNS damage has occurred. Intra-carotid injections can be fatal, particularly with phenothiazine agents[18] (personal observation).

In summary, sedation prior to induction of anaesthesia is recommended. In most horses adequate sedation can only be achieved with α_2-agonist agents but the addition of acepromazine offers many added benefits.

INDUCTION OF ANAESTHESIA

Anaesthesia is most safely and easily induced with injectable agents and indeed induction of anaesthesia with inhalant agents, a technique which has been used in foals, is associated with an increased anaesthetic risk.[4] None of the commonly used induction drugs or protocols (diazepam/ketamine, guaiphenesin/ketamine, guaiphenesin/thiopentone, thiopentone) have an effect on outcome[4] and therefore this choice can be based on the anaesthetist's personal preference, experience and availability of drugs.

MAINTENANCE OF ANAESTHESIA

Anaesthesia may be short and the procedure completed under the influence of the induction agents, or maintained by injectable agents given as repeated boluses, or as infusions, or by inhalant agents including halothane, isoflurane and sevoflurane.

The choice of maintenance agent and technique does have important implications – the use of volatile agents carries a three times higher risk of death than total intravenous (TIVA) maintenance (0.99% versus 0.31%, respectively).[4] Although procedures conducted under TIVA tended to be shorter this did not fully explain the discrepancy in outcome. Intravenous agents cause less cardiovascular depression and a decreased stress response (less adrenocortical activity).[19,20] The cardiovascular depression associated with volatile inhalant agents seems to be implicated in the high incidence of anaesthetic complications in horses. For these reasons TIVA techniques should be used when possible and these have recently been reviewed.[21] The most popular technique is guaiphenesin-ketamine-xylazine ("triple drip") which can be used for procedures up to 2 hours with minimal cardiorespiratory effects.[22,23] Newer techniques that include propofol have been reported and provide remarkable cardiovascular stability for up to 4 hours[9] but the high cost of propofol currently limits its use in clinical practice.

Another approach is to use anaesthetic sparing agents in combination with inhalant agents. Infusions of lignocaine produce a dose-dependent decrease in the minimum alveolar concentration (MAC) of halothane,[24] but unlike other species including human beings, opioids are less consistent at reducing the requirements of inhalant agents in horses.[25] If the procedures involve surgery of the pelvic limb epidural anaesthesia should be considered; morphine and ketamine both reduced the MAC of halothane in the pelvic but not thoracic limbs of ponies.[26]

If inhalant agents are used the question must be is one better than the other? In an attempt to answer this question a large randomized study was undertaken to compare isoflurane and halothane in equine anaesthesia.[5] Overall (>8000 horses) there was no difference in outcome between the two agents; however, the mortality rate was significantly reduced in horses aged 2 to 5 years and the incidence of cardiac arrest was reduced by 60%, especially in high-risk cases if isoflurane was used. This is likely related to a lesser degree of cardiovascular depression reported with isoflurane compared to halothane in horses.[27–29] More recently sevoflurane has been used in equine anaesthesia and although it has not undergone a large head to head clinical trial with other inhalants, its cardiovascular depressant effects are similar to other inhalant agents and are dose related.[30,31]

Regardless of the technique employed, the problems faced by the anaesthetist are similar. Throughout anaesthesia, cardiac rhythm and arterial blood pressure must be closely monitored, even during short procedures. Careful attention to the ECG may show trends that forewarn of serious complications. Severe myopathy resulting in the inability to stand and euthanasia is a complication of the post-anaesthetic period in some equine patients (third cause of death in the CEPEF study[3,4]). It has been shown unequivocally that the initiating factors of this disease originate during anaesthesia, with arterial hypotension (mean arterial blood pressure (MAP), less than 70 mmHg), even for short periods of time, being the most significant contributing factor.[32–35]

CARDIOVASCULAR MONITORING IN THE ANAESTHETIZED PATIENT

Obviously, before one can avert or treat a cardiovascular problem its presence must be detected. Ideally cardiac output (CO) should be measured as this reflects the volume of blood pumped by the heart per minute and available for perfusion of vital organs and tissues. The normal CO of 70 mL/kg/minute in conscious horses can fall by 30–50% in patients anaesthetized with volatile agents especially if mechanically ventilated.[36] Cardiac output measurement is not commonly performed in a clinical setting although newer technologies in both adult horses and foals now make it more feasible.[37-39] A description of the technologies involved is beyond the scope of this chapter but the interested reader is directed to a review by Corley and others.[37]

Much can be learnt about the cardiovascular status of the horse by touch and careful observation. The peripheral pulse should be palpated frequently and is easily felt at the facial artery, digital arteries of the front and hind limbs, or dorsal metatarsal artery. The pulse rate in an anaesthetized adult horse is usually 25–50 bpm. It must be emphasized that it is pulse pressure (PP), the difference between systolic (SBP) and diastolic pressure (DBP), that is being felt when palpating a pulse and that even if it feels strong it does not necessarily equate to an adequate MAP. For example, a horse with a SBP/DBP of 100/40 has a pulse pressure of 60 and a MAP of 60 mmHg using the formula MAP = (SBP + (2 × DBP)/3). An animal with a SBP/DBP of 120/90 has a pulse pressure of only 30 which may feel soft, yet its MAP (100 mmHg) is much better (Fig. 20.1). The relationship between blood pressure and cardiac output must also be considered when interpreting blood pressure values:

$$MAP = cardiac\ output \times systemic\ vascular\ resistance$$

It can be seen from this equation that changes in blood pressure are not always correlated with changes in CO but may reflect changes in vascular resistance and therefore perfusion. However, if MAP and mucous membrane colour are taken into account the anaesthetist should have a good idea of perfusion.

The colour of the mucous membranes and the capillary refill time (CRT) should be assessed as they indicate perfusion of peripheral tissues; however, in horses these can be misleading due to pigmentation and CRT can be measured, albeit prolonged, in a dead horse. When monitoring, one should not rely on a single factor, but build a composite picture of events from several sources.

Electrocardiography is useful for determining rate, rhythm and conduction times but one must be cognizant that an ECG only reflects electrical events and not mechanical function of the heart. The ECG can be obtained using a standard lead system, but during anaesthesia a simple monitor lead such as the base-apex lead may be more practical and less likely to interfere with the surgical site (see Chapter 13). A recorder is useful so that a reference ECG can be obtained at the start of the case for future comparison.

Arterial blood pressure can be measured indirectly (noninvasively) or directly (invasively). Noninvasive methods are attractive, because they are usually less expensive and simple. The Doppler method has been extensively used in horses; this involves placing a piezoelectric probe over an artery, the coccygeal being the most popular. The probe detects blood flow, which is amplified and emitted at an audible frequency from the Doppler unit. A blood pressure cuff and sphygmomanometer are applied proximally; the cuff is inflated until no blood flow is heard then slowly deflated. The first sound occurs when SBP equals cuff pressure. Unfortunately, this technique cannot accurately define MAP, which is the primary determinant of perfusion pressure. In addition, studies show that this method leads to large measurement errors in dorsally recumbent horses.[40] Commercially available oscillometric instruments may have similar limitations and are often unable to measure at the normal slow heart rate of adult horses. The accuracy of an indirect oscillometric monitor has been reported in both awake and anesthetized foals.[41] There was good agreement between this technique (cuff placed around the tail) and direct measurement (greater metatarsal artery) for mean and diastolic blood pressure but less so for systolic blood pressure. Giguere and others also concluded that indirect oscillometric techniques were acceptable for measuring MAP in foals but in that study blood pressure did not correlate with cardiac output.[42] Another disadvantage of these techniques is the frequency of recording; it may take several minutes for the machine to complete its cycle, resulting in a delay in important information reaching the anaesthetist.

In all but the shortest of procedures, direct blood pressure monitoring is recommended. This requires catheterization of a peripheral artery and a site is chosen that gives the anaesthetist free access without interfering with the surgical field. The arterial catheter can be connected to a pressure transducer placed at the level of the atrium (point

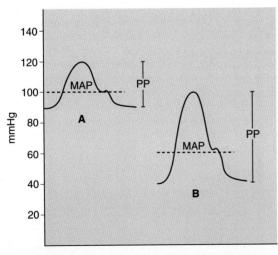

Figure 20.1 The arterial waveform of these two horses shows the importance of direct blood pressure monitoring. Horse B has a pulse pressure (PP) of 60 mmHg and will feel strong on palpation yet the mean arterial pressure (MAP) is only 60 mmHg. Horse A has a PP half that of horse B but its MAP is 100 mmHg. However, waveform A suggests peripheral vasoconstriction which impedes cardiac output whereas waveform B shows a rapid "runoff": blood pressure and cardiac output are not well correlated in anaesthetized horses. See text for details.

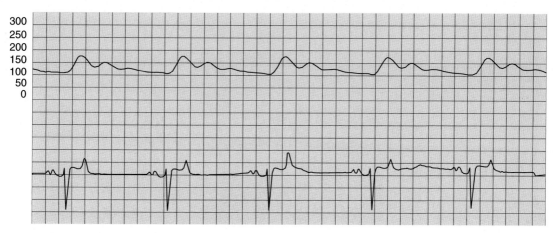

Figure 20.2 Simultaneous recording of the ECG and pulse pressure provides the anaesthetist with continuous information on the electrical and mechanical function of the heart.

of the shoulder in dorsal recumbency, at the level of the xiphoid if in a lateral position) and displayed on an oscilloscope, usually along with the simultaneously recorded ECG (Fig. 20.2). This system will provide beat-by-beat information on systolic, diastolic and mean blood pressure. Interpretation of the arterial wave form may indicate if there is peripheral vasoconstriction; a long slow decline in the waveform suggests resistance to run off (vasoconstriction, waveform A in Fig. 20.1) and a steep and rapid decline would suggest that peripheral resistance is low (waveform B in Fig. 20.1); vasoconstriction and increased afterload may be associated with a lower cardiac output. Pulse contour analysis is an emerging noninvasive technology for assessing cardiac output and has been studied in horses.[43]

An alternative but excellent system employs an aneroid manometer. An inexpensive aneroid manometer can be connected via heparinized-saline filled tubing to the catheter. The needle deflects with each pulse and the upper deflection corresponds to the MAP.

Arterial blood gas monitoring is also recommended in anaesthetized horses because hypoxaemia due to shunting and ventilation-perfusion mismatch is common and will impact on oxygen delivery to vital organs and tissues.[44,45]

INTRAOPERATIVE CARDIOVASCULAR COMPLICATIONS

Hypotension

Hypotension associated with a decreased cardiac output is probably the commonest problem facing the equine anaesthetist. Undetected and untreated hypotension may lead to cardiovascular collapse and serious postoperative consequences including myopathies. Mean arterial blood pressure in awake horses is usually between 105 and 135 mmHg. Below a MAP of 60 mmHg autoregulation of blood flow to vascular beds is lost. Blood pressure must be monitored under anaesthesia and it is desirable to maintain a MAP greater than 70 mmHg to avoid muscle hypoperfusion and postanaesthetic myopathy in adult horses.[35] If only indirect systolic pressure (SAP) can be measured, one must be cognizant of its limitations,[40] but a SAP greater than 90 mmHg, especially in a laterally recumbent animal, should reflect an adequate MAP. There are many possible causes of hypotension (Table 20.1), and often more than one problem is present. These include continued influence of premedicant and induction agents, potent inhalant agents, positive pressure ventilation, hypovolaemia, too deep a plane of anaesthesia and bradycardia. Positive pressure ventilation retards cardiac return and can lead to a drop in cardiac output and blood pressure. If ventilation seems to be the cause, check that the peak inspiratory pressure is ≤20 cmH₂O, and that the expiratory pause is as long as possible. Administration of antibiotics, especially sodium penicillin, may cause a significant drop in arterial blood pressure.[46]

Paradoxically, it is a common observation among anaesthetists that very fit horses appear more susceptible to hypotension. Reasons such as differences in body composition and muscle mass have been suggested but there is no comprehensive scientific study that provides a good explanation; however, if the surgery is elective and the horse is "let-down" for 7–10 days, it usually fares better under anaesthesia.

Table 20.1 Possible causes and specific treatments of hypotension in anaesthetized horses

CAUSE	TREATMENT(S)*
Premedicant agents	
Acepromazine	Usually only seen in hypovolaemic horses – IV fluids, ephedrine
α_2-adrenergic agents	If associated with severe bradycardia and pronounced AV block – glycopyrrolate – atropine
Inhalant agents	Check anaesthetic depth – if plane of anaesthesia is deep decrease vaporizer setting – if depth seems adequate, give IV lignocaine so that vaporizer setting may be decreased
Intermittent positive pressure ventilation	Reduce peak inspiratory pressure Increase length of expiratory pause Return to spontaneous breathing
Bradycardia	Glycopyrrolate Atropine
Hypovolaemia Blood loss	Large volumes of IV fluids – insert additional IV catheters, use a fluid pump – hypertonic saline – colloids
Monitoring error	Recheck calibration of equipment and level of pressure transducer relative to the heart
Intravenous antibiotics	Stop administration, increase IV fluid rate
Change in position of horse	If horse was moved from lateral to dorsal, return it to lateral. Move positions very slowly

*If hypotension persists after specific interventions, pharmacological treatment should be initiated.

Pharmacological treatment of hypotension (Table 20.2)

If the response to specific treatments for hypotension (see Table 20.1) is not rapid, then pharmacological intervention is indicated; it is unwise to delay treatment or allow hypotension to persist for more than 10 minutes. Infusions of the positive inotropes dopamine or dobutamine are the anaesthetist's mainstay for therapy. Both drugs are catecholamines and increase myocardial contractility and cardiac output by their specific agonist action on β_1-adrenoceptors.[47-49] These agents are superior to drugs such as ephedrine, phenylephrine, adrenaline (epinephrine) and calcium chloride because of their specificity, and as they are administered by infusion and have a short duration of action they are easily controlled and titrated to the desired effect. In most cases a good response is seen when either drug is given in the dose range 1–5 μg/kg/minute. The ECG should be observed carefully during the administration of dopamine and dobutamine as cardiac

Table 20.2 Drugs used to treat cardiovascular problems in anaesthetised horses

DRUG	DOSE
Atropine	0.005–0.01 mg/kg IV
Bretrylium tosylate	3–10 mg/kg IV
Dobutamine	1–5 μg/kg/minute IV
Dopamine	1–5 μg/kg/minute IV
Ephedrine	0.03–0.06 mg/kg IV
Adrenaline (epinephrine)	0.01 mg/kg IV
Glycopyrrolate	0.005–0.01 mg/kg IV
Lignocaine	1–2 mg/kg IV
Phenylephrine	0.2–0.4 μg/kg/minute
Procainamide	1 mg/kg/minute (maximum dose – 20 mg/kg)
Propranolol	0.03–2.0 mg/kg IV
(Arginine) Vasopressin	0.25–0.74 mU/kg/minute

All doses are for intravenous use. See also Tables 7.1 and 13.4.

dysrhythmias can occur,[47] especially at higher infusion rates and more commonly with dopamine. If dysrhythmias do occur, the infusion should be stopped and the situation reassessed. Clinically dobutamine is more commonly used in horses because it usually results in an improvement in blood pressure (which is commonly the main method of cardiovascular monitoring) and cardiac output,[48] whereas dopamine may increase cardiac output but create a fall in arterial blood pressure making it difficult to assess the response in a clinical setting.[49] If there is a poor response to the infusion of dopamine or dobutamine, one should investigate why. These agents work poorly outside the normal physiological pH range, so a blood gas can be drawn and if this confirms one's suspicion, steps can be taken to correct the abnormal acid–base balance. It may be that the horse is hypovolaemic and was not fully hydrated prior to induction, or has a "relative" hypovolaemia secondary to vasodilatation or venous pooling. Under these circumstances, a positive inotrope will be ineffective, because no matter how hard the myocardium contracts, there is insufficient blood to eject. In this situation, the usual response to dopamine or dobutamine administration is tachycardia without improvement in mean arterial pressure. Decreased venous return can be precipitated by moving the horse from lateral to dorsal recumbency and venous pooling can occur if there is mechanical obstruction of blood flow in a large amount of intestine. If the cause is obvious, it can be corrected, for example, by returning the horse to a lateral position. If deficient circulating volume is the cause, continue to deliver intravenous fluids (additional intravenous catheters can be placed or colloids (see later) can be infused) and administer an alternative cardiotonic drug; both ephedrine and phenylephrine can be useful. Ephedrine has a direct and indirect action at both α- and β-adrenergic receptors. In normovolaemic halothane anaesthetized horses, doses of 0.06 mg/kg increased systemic blood pressure, and the mode of action appeared to be predominantly via the β-actions on the heart producing an increase in stroke volume.[50] Ephedrine is often effective in hypovolaemic animals and it is likely that in these circumstances, the α-adrenergic actions are beneficial. Phenylephrine is best given as an infusion (0.2–0.4 µg/kg/minute) and titrated to the desired effect. It is a pure α$_1$-agonist and will mobilize blood from the venous capacitance vessels and improve cardiac return. Phenylephrine should only be used if other measures have failed as the intense vasoconstriction adversely affects muscle blood flow and may result in postanaesthetic myopathy.[51]

Arginine vasopressin is currently undergoing multiple studies in research and clinical settings for the treatment of refractory hypotension and shock, both in humans and animal models but little is known about it in horses.[52] Caution is warranted since its use can seriously decrease splanchnic blood flow[53] and in a model of induced hypotension in foals noradrenaline and dobutamine were superior to vasopressin for restoring cardiovascular function and maintaining splanchnic circulation.[54] Although there is little information on the use of infusions of vasopressin for the support of blood pressure in anaesthetized horses a suggested dose is 0.25–0.75 mU/kg/minute and this can be given in conjunction with a positive inotrope such as dobutamine (personal experience).

Another mode of therapy that can be employed when faced with refractory hypotension is infusion of hypertonic saline. A 7.5% solution of saline has beneficial cardiovascular actions under a variety of circumstances. Pretreatment with hypertonic saline prevented anaesthetic-induced hypotension in horses,[55] and was highly effective when used to treat endotoxic shock.[56] The practical appeal of this therapy includes its simplicity, low cost and speed; only 4 mL/kg are required, and 2 L can be administered to an adult horse in a matter of minutes. Physiologically the responses include an increase in cardiac output and systemic blood pressure with a decrease in total peripheral resistance resulting in improved perfusion.[55,56] Hypertonic saline is especially useful during acute haemorrhage if blood is unavailable or there is a delay in obtaining it. Its administration should be followed by crystalloid fluids to restore extracellular fluid. Colloids including hetastarch and dextrans can be given to increase vascular volume and because a greater percentage of the given volume remains in the vascular space for a longer period of time the response to these fluids is more rapid than that of crystalloids.

Hypertension

The equine anaesthetist is so often battling hypotension in their patients that it is perhaps surprising to include hypertension as an intraoperative complication. Application of a tourniquet to the distal limb is a technique used by surgeons to maintain a blood-free surgical site. This can lead to dramatic haemodynamic changes, especially if the tourniquet is on the dependent limb.[57,58] Systolic blood pressure climbs after tourniquet application and SBP values greater than 200 mmHg followed by a rapid drop after removal have been recorded.[57,58] The aetiology of these changes is uncertain but likely reflects tourniquet pain. The potential dangers of hypertension include severe reflex bradycardia, elevated intracranial pressure, increased left ventricular work and rupture of arterial aneurysms. If arterial blood pressure is relied upon as the sole indicator of anaesthetic depth, there is a danger of anaesthetic overdose and dangerously low blood pressure when the tourniquet is removed. If the tourniquet cannot be removed and blood pressure is alarmingly high, acepromazine can be given and sometimes a local anaesthetic block above the tourniquet relieves the haemodynamic response (personal observation).

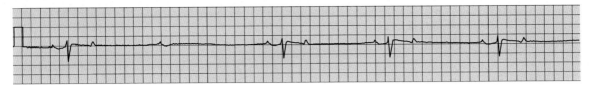

Figure 20.3 ECG demonstrating a second-degree AV block in an anaesthetized horse. The horse had been premedicated with detomidine 30 minutes prior to this recording. The arterial blood pressure was adequate in this horse (systolic, diastolic and mean pressure of 100, 55 and 70 mmHg, respectively) and was not treated and resolved over the next 20 minutes after the start of surgery.

Dysrhythmias

Isolated premature atrial depolarizations and sinus arrhythmias are usually benign and rarely require treatment; however, if these occur potential contributing factors such as acid–base and electrolyte imbalances, hypoxaemia or abnormal carbon dioxide levels should be investigated. The most common intraoperative rhythm disturbance is first- or second-degree AV block (Fig. 20.3). This may have originated from administration of α-adrenergic premedicant agents whose effects have persisted through the induction phase, or may arise spontaneously. AV blocks may or may not require treatment; the decision depends on whether there is concurrent hypotension, the overall heart rate, frequency of dropped beats and duration of the pause between beats. Glycopyrrolate is the anticholinergic of choice to treat severe bradycardia during anaesthesia as it is less arrhythmogenic, causes less tachycardia, does not cross into the CNS and has fewer gastrointestinal effects when compared to atropine. Its onset of action is slower, so perhaps if the bradycardia or AV block was considered life threatening, atropine would be the first drug of choice.

The administration of atropine or glycopyrrolate will often be effective but sometimes β-adrenergic drugs such as dobutamine or ephedrine are needed (see Table 20.2).

Great care must be taken if atropine and dobutamine are used together; in the presence of atropine, the arrhythmogenic dose of dobutamine is decreased by approximately 60% and administration of an anticholinergic to horses given dobutamine can precipitate serious supraventricular tachycardia.[59,60]

Ventricular premature depolarizations (VPDs) should be taken seriously as they usually reflect a more sinister cardiac abnormality. VPDs can be a sign of myocarditis, myocardial hypoxia or ischaemia. They can also arise during treatment with sympathomimetic agents. Adrenaline is used by some surgeons to control haemorrhage and if rapidly absorbed may cause ectopic ventricular activity; therefore, only low concentrations and small volumes should be used for this purpose and other methods of haemostasis tried first.

Ideally, the cause of VPDs should be identified and specific therapy initiated. Look for factors that may enhance abnormal electrical activity such as hypercarbia and hypoxia and take steps to correct these; if halothane is being used, it may help to switch to isoflurane or sevoflurane that are less likely to sensitize the myocardium to catecholamine-induced dysrhythmias. If myocardial hypoxia secondary to profound hypotension is suspected, then treatment should focus on improving the patient's haemodynamic status as described above. If an infusion of dopamine appears to be the culprit, stopping this will quickly resolve the problem due to dopamine's short half-life. If an inciting cause is not identified or corrected, antiarrhythmic drugs may be indicated. Lignocaine can be given at 1–2 mg/kg intravenously as a slow bolus and, if needed, can be continued as an infusion. If lignocaine is ineffective, procainamide or propranolol can be tried (see Table 20.2). One caveat of administering antiarrhythmic drugs is that they must not be given to horses that have VPDs in conjunction with sinus arrest or AV block, as this can lead to cardiac collapse; these cases require an agent that will speed conduction such as glycopyrrolate or atropine.

Hypoxaemia (PaO$_2$ < 8 kPa, 60 mmHg) and ventilation-perfusion mismatch is common in anaesthetized horses[44,45] and can contribute to dysrhythmias. Clinically the simplest way to treat these patients is with aerosolized salbutamol[61] which results in an improvement in PaO$_2$ within 20 minutes in most horses with no adverse cardiovascular effects.

Electrolyte disturbances

The most important electrolyte for normal cardiovascular function is potassium (see Chapter 6). Hyperkalaemia is the most problematic and common disturbance encountered in the perioperative period. This may be a pre-existing condition, for example, in foals with uroperitoneum; in these cases potassium levels should be stabilized prior to anaesthesia. A more problematic case scenario involves horses with hyperkalaemic periodic paralysis (HYPP) that has become a widespread disease in the equine community. This hereditary disease[62] is described in Quarter horses, Appaloosas and Paints and is characterized by periods of profound muscle weakness, fasciculations, respiratory stridor and collapse.[63-66] Usually it is accompanied by hyperkalaemia but a normokalaemic variant may occur.[67] The anaesthetic complications associated with this disease have been reported and some outcomes have been fatal[68–70] and owners of these horses should be informed of the increased risks. Although there is a genetic test for this disease, not all horses are tested; therefore the anaesthetist may be unaware of their status. Some horses may be symptom-free without treatment and some may be receiving treatment for the disease, usually oral acetazolamide. One of the trigger factors for an attack is stress; therefore, in a perioperative setting all horses with this disease should be considered likely to trigger and the anaesthetist must recognize the signs under anaesthesia, monitor for it and be ready to treat. Sudden and dramatic increases in potassium can occur without warning and some horses may undergo several uneventful anaesthetics yet trigger on another occasion (personal experience). Physical signs under anaesthesia usually include muscle fasciculations and this may be mistaken for the horse waking up. Horses with HYPP scheduled for an elective procedure but not under medical management should be started on treatment at least 2 days before anaesthesia; the most common drug used is acetazolamide.[66]

The electrocardiographic changes associated with increasing plasma potassium levels have been documented[71,72] and described in horses with HYPP.[73] Normal reference ranges for plasma K^+ values depend on the individual laboratory or measurement system used so should be established by each clinic; however, the normal range falls between 3.0 and 4.5 mmol/L. An increase in plasma K^+ decreases the cell resting membrane potential, decreases the rate of phase 0 depolarization and shortens the action potential. In research ponies given intravenous potassium chloride the ECG changes are described as follows[71]; at plasma levels >4.5 mmol/L the P wave amplitude begins to change and at >6.5 mmol/L P wave duration increases; the P wave may reverse between 8.6 and 9.7 mmol/L and usually disappears between 9.4 and 12.6 mmol/L. The QRS complex is usually unaffected by plasma K^+ values below 7.5 mmol/L but above this it begins to widen; ST elevation may be seen with merging of the QRS with the T wave resulting in a slow sinusoidal waveform. At plasma K^+ values over 7.5 mmol/L the height of the T wave increases. Periods of cardiac arrest lasting >60 seconds may occur at values >9 mmol/L followed by a terminal arrhythmia which may be complete arrest or ventricular fibrillation. Periods of bradycardia and second-degree AV block may be seen at any time during a hyperkalaemic crisis but do not respond to anticholinergic therapy because the problem is at the cellular level not the receptor level. If the blood pressure is being monitored as plasma K^+ rises hypotension is usually present.

Horses with HYPP should be adequately sedated as described earlier to decrease stress, and acepromazine is highly recommended because of its anti-arrhythmic and anaesthetic sparing effects, however there is no strong indication for a specific premedication or induction protocol in these patients. Isoflurane or sevoflurane should be used in preference to halothane because they do not sensitize the heart to catecholamine-induced dysrhythmias and produce less cardiovascular depression.[27–29] Potassium-free fluids should be used and therefore 0.9% sodium chloride is a good choice.

MONITORING HYPP PATIENTS

A preinduction blood gas and electrolyte analysis should be performed to establish a baseline and repeated every 30 minutes during the procedure or immediately if clinical signs appear or a change in heart rate or ECG is noted. Portable and relatively inexpensive point-of-care analysers have facilitated these measurements and have been evaluated for use in horses.[74] The pH should be kept as close to normal (7.40) as possible since acidosis can promote movement of potassium from intracellular locations to the blood. Under anaesthesia, respiratory acidosis is common so ventilation should be assisted to maintain normocapnia ($PaCO_2$ of 5.3–6.0 kPA, 40–45 mmHg). The ECG must be monitored continuously for signs of increasing plasma potassium levels as outlined above. An emergency kit containing dextrose, sodium bicarbonate, 23% calcium borogluconate and insulin with precalculated doses should be available so that treatment can be quickly initiated (see Table 20.3 for doses). Sodium bicarbonate should not be used if the $PaCO_2$ is increased or cannot be controlled because sodium bicarbonate will liberate CO_2 and worsen the respiratory acidosis; it can be used if metabolic acidosis is present as correcting the pH will drive K^+ into cells. Calcium-containing solutions will counteract the cellular effects of K^+ and will "buy time" until plasma K^+ values can be decreased by increasing the fluid administration rate (dilutional effect) and administering dextrose and if needed insulin, which drive K^+ back into cells. Treatment should be initiated if changes in the ECG compatible with hyperkalaemia occur even before a confirmatory electrolyte analysis is performed as plasma levels can climb to fatal levels very quickly. An increase of >1 mmol/L over baseline potassium values warrants caution and levels >5.5 mmol/L should be treated.

Table 20.3 Recommended treatment for hyperkalaemia

DRUG	DOSE (IV)
Calcium borogluconate (23%)	0.2–0.4 mL/kg
Sodium bicarbonate	1–2 mEq/kg
Insulin (regular/soluble)	0.05–0.15 IU/kg
Dextrose	0.5–1.0 g/kg
	2 g per unit of insulin

Reflex vagal responses

Sudden bradycardia or asystole can occur in response to specific manipulations including traction on the bladder, spermatic cord or ovarian pedicle, and by joint distension; however, clinically their occurrence is unpredictable. Stimulation via the ovarian pedicle and spermatic cord are often accompanied by sudden peripheral vasoconstriction and hypertension that are the likely cause of the bradycardia. These nociceptive responses are mediated through a vagal reflex. It is difficult for a surgeon to perform an ovariectomy without applying traction to the ovarian pedicle; however, a lignocaine block may help to obtund the response and the use of local anaesthetics is also recommended for castration. If these procedures cause acute bradycardia or asystole occurs a normal rhythm can frequently be restored simply by having the surgeon stop the manipulation. If this is not sufficient, or it reoccurs each time the surgeon tries to continue, an anticholinergic may be given (see Table 20.2) and an appropriate anaesthetic block performed.

Cardiac complications during ophthalmic surgery in foals and adult horses have been reported[75,76] but are not as common as in humans. The oculocardiac reflex resulting in acute bradycardia, asystole or atrioventricular block can be initiated by increased intraocular pressure, pressure on the globe or traction on extraocular muscles. Although mediated through a vagal reflex, pretreatment with an anticholinergic does not guarantee inhibition of the response; this fact in combination with the known complications of anticholinergics in horses precludes their routine use in ophthalmic patients. In an attempt to avoid these complications and to provide a more reliable inhibition of the oculocardiac reflex, Raffe and others[76] performed retrobulbar blocks in horses scheduled for eye surgery. This technique significantly reduced the cardiovascular complications related to enucleation and cataract surgery; 4 of 25 horses in the control group developed cardiovascular complications (3 second-degree AV block, 1 cardiac arrest) whereas only one of the 12 horses in the retrobulbar group developed problems and this was a brief period of AV block which responded quickly to atropine administration. In addition this technique provided a more stable field for the surgeon and potentially better postoperative pain relief. The block must be performed carefully to avoid damage to retrobulbar structures and the heart rate and blood pressure must be monitored carefully because the procedure itself may cause a reflex vagal block. An auriculopalpebral block may be beneficial as it will prevent the palpebral response, relax the extraocular muscles which should provide better surgical conditions and potentially reduce the chance of pressure on the globe.

All horses undergoing ophthalmic procedures should have their heart rate and blood pressure closely and continuously monitored. An audible monitor of pulse rate, such as a Doppler, is strongly recommended. If a problem arises, the surgeon should stop and the situation assessed. Less aggressive manipulation, anticholinergic agents or a local anaesthetic block may be required before the procedure can be continued. Sudden onset of bradycardia with no obvious explanation should always be taken seriously as it can be the harbinger of impending cardiac arrest.[77,78] Treatment would include turning off the inhalant anaesthetic if being used, providing 100% oxygen and administration of intravenous atropine.

Cardiac arrest or collapse

Cardiac arrest represents the most serious cardiovascular complication that an anaesthetist can face. The results of the Confidential Enquiry into Perioperative Equine Fatalities revealed that approximately one-third of unexpected deaths are a consequence of cardiac arrest.[4,5] This occurs most commonly during the surgical procedure (78%) but can also happen at induction (13%) or during recovery (8%).

Sometimes the cause of cardiac arrest can be determined, for example, hyperkalaemia or sudden catastrophic haemorrhage is not totally unexpected as in the case of a severely compromised patient with colon torsion and endotoxaemia. However, it can occur unexpectedly and without warning in healthy horses during elective surgery and without warning even in horses that are being adequately monitored.[77–80]

Cardiovascular collapse can occur when horses are moved from one lateral position to the other: the aetiology of this phenomenon is unknown but may be related to redistribution of drugs and blood volume and is well recognized by anaesthetists. It is recommended to avoid this manoeuvre but when mandated by the surgical procedure, the move should be done slowly and with careful monitoring of the heart rate and blood pressure.

Performing cardiopulmonary resuscitation (CPR) on a horse sounds somewhat daunting but should not be thought of as futile; there are reports of successful outcomes[77,78,80] when the arrest was recognized early and treated aggressively.

Diagnosis depends on monitoring arterial blood pressure and electrical activity of the heart. It should be emphasized that the horse can still have a palpebral reflex and be breathing spontaneously when cardiac function has ceased[77] (personal experience). When functional cardiac activity stops, there is no detectable peripheral pulse and if blood pressure is being monitored directly there is no visible arterial wave form. The ECG may show asystole (flat line), ventricular fibrillation (erratic wave forms) or a somewhat normal electrical pattern (pulseless electrical activity). It is unclear from the literature which type of arrest is most common in the horse but asystole[77,78,80] and fibrillation[80] have both been reported.

The goal of CPR is to restore blood flow to organs that cannot tolerate oxygen deprivation, most importantly the brain and myocardium. In addition, if some blood flow can be maintained, even if it is suboptimal, for short periods of time, there is a chance of delivering cardiovascular stimulants to the myocardium and vascular beds.[81]

As in all species the "ABCDs" of CPR should be immediately initiated. **Airway** – if not already in place an airway must be established with an endotracheal tube. **Breathing** – some horses may continue to breathe even after cardiac function has ceased, but if apnoea has occurred breaths can be administered using a demand valve attached to a source of oxygen, or by manually compressing the rebreathing bag on the anaesthetic machine, making sure that the vaporizer has been turned off and the circuit flushed with oxygen. **Circulation** should be assessed and supported. In research ponies weighing between 103 and 173 kg, cardiac arrest occurred after endotoxin administration but external thoracic compressions at a rate of 20/minute maintained systolic and diastolic aortic blood pressure above 50% of baseline values and resuscitation was successful in 6 out of 8 animals.[80] Hubbell and others[81] reported that thoracic compression at a rate of 80/minute can produce a cardiac output of approximately 8 L/minute and a mean arterial blood pressure of approximately 49 mmHg in adult horses weighing an average of 445 kg. This cardiac output is only half that reported for horses in a deep surgical plane of anaesthesia and is not life sustaining, but may be sufficient for distribution of emergency drugs to the myocardium and vascular tissues. Rates of 40 and 60 compressions per minute only produced a mean cardiac output of 5.5 and 6 L, respectively. These investigators performed thoracic compression on horses in left lateral recumbency by delivering a blow just behind the elbow with their knee; however, it is unlikely they were directly compressing the heart and more likely that they were causing an increase in intrathoracic pressure. The heavier the resuscitator the better the cardiac output, but this procedure is exhausting and can usually only be sustained for brief periods; therefore appropriate emergency drugs must be available and quickly administered.

Drugs

If the arrest was preceded by profound bradycardia or AV block, atropine or glycopyrrolate are appropriate choices. Asystole may respond to intravenous adrenaline. Drug treatments for CPR in horses are extrapolated from other species or based on isolated case reports. However, in most cases veterinary surgeons will base their therapy on the American Heart Association guidelines which are frequently reviewed (http://www.americanheart.org). The recommended vasopressors are adrenaline and vasopressin. The suggested dose of adrenaline is 0.01 mg/kg and this dose has been successfully used in horses[78] and can be given in repeated boluses while external thoracic compressions and oxygen are administered. A consequence of successful resuscitation with adrenaline is a period of tachycardia and hypertension which is usually transient; however, if there is prolonged ectopic ventricular activity lignocaine (1–2 mg/kg IV) can be administered. Since the use of vasopressin is a relatively new recommendation there is not a lot of information on its use in adult horses for the treatment of cardiac arrest.[52] There are no established doses for cardiac arrest in horses. Ventricular fibrillation is particularly serious in the adult horse because unlike small mammals, large hearts rarely revert to sinus rhythm spontaneously and there is no practical way of electrically defibrillating such a large myocardial mass (see chapter 14). Commercially available defibrillators deliver up to 360 joules; it has been calculated that over 8000 joules would be required in an adult 500 kg horse with a heart weight of approximately 3.8 kg.[82] However, thoracic compression and ventilation with oxygen should be tried. Methods for chemical defibrillation with bretylium tosylate[83] have been described but their efficacy in horses is not well documented and such drugs are unlikely to be readily available.

CONCLUSIONS

General anaesthesia in horses remains a "risky game"[1] to play; however, the key to success is thorough evaluation of the situation, identification of risk factors, paying attention to detail, constant vigilance, careful monitoring techniques and having a plan to deal with any adverse change in cardiovascular function. The inclusion of acepromazine and less reliance on inhalant agents should decrease the cardiovascular complications associated with anaesthesia in horses.

REFERENCES

1. Johnston GM. The risks of the game: the confidential enquiry into perioperative equine fatalities. Br Vet J 1995;151(4):347–350.

2. Johnston GM, Steffey E. Confidential enquiry into perioperative equine fatalities (CEPEF). Vet Surg 1995;24(6):518–519.

3. Johnston GM, Taylor PM, Holmes MA, Wood JL. Confidential enquiry of perioperative equine fatalities (CEPEF-1): preliminary results. Equine Vet J 1995;27(3):193–200.

4. Johnston GM, Eastment JK, Wood JLN, Taylor PM. The confidential enquiry into perioperative equine fatalities (CEPEF): mortality results of Phases 1 and 2. Vet Anaesth Analg 2002;29:159–170.

5. Johnston GM, Eastment JK, Taylor PM, Wood JL. Is isoflurane safer than halothane in equine anaesthesia? Results from a prospective multicentre randomised controlled trial. Equine Vet J 2004;36(1):64–71.

6. Brodbelt D. Perioperative mortality in small animal anaesthesia. Vet J 2009;182(2):152–161.

7. Ducharme NG, Fubini SL. Gastrointestinal complications associated with the use of atropine in horses. J Am Vet Med Assoc 1983;182(3):229–231.

8. Yamashita K, Muir WW 3rd, Tsubakishita S, et al. Clinical comparison of xylazine and medetomidine for premedication of horses. J Am Vet Med Assoc 2002;221(8):1144–1149.

9. Bettschart-Wolfensberger R, Bowen IM, Freeman SL, Weller R, Clarke KW. Medetomidine-ketamine anaesthesia induction followed by medetomidine-propofol in ponies: infusion rates and cardiopulmonary side effects. Equine Vet J 2003;35(3):308–313.

10. Muir WW, Werner LL, Hamlin RL. Effects of xylazine and acetylpromazine upon induced ventricular fibrillation in dogs anesthetized with thiamylal and halothane. Am J Vet Res 1975;36(9):1299–1303.

11. Steffey EP, Kelly AB, Farver TB, Woliner MJ. Cardiovascular and respiratory effects of acetylpromazine and xylazine on halothane-anesthetized horses. J Vet Pharmacol Ther 1985;8(3):290–302.

12. Doherty TJ, Geiser DR, Rohrbach BW. Effect of acepromazine and butorphanol on halothane minimum alveolar concentration in ponies. Equine Vet J 1997;29(5):374–376.

13. Marntell S, Nyman G, Funkquist P, Hedenstierna G. Effects of acepromazine on pulmonary gas exchange and circulation during sedation and dissociative anaesthesia in horses. Vet Anaesth Analg 2005;32(2):83–93.

14. Muir WW. Drugs used to produce standing chemical restraint in horses. Veterinary Clinics of North America Large Animal Practice 1981;3:17–44.

15. England GC, Clarke KW, Goossens L. A comparison of the sedative effects of three alpha 2-adrenoceptor agonists (romifidine, detomidine and xylazine) in the horse. J Vet Pharmacol Ther 1992;15(2):194–201.

16. Yamashita K, Tsubakishita S, Futaok S, Ueda I, Hamaguchi H, Seno T, et al. Cardiovascular effects of medetomidine, detomidine and xylazine in horses. J Vet Med Sci 2000;62(10):1025–1032.

17. Steffey EP, Pascoe PJ, Woliner MJ, Berryman ER. Effects of xylazine hydrochloride during isoflurane-induced anesthesia in horses. Am J Vet Res 2000;61(10):1225–1231.

18. Gabel AA, Koestner A. The effects of intracarotid artery injection of drugs in domestic animals. J Am Vet Med Assoc 1963;142:1397–1403.

19. Taylor PM, Kirby JJ, Shrimpton DJ, Johnson CB. Cardiovascular effects of surgical castration during anaesthesia maintained with halothane or infusion of detomidine, ketamine and guaifenesin in ponies. Equine Vet J 1998;30(4):304–309.

20. Taylor PM. Equine stress responses to anaesthesia. Br J Anaesth 1989;63(6):702–709.

21. Bettschart-Wolfensberger R. Modern injection anesthesia for horses. In: Auer JA, Stick JA, editors. Equine Surgery. 3rd ed. St Louis: Saunders Elsevier; 2006. p. 223–226.

22. Greene SA, Thurmon JC, Tranquilli WJ, Benson GJ. Cardiopulmonary effects of continuous intravenous infusion of guaifenesin, ketamine, and xylazine in ponies. Am J Vet Res 1986;47(11):2364–2367.

23. Young LE, Bartram DH, Diamond MJ, Gregg AS, Jones RS. Clinical evaluation of an infusion of xylazine, guaifenesin and ketamine for maintenance of anaesthesia in horses. Equine Vet J 1993;25(2):115–119.

24. Doherty TJ, Frazier DL. Effect of intravenous lidocaine on halothane minimum alveolar concentration in ponies. Equine Vet J 1998;30(4):300–303.

25. Steffey EP, Eisele JH, Baggot JD. Interactions of morphine and isoflurane in horses. Am J Vet Res 2003;64(2):166–175.

26. Doherty TJ, Geiser DR, Rohrbach BW. Effect of high volume epidural morphine, ketamine and butorphanol on halothane minimum alveolar concentration in ponies. Equine Vet J 1997;29(5):370–373.

27. Grubb TL, Benson GJ, Foreman JH, Constable PD, Thurmon JC, Olson WO, et al. Hemodynamic effects of ionized calcium in horses anesthetized with halothane or isoflurane. Am J Vet Res 1999;60(11):1430–1435.

28. Raisis AL, Blissitt KJ, Henley W, Rogers K, Adams V, Young LE. The effects of halothane and isoflurane on cardiovascular function in laterally recumbent horses. Br J Anaesth 2005;95(3):317–325.

29. Raisis AL, Young LE, Blissitt KJ, Brearley JC, Meire HB, Taylor PM, et al. A comparison of the haemodynamic effects of isoflurane and halothane anaesthesia in horses. Equine Vet J 2000;32(4):318–326.

30. Grosenbaugh DA, Muir WW. Cardiorespiratory effects of sevoflurane, isoflurane, and halothane anesthesia in horses. Am J Vet Res 1998;59(1):101–106.

31. Steffey EP, Mama KR, Galey FD, Puschner B, Woliner MJ. Effects of sevoflurane dose and mode of ventilation on cardiopulmonary function and blood biochemical variables in horses. Am J Vet Res 2005;66(4):606–614.

32. Grandy JL, Steffey EP, Hodgson DS, Woliner MJ. Arterial hypotension and the development of postanesthetic myopathy in halothane-anesthetized horses. Am J Vet Res 1987;48(2):192–197.

33. Lindsay WA, Robinson GM, Brunson DB, Majors LJ. Induction

of equine postanesthetic myositis after halothane-induced hypotension. Am J Vet Res 1989;50(3):404–410.

34. Richey MT, Holland MS, McGrath CJ, Dodman NH, Marshall DB, Court MH, et al. Equine post-anesthetic lameness: a retrospective study. Vet Surg 1990;19(5): 392–397.

35. Duke T, Filzek U, Read MR, Read EK, Ferguson JG. Clinical observations surrounding an increased incidence of postanesthetic myopathy in halothane-anesthetized horses. Vet Anaesth Analg 2006;33(2): 122–127.

36. Steffey EP, Dunlop CI, Farver TB, Woliner MJ, Schultz LJ. Cardiovascular and respiratory measurements in awake and isoflurane-anesthetized horses. Am J Vet Res 1987;48(1):7–12.

37. Corley KT, Donaldson LL, Durando MM, Birks EK. Cardiac output technologies with special reference to the horse. J Vet Intern Med 2003;17(3):262–272.

38. Corley KT, Donaldson LL, Furr MO. Comparison of lithium dilution and thermodilution cardiac output measurements in anaesthetised neonatal foals. Equine Vet J 2002;34(6):598–601.

39. Giguere S, Bucki E, Adin DB, Valverde A, Estrada AH, Young L. Cardiac output measurement by partial carbon dioxide rebreathing, 2-dimensional echocardiography, and lithium-dilution method in anesthetized neonatal foals. J Vet Intern Med 2005;19(5):737–743.

40. Bailey JE, Dunlop CI, Chapman PL, Demme WC, Allen SL, Heath RB, et al. Indirect Doppler ultrasonic measurement of arterial blood pressure results in a large measurement error in dorsally recumbent anaesthetised horses. Equine Vet J 1994;26(1):70–73.

41. Nout YS, Corley KT, Donaldson LL, Furr MO. Indirect oscillometric and direct blood pressure measurements in anesthetized and conscious neonatal foals. JJ Vet Emerg Crit Care 2002;12(2):75–80.

42. Giguere S, Knowles HA, Valverde A, Bucki E, Young L. Accuracy of indirect measurement of blood pressure in neonatal foals. JJ Vet Intern Med 2005;19(4):571–576.

43. Hallowell GD, Corley KT. Use of lithium dilution and pulse contour analysis cardiac output determination in anaesthetized horses: a clinical evaluation. Vet Anaesth Analg 2005;32(4): 201–211.

44. Whitehair KJ, Willits NH. Predictors of arterial oxygen tension in anesthetized horses: 1,610 cases (1992–1994). J Am Vet Med Assoc 1999;215(7):978–981.

45. Day TK, Gaynor JS, Muir WW 3rd, Bednarski RM, Mason DE. Blood gas values during intermittent positive pressure ventilation and spontaneous ventilation in 160 anesthetized horses positioned in lateral or dorsal recumbency. Vet Surg 1995;24(3):266–276.

46. Hubbell JA, Muir WW, Robertson JT, Sams RA. Cardiovascular effects of intravenous sodium penicillin, sodium cefazolin, and sodium citrate in awake and anesthetized horses. Vet Surg 1987;16(3): 245–250.

47. Swanson CR, Muir WW 3rd, Bednarski RM, Skarda RT, Hubbell JA. Hemodynamic responses in halothane-anesthetized horses given infusions of dopamine or dobutamine. Am J Vet Res 1985;46(2):365–370.

48. Young LE, Blissitt KJ, Clutton RE, Molony V. Temporal effects of an infusion of dobutamine hydrochloride in horses anesthetized with halothane. Am J Vet Res 1998;59(8):1027–1032.

49. Young LE, Blissitt KJ, Clutton RE, Molony V. Haemodynamic effects of a sixty minute infusion of dopamine hydrochloride in horses anaesthetised with halothane. Equine Vet J 1998;30(4):310–316.

50. Grandy JL, Hodgson DS, Dunlop CI, Chapman PL, Heath RB. Cardiopulmonary effects of ephedrine in halothane-anesthetized horses. J Vet Pharmacol Ther 1989;12(4): 389–396.

51. Lee YH, Clarke KW, Alibhai HI, Song D. Effects of dopamine, dobutamine, dopexamine, phenylephrine, and saline solution on intramuscular blood flow and other cardiopulmonary variables in halothane-anesthetized ponies. Am J Vet Res 1998;59(11):1463–1472.

52. Corley KT. Inotropes and vasopressors in adults and foals. Vet Clin North Am Equine Pract 2004;20(1):77–106.

53. Woolsey CA, Coopersmith CM. Vasoactive drugs and the gut: is there anything new? Curr Opin Crit Care 2006;12(2):155–159.

54. Valverde A, Giguère S, C. S, SA. Effects of dobutamine, norepinephrine, and vasopressine on cardiovascular function in anesthetized neonatal foals with induced hypotension. In: Proceedings of the 30th Annual Meeting of the American College of Veterinary Anesthesiologists. Atlanta, Georgia, 20–21 Oct, 2005. p. 31.

55. Dyson DH, Pascoe PJ. Influence of preinduction methoxamine, lactated Ringer solution, or hypertonic saline solution infusion or postinduction dobutamine infusion on anesthetic-induced hypotension in horses. Am J Vet Res 1990;51(1):17–21.

56. Bertone JJ, Gossett KA, Shoemaker KE, Bertone AL, Schneiter HL. Effect of hypertonic vs isotonic saline solution on responses to sublethal Escherichia coli endotoxemia in horses. Am J Vet Res 1990;51(7):999–1007.

57. Copland VS, Hildebrand SV, Hill T 3rd, Wong P, Brock N. Blood pressure response to tourniquet use in anesthetized horses. J Am Vet Med Assoc 1989;195(8): 1097–1103.

58. Abrahamsen E, Hellyer PW, Bednarski RM, Hubbell JA, Muir WW 3rd. Tourniquet-induced hypertension in a horse. J Am Vet Med Assoc 1989;194(3):386–388.

59. Light GS, Hellyer PW. Effects of atropine on the arrhythmogenic dose of dobutamine in xylazine-thiamylal-halothane-anesthetized horses. Am J Vet Res 1993;54(12): 2099–2103.

60. Light GS, Hellyer PW, Swanson CR. Parasympathetic influence on the arrhythmogenicity of graded dobutamine infusions in halothane-anesthetized horses. Am J Vet Res 1992;53(7):1154–1160.

61. Robertson SA, Bailey JE. Aerosolized salbutamol (albuterol) improves PaO$_2$ in hypoxaemic anaesthetised horses: a prospective clinical trial in 81 horses. Vet Anaesth Analg 2002;29:212–218.

62. Spier SJ, Carlson GP, Harrold D, Bowling A, Byrns G, Bernoco D. Genetic study of hyperkalemic periodic paralysis in horses. J Am Vet Med Assoc 1993;202(6): 933–937.

63. Meyer TS, Fedde MR, Cox JH, Erickson HH. Hyperkalaemic periodic paralysis in horses: a review. Equine Vet J 1999;31(5): 362–367.

64. Nollet H, Deprez P. Hereditary skeletal muscle diseases in the horse: a review. Vet Q 2005;27(2): 65–75.

65. Carr EA, Spier SJ, Kortz GD, Hoffman EP. Laryngeal and pharyngeal dysfunction in horses homozygous for hyperkalemic periodic paralysis. J Am Vet Med Assoc 1996;209(4):798–803.

66. Spier SJ, Carlson GP, Holliday TA, Cardinet GH 3rd, Pickar JG. Hyperkalemic periodic paralysis in horses. J Am Vet Med Assoc 1990;197(8):1009–1017.

67. Stewart RH, Bertone JJ, Yvorchuk-St Jean K, Reed SM, Neil WH Jr. Possible normokalemic variant of hyperkalemic periodic paralysis in two horses. J Am Vet Med Assoc 1993;203(3):421–424.

68. Robertson SA, Green SL, Carter SW, Bolon BN, Brown MP, Shields RP. Postanesthetic recumbency associated with hyperkalemic periodic paralysis in a quarter horse. J Am Vet Med Assoc 1992;201(8):1209–1212.

69. Bailey JE, Pablo L, Hubbell JA. Hyperkalemic periodic paralysis episode during halothane anesthesia in a horse. J Am Vet Med Assoc 1996;208(11): 1859–1865.

70. Carpenter RE, Evans AT. Anesthesia case of the month: hyperkalemia. J Am Vet Med Assoc 2005;226(6): 874–876.

71. Glazier DB, Littledike ET, Evans RD. Electrocardiographic changes in induced hyperkalemia in ponies. Am J Vet Res 1982;43(11): 1934–1937.

72. Epstein V. Relationship between potassium administration, hyperkalaemia and the electrocardiogram: an experimental study. Equine Vet J 1984;16(5): 453–456.

73. Castex AM, Bertone JJ. ECG of the month: sinus tachycardia and hyperkalemia in a horse. J Am Vet Med Assoc 1989;194(5): 654–655.

74. Grosenbaugh DA, Gadawski JE, Muir WW. Evaluation of a portable clinical analyzer in a veterinary hospital setting. J Am Vet Med Assoc 1998;213(5): 691–694.

75. Short CE, Rebhun WC. Complications caused by the oculocardiac reflex during anesthesia in a foal. J Am Vet Med Assoc 1980;176(7):630–631.

76. Raffe MR, Bistner SI, Crimi AJ, Ruff J. Retrobulbar block in combination with general anesthesia for equine ophthalmic surgery. Vet Surg 1986;15(1): 139–141.

77. Kellagher RE, Watney GC. Cardiac arrest during anaesthesia in two horses. Vet Rec 1986;119(14): 347–349.

78. McGoldrick TM, Bowen IM, Clarke KW. Sudden cardiac arrest in an anaesthetised horse associated with low venous oxygen tensions. Vet Rec 1998;142(22):610–611.

79. Young SS, Taylor PM. Factors influencing the outcome of equine anaesthesia: a review of 1,314 cases. Equine Vet J 1993;25(2): 147–151.

80. Frauenfelder HC, Fessler JF, Latshaw HS, Moore AB, Bottoms GD. External cardiovascular resuscitation of the anesthetized pony. J Am Vet Med Assoc 1981;179(7):673–676.

81. Hubbell JA, Muir WW, Gaynor JS. Cardiovascular effects of thoracic compression in horses subjected to euthanasia. Equine Vet J 1993;25(4):282–284.

82. Witzel DA, Geddes LA, Hoff HE, McFarlane J. Electrical defibrillation of the equine heart. Am J Vet Res 1968;29(6):1279–1285.

83. Klein L. Anesthetic complications in the horse. Vet Clin North Am Equine Pract 1990;6(3):665–692.

Chapter | **21** |

Cardiovascular complications in the intensive care patient

Celia M Marr and Virginia B Reef

INTRODUCTION

Critically ill horses commonly develop cardiovascular complications, often associated with systemic inflammatory response syndrome (SIRS), multiple organ dysfunction syndrome (MODS) or electrolyte and acid–base disturbances that are seen in a variety of systemic conditions, most notably in the adult horse with gastrointestinal diseases and in foals with neonatal septicaemia or perinatal asphyxia syndrome. Equally, a wide range of primary cardiac disorders should be considered in horses presenting as emergencies with signs of recent onset heart failure: horses that experience sudden-onset disruption of valvular integrity can develop dramatic and fulminant signs of heart failure and horses with pericarditis or myocardial lesions such as bacterial myocarditis and cardiomyopathy also tend to present as emergencies with signs of recent onset heart failure (see Chapters 17 and 19). The clinician should also be careful not to overlook the potential for primary cardiovascular disease in animals presenting with signs of shock, pain and distress and it is important to note that horses with intrathoracic disease and certain cardiac dysrhythmias may initially display signs that are confused with colic of gastrointestinal origin. Primary cardiac diseases of the horse are extensively described in the other chapters in this book, while this chapter will focus on cardiovascular complications that are encountered commonly in the intensive care unit (ICU).

PREVALENCE AND RISK FACTORS FOR CARDIOVASCULAR COMPLICATIONS IN THE ICU

Although there are no specific data on the prevalence of cardiac problems in equine ICU, endotoxaemia is undoubtedly the major pathological state which underlies a large proportion of secondary cardiac problems seen in critically ill adult horses, while in the foal septicaemia, perinatal asphyxia and prematurity/dysmaturity are common underlying primary problems. Endotoxaemia can be associated with a range of forms of gram-negative sepsis and in adults the gastrointestinal tract is its most frequent source, while peritonitis, metritis, pleuropneumonia and neonatal septicaemia are also common potential causes. Mild fibrinous pericarditis, right atrial and ventricular enlargement, myocardial depression and ventricular tachycardia have been documented in streptococcal toxic shock with multiple organ dysfunction in a horse.[1] Streptococcal toxic shock was previously associated specifically with *Streptococcus pyogenes* infection in humans but it is now recognized in association with a wide range of *Streptococcal* species in both human beings[2] and dogs.[3] In the last 20 years, there has been a marked increase in the frequency of diagnosis of the condition in human beings[2]

DOI: 10.1016/B978-0-7020-2817-5.00026-2

and it may become more important in horses in the future.[1]

CARDIOVASCULAR MONITORING IN THE ICU

Electrocardiography (ECG)

Clinical examination remains the most important diagnostic tool available to the equine clinician. However, in critical patients, dysrhythmias can easily go undetected on both clinical examination and using short ECG rhythm strips because dysrhythmias frequently occur intermittently and particularly in the case of monomorphic ventricular tachycardia, are often very regular and difficult to appreciate on auscultation alone. A variety of ambulatory and telemetric ECG systems are available for use in horses (see Chapter 10). Telemetric systems have the major advantage in the ICU that the clinician can identify arrhythmic episodes immediately and take appropriate action; thus, radiotelemetric ECG is the technique of choice for monitoring horses with unstable dysrhythmias and those receiving potentially pro-arrhythmic drugs.

Haemodynamic monitoring

Indirect techniques are the most accessible method for blood pressure measurement in conscious horses. The coccygeal artery is used most often in both foals and adult horses. The cuff width should be 0.2–0.26 times the tail circumference because blood pressure is underestimated if the cuff is too wide and overestimated if it is too narrow.[4] The inflation bladder must be centred over the artery and the cuff fitted tightly[5] to avoid inaccuracy in blood pressure measurement.[6,7] The indirect blood pressure in healthy adult horses is 111.8 ± 13.3 mmHg in systole and 67.7 ± 13.8 mmHg in diastole.[8] A number of studies have reported noninvasive blood pressures in healthy foals as around 80–125 mmHg in systole and 60–80 mmHg in diastole.[9,10] However, the mean arterial pressure is the more important determinant of organ perfusion than the systolic or diastolic pressures and supportive intervention should be considered if the mean arterial pressures fall below 60,[5,11] particularly if there are other clinical signs of poor perfusion such as abnormal mucous membranes, capillary refill time, heart rate, extremity temperature, pulse quality and urine output.[12] Furthermore, while its simplicity and noninvasive nature are an undoubted advantage, the clinician should remain aware of limitations in the accuracy of indirect blood pressure measurement and therefore it is best applied as a means to identify trends within an individual patient, rather than to compare between horses.

In human ICUs, direct measurement of pulmonary artery and capillary wedge pressure is considered the most reliable means to document pulmonary hypertension and invasive measurements of cardiac output and other haemodynamic variables are widely used in monitoring and therapeutic planning. However, while technically feasible, cardiac catheterization to allow direct measurement of pulmonary artery pressure or facilitate cardiac output measurement is still rarely employed in equine patients. (PH) Nevertheless, practical means to measure cardiac output and other haemodynamic indices, such as lithium dilution, are becoming more widely available and are likely to be used in equine critical patients with increasing frequency.[13,14] Monitoring of the cardiac output, stroke volume and systemic vascular resistance can allow the clinician to distinguish whether the cardiovascular status is compromised by reduced circulating volume, vascular tone, cardiac output or a combination of these and in doing so, select the most appropriate treatment and monitor the effects of vasopressors, inotropes and volume expansion.[5,11]

Echocardiography

Echocardiography is the most valuable diagnostic aid for assessment of cardiac structure in horses and thus is the technique of choice in horses presenting with cardiac murmurs, and it is useful in ruling in or out structural heart disease in horses presenting with cardiac dysrhythmias. In the ICU setting, although echocardiography has the potential to assess cardiac output and pulmonary hypertension (see Chapter 9), it is less accurate than the gold-standard direct methods. On the other hand, its noninvasive nature is particularly attractive. Due to limitations in their accuracy, echocardiographic measurements of haemodynamic indices should be used primarily to identify trends within patients rather than taken as absolute measurements. Furthermore, the distributive shock that occurs with endotoxaemia and SIRS is principally due to dysregulation of systemic vascular function and accompanied by microthrombosis and possibly a direct myocardial depressant mechanism. Echocardiography is not a particularly useful tool for identifying these haemodynamic alterations when compared to measurement of cardiac output by thermodilution or lithium dilution, although horses and foals with endotoxaemia or septicaemia often have nonspecific echocardiographic signs of global cardiac dysfunction such as reduced fractional shortening, spontaneous contrast and poor ventricular wall movement. Hypovolaemic patients can have reduced cardiac chamber size and in septicaemic patients mild pericardial effusions are fairly common.[1]

SPECIFIC FORMS OF CARDIAC COMPLICATIONS IN INTENSIVE CARE PATIENTS

Circulatory collapse

Circulatory collapse, or shock, can arise from reduced cardiac output, reduction of circulating volume, dysregulation of vasomotor tone or a combination of these factors. Acute heart failure is described in Chapter 19. Endotoxaemia, sepsis and SIRS are classified as forms of distributive shock as they are characterized by widespread systemic vasodilation although both hypovolaemia and myocardial depression can contribute to the pathogenesis. Hypovolaemia can be due to severe haemorrhage or sequestration of fluid into the body cavities or into the gastrointestinal or urogenital tracts. The main goals of therapy in circulatory collapse are to restore and maintain the circulating volume and to attempt to increase vasomotor tone and cardiac output with pressor and ionotropic agents (see Chapter 7). Clearly, treatment aimed at addressing and correcting the predisposing condition is critical. Global myocardial depression is difficult to document in equine critical care patients but the techniques described above can be very helpful in identifying cardiac abnormalities that accompany circulatory collapse.

Cardiac dysrhythmias

In horses, dysrhythmias occurring secondary to other systemic diseases, particularly gastrointestinal disease,[15,16] are encountered more frequently than rhythm disturbances associated with primary myocardial pathology. In a group of 67 horses with duodenitis/proximal jejunitis, six horses (9%) had dysrhythmias detected by auscultation and conventional electrocardiography.[15] The prevalence of dysrhythmias in the postoperative period following abdominal surgery is not known but is likely to be higher than may be appreciated on auscultation alone: in one survey of horses with ventricular dysrhythmias, 4 of 21 cases had recently undergone colic surgery[16] and ambulatory ECGs obtained from fifty horses within 3 days of exploratory celiotomy demonstrated that 11 horses (22%) had isolated supraventricular premature depolarizations while 8 horses (16%) had ventricular dysrhythmias, including 4 (8%) with idioventricular rhythms or paroxysmal monomorphic ventricular tachycardia.[17] In all but one of these cases the dysrhythmias were self-limiting, no specific treatment was required and the dysrhythmia had not been recognized on auscultation. Occasionally, more clinically significant dysrhythmias are encountered in the postoperative period following colic surgery, and in this instance clinical signs of reduced cardiac output and

marked tachycardias may be apparent. A high index of suspicion is required and the clinician should consider an ECG assessment in all horses that have heart rates that are higher than might otherwise be suspected given the degree of pain or in horses showing weakness, pallor and other signs of low cardiac output.

Causes of dysrhythmias secondary to gastrointestinal disease include the direct effects of endotoxin on the myocardium, autonomic imbalance resulting from gastrointestinal distension and metabolic, electrolytic or acid–base imbalances.[15] Ideally, underlying and contributory factors should be addressed first. The decision to institute specific antidysrhythmic therapy is generally based on assessment of whether it is likely that the dysrhythmia will destabilize into a life-threatening state. In general, ventricular dysrhythmias are much more likely to require antidysrhythmic therapy than supraventricular dysrhythmias, and commonly applied guidelines suggest that antidysrhythmics should be considered where the heart rate is rapid (greater than 100 bpm), the dysrhythmia is polymorphic and R on T phenomenon is present (see Fig. 13.17). However, the most important thing to consider is the clinical status of the animal, and the decision of whether to utilize antidysrhythmics should be based on the presence or absence of signs of low cardiac output. Strong evidence to support decisions on which specific antidysrhythmic agents to use in equine patients is lacking but procainamide, lignocaine and quinidine gluconate are popular first choices in ventricular tachycardia. Magnesium sulphate has been successful, and can be used alone, or in combination with other antidysrhythmic agents. Further details of these and other antidysrhythmics are described in more detail in Chapter 13. (VT)

The electrolytes that are most commonly associated with dysrhythmias are potassium, calcium and magnesium and the role of these electrolytes in arrhythmiogenesis is discussed in detail in Chapter 6. Hypokalaemia, hypocalcaemia and hypomagnesaemia are common in horses with sepsis and endotoxaemia,[18] thus monitoring and addressing electrolyte imbalances in critically ill horses is an important priority.

Hypokalaemia

Hypokalaemia is commonly found in ill animals and causes include endotoxaemia,[18] anorexia, diarrhoea and starvation.[19] It is frequently present in horses with heat exhaustion along with hypochloraemia, hypocalcaemia and metabolic alkalosis. Hypokalaemia leads to prolongation of the Q–T interval and both supraventricular and ventricular dysrhythmias can be seen in horses with hypokalaemia. Supraventricular tachycardia, ventricular tachycardia, torsades de pointes and ventricular fibrillation can all occur with severe hypokalaemia. If severe hypokalaemia is present, the calculated potassium deficit

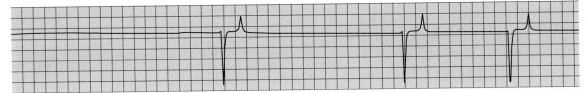

Figure 21.1 An ECG recorded from a 6-year-old Thoroughbred gelding with septic peritonitis and hyperkalaemia due to renal failure associated with aminoglycoside toxicity and endotoxaemia. The P waves are absent and the T waves are tall and peaked.

should be replaced slowly intravenously at a maximum rate of 0.5 mEq/kg/hour while monitoring serum potassium concentrations.

Hyperkalaemia

Hyperkalaemia is uncommon in horses except in foals with uroperitoneum. Hyperkalaemia is occasionally detected in adult horses, primarily those with acute renal failure or in Quarter horses with hyperkalaemic periodic paralysis (HYPP); this condition is described in more detail in Chapter 20. Cardiac dysrhythmias may or may not be detected on auscultation in hyperkalaemia but an ECG should be obtained in horses or foals with a plasma potassium equal to or greater than 6 mEq/L. Tall peaked T waves are detected with plasma potassium values equal to or greater than 6.2 mEq/L (Fig. 21.1). Progressive slowing of conduction and decreased excitability occur with hyperkalaemia and may result in cardiac arrest or ventricular fibrillation. Broadening and flattening of the P waves, prolonged P–R intervals and bradycardia are a reflection of this on the ECG. Atrial arrest or atrial standstill develops with progressive hyperkalaemia. Supraventricular and ventricular premature depolarizations and ventricular tachycardia have also been reported. Widened QRS complexes are further indications of severe, near lethal hyperkalaemia.

In uroperitoneum, treatment for hyperkalaemia must be aggressive because these foals are at high risk for the development of cardiac dysrhythmias, particularly under general anaesthesia during surgical repair of the ruptured bladder, urachus or ureter (see Table 20.3). Sodium deficit should be replaced slowly at the rate of 0.5 mEq/hour with 0.45–0.9% saline intravenously. Sodium bicarbonate (1 mEq/kg intravenously) will help drive potassium intracellularly. Intravenous dextrose and insulin may also help drive the potassium intracellularly. The addition of 5 ml of the foal's blood to the fluid will help prevent the insulin from adhering to the fluid administration bag. If severe cardiac dysrhythmias are detected calcium gluconate can be administered slowly, over a 10-minute period, intravenously to effect (see Table 20.3). Calcium gluconate should be discontinued if bradycardia occurs. Drainage of the uroperitoneum should be performed in foals with

uroperitoneum in conjunction with intravenous fluid replacement therapy. Surgical correction of the uroperitoneum should only be undertaken following medical stabilization of the foal.

In horses with HYPP experiencing an acute episode, a blood sample should be obtained to measure serum potassium concentration, which is often in excess of 6 mEq/L. Calcium borogluconate, sodium bicarbonate, dextrose and insulin may be used as indicated above (see Table 20.3). If insulin is used blood glucose concentration should be monitored for the following 24 hours. Acute episodes in horses with HYPP may be prevented through careful management of affected horses. Horses with HYPP should be fed diets low in potassium (timothy hay and Bermuda grass hay, no molasses) and kept in a regular exercise programme. Kaliuretic diuretics such as acetazolamide (2–4 mg/kg PO q.i.d.) or hydrochlorothiazide (250 mg IM or IV q.i.d.) have been effective in affected horses in reducing the frequency and severity of clinical signs.

Hypomagnesaemia

Magnesium deficiency usually occurs with hypokalaemia. Serious ventricular dysrhythmias are most likely in patients with significant hypomagnesaemia, but supraventricular tachycardia and AF also occur in patients with severe hypomagnesaemia. Prolongation of the P–R interval, widening of the QRS complex, ST segment depression and peaked T waves may all be detected on the ECG of a horse with hypomagnesaemia. For correction of hypomagnesaemia, a dose of 4–16 mg/kg over 4 hours is generally recommended but magnesium sulphate has also be used as an antidsyrhythmic in horses with unstable ventricular dysrhythmias[20] at the higher dose of 2.2–4.4 mg/kg IV slowly, repeated at 5-minute intervals to total dose of 55 mg/kg.

Hypocalcaemia

Hypocalcaemic tetany, lactation tetany, transport tetany or eclampsia is uncommon in horses. Hypocalcaemia may also be seen following prolonged or strenuous exercise, prolonged transport, in horses with diarrhoea or cantharidin (blister beetle) toxicosis and in horses fed a diet deficient in calcium; diets concurrently deficient in magnesium will increase this risk. In horses with lactation tetany, the clinical episode often occurs following peak lactation, approximately 60–100 days post partum. Ionized calcium should be measured in horses with suspected hypocalcaemia. If ionized calcium cannot be measured in horses with hypoalbuminaemia the following formula is a better reflection of the horse's calcium status:

$$\text{corrected calcium} = \text{measured calcium (mg/dL)} - \text{albumin (g/dL)} + 3.5$$
(to convert mmol/L to mg/dL multiply by 4.01)

There are two different clinical syndromes in horses with hypocalcaemia. Horses with low serum total calcium (5–8 mg/dL; 1.25–2 mmol/L) and low serum magnesium present with tachycardia, synchronous diaphragmatic flutter, laryngospasm, loud laboured breathing, trismus, protrusion of the nictitans, dysphagia, goose-stepping or stiff hind limb gait and ataxia. Rhabdomyolysis, convulsions, coma and death may ensue. Horses with even lower serum total calcium (<5 mg/dL; 1.25 mmol/L) and normal serum magnesium concentrations usually present with flaccid paralysis, mydriasis, stupor and recumbency. Ionized plasma calcium concentration influences myocardial contractility and the Q–T interval. Electrocardiographic abnormalities other than tachycardia are rarely seen with hypocalcaemia although supraventricular or ventricular premature depolarizations or ventricular tachycardia are occasionally detected. Cardiac arrest or ventricular standstill may occur. The treatment of horses with hypocalcaemia should include a slow, over 10–20 minutes, intravenous infusion of calcium gluconate (4 mg/kg) to effect. The horse's ration should be analysed to ensure an adequate calcium:phosphorus ratio in the diet (1.3 : 2.1) and adequate magnesium in the diet. Concurrent hypomagnesaemia may also require treatment.

Mild to moderate hypocalcaemia is commonly seen in critically ill horses with sepsis and endotoxaemia.[18] However, supplementation of calcium in these patients is controversial. Low ionized calcium was a risk factor that increased the odds of development of ileus and of non-survival in a large study of horses with enterocolitis and severe gastrointestinal disorders while calcium supplementation increased the odds of survival.[21] However, calcium administration did not improve haemodynamics and survival in endotoxaemic pigs[22] and administration of calcium has been shown to exacerbate endotoxaemia and increase mortality in rodent models.[23,24] Thus clear recommendations are lacking but currently in endotoxaemic horses, calcium is usually supplemented if the ionized concentration is less than 3.6 mg/dL or 0.9 mmol/L.

Hypercalcaemia

Hypercalcaemia is uncommon in horses but is detected in those with chronic renal failure, lymphosarcoma, paraneoplastic syndromes, hypervitaminosis D and the inges-

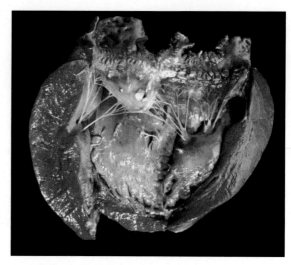

Figure 21.2 Calcification of the endocardium in a 7-year-old Thoroughbred gelding with hypercalcaemia of malignancy and splenic lymphoma.

tion of *Cestrum diurnum*. Hypercalcaemia results in soft tissue mineralization and mineralization of the heart and blood vessels especially the aorta, pulmonary artery, coronary arteries and endocardium (Fig. 21.2). With hypercalcaemia the heart rate initially slows and sinus arrhythmia and partial AV block are detected. Premature depolarizations are a common finding in horses with hypercalcaemia and supraventricular or ventricular tachycardia may be present. Terminally cardiac arrest, ventricular fibrillation or ventricular standstill occurs.

Emergency treatment is indicated in horses with hypercalcaemia in the 15–20 mg/dL or 3.75–5 mmol/L range, particularly if cardiac dysrhythmia is present. The extracellular fluid volume should be expanded with 0.9% saline intravenously, also increasing the glomerular filtration rate. Potassium supplementation of the intravenous fluids should be administered if indicated. A calciuretic diuretic such as frusemide should be administered at 2–4 mg/kg every 12 hours with intravenous fluids at 5 mL/kg/hour. Corticosteroids may reduce calcium concentrations and decrease the likelihood of soft tissue and cardiac mineralization by decreasing calcium loss from bone, decreasing intestinal calcium absorption and increasing renal excretion of calcium. Steroid-responsive hypercalcaemias include lymphoma, lymphosarcoma, leukaemia, multiple myeloma, thymoma, vitamin D toxicity, granulomatous disease and hyperadrenocorticism. Treatment with salmon calcitonin may be indicated if severe prolonged hypercalcaemia is present. The underlying cause of the hypercalcaemia should be determined and removed or treated, if possible. All exogenous supplements containing calcium, phosphorus and vitamin D should be discontinued and horses removed from *Cestrum diurnum*-infected pasture.

Haemothorax, haemopericardium and haemoperitoneum

(VT)

Haemoperitoneum can be idiopathic or arise secondary to trauma, neoplasia, mesenteric injury, systemic amyloidosis and disseminated intravascular coagulopathy (DIC) and, in periparturient broodmares, it can follow injury to the uterus or rupture of the uterine artery.[25-31] Affected horses present with signs of abdominal discomfort and shock if the haemorrhage is severe. Because splenic contraction can temporarily support the packed cell volume with recent haemorrhage, it is not necessarily a very accurate guide to the degree of acute haemorrhage and the heart rate probably serves as a better guide to the severity of haemorrhagic shock: if the heart rate is greater than 80 bpm, emergency blood transfusion should be considered and if this is not available, the administration of hypertonic saline and colloids such as hetastarch are indicated. Horses with haemoperitoneum frequently develop ventricular and supraventricular dysrhythmias[31] so that continuous ECG monitoring of these patients is prudent. The prognosis varies with the underlying cause. Most horses with idiopathic haemoperitoneum respond successfully to supportive management. Horses with underlying neoplasia generally have a poor prognosis, except in the case of ovarian granulosa cell tumor where the tumor can be removed successfully.[29] Broodmares with rupture of the uterine artery are usually managed medically and the prognosis for survival is good with reasonable future fertility: 84% and 49%, respectively, in a recent large case series.[31] If they can be identified at surgery, uterine tears should be repaired but in addition to haemorrhage these mares also usually have septic peritonitis and require extremely intensive care if they are to survive.

Haemothorax and haemopericardium can also arise as a result of neoplasia and trauma, including iatrogenically during lung biopsy and bone marrow aspiration.[32,33] Thoracic trauma occurs commonly during parturition.[34,35] Ultrasonography is more sensitive than radiography in demonstrating rib fractures in newborn foals.[36] In the majority of cases the ribs are not displaced, the foal displays only relatively mild discomfort and the nondisplaced ribs will repair with time without surgical intervention. If multiple ribs are involved and the fragments are displaced, there is a significant risk of trauma to the underlying structures, particularly the heart. Haemothorax does not necessarily require drainage for successful resolution[32] but in foals with unstable rib fractures, surgical stabilization is necessary to prevent fatal cardiac injury and/or severe intrathoracic haemorrage.[37,38] Similarly haemopericardium does not necessarily require drainage and may resolve with conservative management. Pericardial drainage should only be considered if cardiac tamponade is present (see Chapter 17).

Thrombophlebitis

(AF)

Thrombophlebitis is defined as vein thrombosis with mural inflammation and is a common complication of intravenous catheterization.[39] The prevalence of jugular thrombosis in horses being treated for a variety of gastrointestinal diseases has ranged from 6% to 22%.[17,40,41] There are numerous proven and putative positive risk factors for thrombophlebitis including use of home-produced fluid solutions, fever, colic, diarrhoea, irritant drugs, rapid infusion rate and prolonged intravenous treatment.[39,42,43] Both catheter material and design contribute: flexible, polyurethane over-the-wire catheters have less risk than the more rigid polyurethane over-the-needle catheters while Teflon or polytetrafluoroethylene catheters are likely to carry the greatest risk.[43] Jugular thrombophlebitis can be septic or nonseptic. Micro-organisms most commonly isolated from the tips of intravenous catheters are coagulase-negative *Staphylococcus* species, *Corynebacterium* species, *Enterobacter* species and *Streptococcus* species.[42]

Swelling or palpable thickening of the jugular vein with variable degrees of perivenous swelling is characteristic of thrombophlebitis. Heat, pain and discharge from the site of venepuncture suggest sepsis. Acute onset, severe thrombophlebitis can cause obstruction to venous drainage of the head and there may be swelling in the supraorbital area, muzzle and cheek on the affected side. Bilateral thrombosis can be associated with swelling of the tongue and airway obstruction. Chronic thrombophlebitis can lead to distension of the veins of the face and discharging abscesses. Diagnostic ultrasonography is useful to characterize the nature and extent of thrombophlebitis. Nonseptic thrombi are usually uniformly echogenic and fairly small (Fig. 21.3). Septic thrombophlebitis is heterogeneous with numerous anechoic areas representing areas of fluid accumulation or necrosis and hyperechoic areas representing reverberation artifacts representing gas formation (Fig. 21.4). The patency of the vein should be assessed (see Figs. 21.3 and 21.4). Leukocytosis, neutrophilia and hyperfibrinogenaemia are common but nonspecific findings in septic thrombophlebitis. If DIC is suspected, platelet count, prothrombin time, activated partial thromboplastin time, fibrinolytic degradation products and antithrombin III should be measured, with abnormalities of four out of five of these being indicative of DIC. The tips of catheters removed from the affected vein should be sterilely inserted into thioglycolate broth for bacterial culture. Blood cultures, swabs discharging tracts at the catheter insertion site and aspirates of fluid pockets obtained in a sterile manner can be submitted for bacterial culture and antimicrobial sensitivity testing.

Intravenous catheters should be removed promptly and, if possible, further intravenous therapy should be

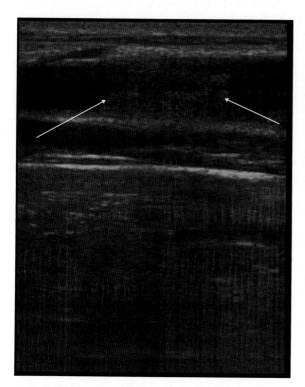

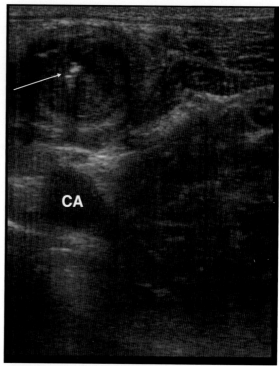

Figure 21.3 An ultrasonogram of a small, nonseptic jugular thrombus (between arrows) that has uniform echogenicity and is partially obstructing the vessel from a 3-year-old Thoroughbred colt that has recently had an intravenous catheter removed.

Figure 21.4 An ultrasonogram of a septic jugular thrombus that is completely occluding the vessel and is heterogeneous, with hyperechoic areas (arrow) and reverberation artifacts typical of gas formation from a 5-month-old Thoroughbred filly that has recently received intravenous fluids and drugs via an intravenous catheter. CA, carotid artery.

avoided if there are signs of thrombophlebitis. However, if this in unavoidable, it is prudent to place a catheter at an alternative site such as the lateral thoracic or cephalic rather than the opposite jugular vein. Bilateral jugular thrombophlebitis leads to problems with venous drainage of the head and upper respiratory tract obstruction may ensue. Penicillin with an aminoglycoside, enrofloxacin, cephalosporins and trimethoprim sulphonamides are appropriate choices prior to availability of results of anti-microbial sensitivity. The presence of gas echoes may indicate anaerobic infection and the inclusion of metrinidazole should be considered. Generally, parenteral administration is preferred in the acute stages but some cases of chronic septic thrombophlebitis may require several weeks of antimicrobial therapy and therefore oral administration of enrofloxacin, with or without metronidazole, or a combination of trimethoprim-sulphonamide and rifampin may be more practical. Horses with head swelling should be tied with the head up, ideally with the option of resting on straw bales or some other suitable support. Oral aspirin (18 mg/kg PO every other day) and topical treatments such as hot-packing may be helpful.

Reconstructive surgery using saphenous vein grafts has been reported to be effective in horses with permanent thrombophlebitic stenosis.[44]

The majority of cases resolve uneventfully although jugular thrombophlebitis can occasionally prolong treatment and delay hospital discharge in gastrointestinal patients. Septic jugular thrombosis can be associated with a variety of serious complications including infective endocarditis,[45] temporary or permanent damage to the sympathetic and/or recurrent laryngeal nerves, and upper airway oedema that affects the horse's athletic performance. In most individuals, even with complete loss of the jugular vein, a collateral circulation will develop to allow adequate drainage of the head.

The severity of thrombophlebitis can be minimized with early identification and appropriate treatment of the coagulation disturbances associated with gastrointestinal disease and SIRS, careful selection, insertion and use of intravenous catheters, avoiding home-made intravenous fluid solutions, diluting irritant drugs appropriately and avoiding needle sticks in veins that are, or recently have been, catheterized. Catheters should be flushed frequently with heparinized saline when not in continuous use and Teflon over-the-needle catheters should be left in place for no more than 72 hours while polyurethane over-the-needle catheters can be maintained for up to 5 days. The more flexible, polyurethane over-the-wire catheters can be left in place for considerably longer provided that no perivenous reaction occurs. Fluid lines should be changed every 24 hours in high-risk patients. It can be helpful to cover the catheter with bandage material in foals or horses that are frequently recumbent but this is not done routinely in adult horses in many veterinary hospitals.[43]

Arterial thrombosis

Arterial thrombosis associated with sepsis is rare but has been documented in association with neonatal septiacemia affecting the aorto-iliac quadrification (saddle thrombus),[46,47] digital,[48,49] metacarpal and metatarsal arteries,[49] and in the major vessels of the metatarsal and metacarpal regions in older animals with enterocolitis.[49] An additional case of brachial artery thrombosis in a foal with an atrial septal defect has been reported and it was suggested that the condition may have arisen following embolism from an atrial thrombus.[50] In septicaemia and endotoxaemia, abnormalities of haemostatsis and/or fibrinolytic pathways may lead to the condition. Thrombocytopaenia and deficiencies in antithrombin III, due either to excessive consumption or loss via the gastrointestinal tract in protein-losing enteropathy, have been documented in affected cases.[48,49] Activation of procoagulants by endotoxin, dehydration, hypoxia and acidosis may also contribute to the pathogenesis.[49] Clinical examination reveals that the affected limb(s) are cold and there may be partial or complete sloughing of the hoof. Arterial thrombosis can be documented using Doppler ultrasonography, nuclear scintigraphy[47] and contrast angiography.[50] Attempts to remove the thrombus by surgical embolectomy[50] and using tissue plasminogen activator[47] and urokinase[48] have not yet produced successful results.

Cardiac murmurs in colic patients

The clinician should consider heart disease a potential cause of signs that can be confused with abdominal pain. However, loud cardiac murmurs are frequently identified in horses with colic that subsequently disappear when the gastrointestinal signs resolve. Currently, the causes of such murmurs remain unclear. Using intact aortic valves, suspended by isometric force transducers, it is possible to quantify the forces exerted by the cusps in response to various mediators; equine aortic valves contract in response to angiotensin II, endothelin, thomboxane and α-adrenoreceptor agonists.[51] The physiological and pathological relevance of modification of valve tone in response to vasoactive mediators is currently unknown; however, it may be of relevance to the equine colic patient, as many of these vasoactive mediators are likely to be released in association with SIRS.

REFERENCES

1. Dolente BA, Seco OM, Lewis ML. Streptococcal toxic shock in a horse. J Am Vet Med Assoc 2000;217(1):64–67, 30.

2. Stevens DL. Streptococcal Toxic-Shock Syndrome: spectrum of disease, pathogenesis, and new concepts in treatment. Emerg Infect Dis 1995;1(3):69–78.

3. Miller CW, Prescott JF, Mathews KA. Streptococcal toxic shock syndrome in dogs. J Am Vet Med Assoc 1996;209:1421–1426.

4. Latshaw H, Fessler JF, Whistler SJ, et al. Indirect measurement of mean blood pressure in the normotensive and hypotensive horse. Equine Vet J 1979;11(3): 191–194.

5. Corley K. Monitoring and treating haemodynamic disturbances in critically ill neonatal foals. Part 1: Haemodynamic monitoring. Equine Vet Educ 2002;14:270–279.

6. Kvart C. An ultrasonic method for indirect blood pressure measurement in the horse. J Equine Med Surg 1979;3:16–23.

7. Parry BW, Anderson GA. Importance of uniform cuff application for equine blood pressure measurement. Equine Vet J 1984;16(6):529–531.

8. Johnson JH, Garner HE, Hutcheson DP. Ultrasonic measurement of arterial blood pressure in conditioned thoroughbreds. Equine Vet J 1976;8(2):55–57.

9. Holdstock NB, Ousey JC, Rossdale PD. Glomerular filtration rate, effective renal plasma flow, blood pressure and pulse rate in the equine neonate during the first 10 days post partum. Equine Vet J 1998;30(4):335–343.

10. Vaala W, House, JK. Supportive care of the abnormal newborn. In: Smith B, editor. Large Animal Internal Medicine. 3rd ed. St Louis: Mosby; 2002. p. 294–302.

11. Corley K. Monitoring and treating haemodynamic disturbances in critically ill neonatal foals. Part 2: Assessment and treatment. Equine Vet Educ 2002;14:328–336.

12. Magdesian KG. Monitoring the critically ill equine patient. Vet Clin North Am Equine Pract 2004;20(1):11–39.

13. Linton RA, Young LE, Marlin DJ, et al. Cardiac output measured by lithium dilution, thermodilution, and transesophageal Doppler

echocardiography in anesthetized horses. Am J Vet Res 2000;61(7): 731–737.

14. Corley KT, Donaldson LL, Durando MM, et al. Cardiac output technologies with special reference to the horse. J Vet Intern Med 2003;17(3):262–272.

15. Cornick JL, Seahorn TL. Cardiac arrhythmias identified in horses with duodenitis/proximal jejunitis: six cases (1985–1988). J Am Vet Med Assoc 1990;197(8): 1054–1059.

16. Reimer JM, Reef VB, Sweeney RW. Ventricular arrhythmias in horses: 21 cases (1984–1989). J Am Vet Med Assoc 1992;201(8): 1237–1243.

17. Protopapas K. Studies on metabolic disturbances and other post-operative complications following equine colic surgery. D Vet Med thesis, University of London; 2000.

18. Toribio RE, Kohn CW, Hardy J, et al. Alterations in serum parathyroid hormone and electrolyte concentrations and urinary excretion of electrolytes in horses with induced endotoxemia. J Vet Intern Med 2005;19(2): 223–231.

19. MacIntire D. Disorders of potassium, phosphorus and magnesium in critical illness. Comp Contin Educ Pract Vet 1997;19:41–48.

20. Marr CM, Reef VB. ECG of the month. J Am Vet Med Assoc 1991;198(9):1533–1534.

21. Delesalle C, Dewulf J, Lefebvre RA, et al. Use of plasma ionized calcium levels and Ca^{2+} substitution response patterns as prognostic parameters for ileus and survival in colic horses. Vet Q 2005;27(4):157–172.

22. Carlstedt F, Eriksson M, Kiiski R, et al. Hypocalcemia during porcine endotoxemic shock: effects of calcium administration. Crit Care Med 2000;28(8):2909–2914.

23. Malcolm DS, Zaloga GP, Holaday JW. Calcium administration increases the mortality of endotoxic shock in rats. Crit Care Med 1989;17(9):900–903.

24. Zaloga GP, Sager A, Black KW, et al. Low dose calcium administration increases mortality

25. Dechant JE, Nieto JE, Le Jeune SS. Hemoperitoneum in horses: 67 cases (1989–2004). J Am Vet Med Assoc 2006;229(2):253–258.

26. Pusterla N, Fecteau ME, Madigan JE, et al. Acute hemoperitoneum in horses: a review of 19 cases (1992–2003). J Vet Intern Med 2005;19(3):344–347.

27. Alexander GR, Tweedie MA, Lescun TB, et al. Haemoperitoneum secondary to granulosa cell tumour in two mares. Aust Vet J 2004; 82(8):481–484.

28. Gatewood DM, Douglass JP, Cox JH, et al. Intra-abdominal hemorrhage associated with a granulosa-thecal cell neoplasm in a mare. J Am Vet Med Assoc 1990;196(11):1827–1828.

29. Green SL, Specht TE, Dowling SC, et al. Hemoperitoneum caused by rupture of a juvenile granulosa cell tumor in an equine neonate. J Am Vet Med Assoc 1988;193(11): 1417–1419.

30. Roby KA, Beech J, Bloom JC, et al. Hepatocellular carcinoma associated with erythrocytosis and hypoglycemia in a yearling filly. J Am Vet Med Assoc 1990;196(3): 465–467.

31. Arnold CE, Payne M, Thompson JA, et al. Periparturient hemorrhage in mares: 73 cases (1998–2005). J Am Vet Med Assoc 2008;232(9): 1345–1351.

32. Perkins G, Ainsworth DM, Yeager A. Hemothorax in 2 horses. J Vet Intern Med 1999;13(4):375–378.

33. Gruys E, Kok HA, Van Der Werff YD. [Dyspnoea due to intrathoracic haemorrhage and haemangiosarcoma in a horse (author's transl)]. Tijdschr Diergeneeskd 1976;101(6): 310–312.

34. Schambourg MA, Laverty S, Mullim S, et al. Thoracic trauma in foals: post mortem findings. Equine Vet J 2003;35(1):78–81.

35. Jean D, Laverty S, Halley J, et al. Thoracic trauma in newborn foals. Equine Vet J 1999;31(2):149–152.

36. Jean D, Picandet V, Macieira S, et al. Detection of rib trauma in newborn foals in an equine critical care unit: a comparison of

ultrasonography, radiography and physical examination. Equine Vet J 2007;39(2):158–163.

37. Bellezzo F, Hunt RJ, Provost R, et al. Surgical repair of rib fractures in 14 neonatal foals: case selection, surgical technique and results. Equine Vet J 2004;36(7):557–562.

38. Kraus BM, Richardson DW, Sheridan G, et al. Multiple rib fracture in a neonatal foal using a nylon strand suture repair technique. Vet Surg 2005;34(4): 399–404.

39. Traub-Dargatz JL, Dargatz DA. A retrospective study of vein thrombosis in horses treated with intravenous fluids in a veterinary teaching hospital. J Vet Intern Med 1994;8(4):264–266.

40. Lankveld DP, Ensink JM, van Dijk P, et al. Factors influencing the occurrence of thrombophlebitis after post-surgical long-term intravenous catheterization of colic horses: a study of 38 cases. J Vet Med A Physiol Pathol Clin Med 2001;48(9):545–552.

41. Darbareiner RM, White NA. Large colon impaction in horses;147 cases (1985–1991). J Am Vet Med Assoc 1995;199(3): 370–373.

42. Ettlinger JJ, Palmer JE, Benson C. Bacteria found on intravenous catheters removed from horses. Vet Rec 1992;130(12):248–249.

43. Divers TJ. Prevention and treatment of thrombosis, phlebitis and laminitis in horses with gastrointestinal disease. Vet Clin North Am Equine Pract 2003;19: 779–790.

44. Rijkenhuizen AB, Van Swieten HA. Reconstruction of the jugular vein in horses with post thrombophlebitis stenosis using saphenous vein graft. Equine Vet J 1998;30(3):236–239.

45. Maxson AD, Reef VB. Bacterial endocarditis in horses: ten cases (1984–1995). Equine Vet J 1997;29(5):394–399.

46. Moore LA, Johnson PJ, Bailey KL. Aorto-iliac thrombosis in a foal. Vet Rec 1998;142(17):459– 462.

47. Duggan VE, Holbrook TC, Dechant JE, et al. Diagnosis of aorto-iliac thrombosis in a quarter horse foal

using Doppler ultrasound and nuclear scintigraphy. J Vet Intern Med 2004;18(5):753–756.

48. Forrest LJ, Cooley AJ, Darien BJ. Digital arterial thrombosis in a septicemic foal. J Vet Intern Med 1999;13(4):382–385.

49. Brianceau P, Divers TJ. Acute thrombosis of limb arteries in horses with sepsis: five cases (1988–1998). Equine Vet J 2001;33(1):105–109.

50. Spier SJ. Arterial thrombosis as the cause of lameness in a foal. J Am Vet Med Assoc 1985;187(2): 164–165.

51. Bowen IM, Marr CM, Chester AH, et al. In-vitro contraction of the equine aortic valve. J Heart Valve Dis 2004;13(4):593–599.

Appendix: Website Index

Appendix: Website Index

Features of interest	Short name	Case No
Dexamethasone: therapeutic use	PC	1, case series
Dexamethasone: therapeutic use	RCT	2
Dexamethasone: therapeutic use	VT	2
Digoxin: therapeutic use	AF	3
Digoxin: therapeutic use	VMD	4
Digoxin: therapeutic use	VT	2
Dilated cardiomyopathy: echo	VMD	6
Doppler echocardiography aliasing: echo	RCT	1
Doppler echocardiography aliasing: echo	VMD	5
Doppler echocardiography aliasing: echo	VSD	2,3
Double-apex sign: echo	VSD	3
Ductus arteriosus, patent: auscultation	EA	6
Echocardiography: standard imaging planes	ET	NA
Electrocardioversion, treatment of atrial fibrillation: transvenous technique	AF	3
Enalapril: therapeutic use	AF	2
Enalapril: therapeutic use	IE	1
Enalapril: therapeutic use	VT	2
Endocardial cushion defect: echo	CCC	3
Endocardial cushion defect: pathology	CCC	3
Exercise-induced pulmonary haemorrhage: endoscopy	AF	6
Exercise-induced pulmonary haemorrhage: endoscopy	AR	1
Exercising electrocardiography	AF	5, 7
Exercising electrocardiography	AR	1, 4
Exercising electrocardiography	SFP	1, 2, 4
Exercising electrocardiography	VSD	1
Flail cusp: echo	RCT	1, 2, 3, 4
Foramen ovale: echo	CCC	4
Foramen ovale: echo	VMD	2
Furosemide/frusemide: therapeutic use	PH	2
Furosemide/frusemide: therapeutic use	VMD	4
Haemangiosarcoma: echo	CN	2, 3
Haemangiosarcoma: pathology	CN	2
Haemopericardium: echo	HP	1, 4
Haemoperitoneum: ultrasonography	VT	1
Haemothorax: computed tomography	HP	3
Haemothorax: ultrasonography	CN	3
Harmonics: echo	AR	2
Hepatic congestion: ultrasonography	PC	1, case series
Hepatic congestion: ultrasonography	VMD	6
Hyoplastic aorta: echo	VSD	6
Hyoplastic aorta: pathology	VSD	6
Interstitial pneumonia: pathology	RCT	4
Interstitial pneumonia: ultrasonography	RCT	4
Interstitial pneumonia: radiography	RCT	4
Intracardiac echocardiography	VSD	5
Jugular thrombosis, septic: clinical signs	AF	4
Jugular thrombosis, septic: ultrasonography	AF	4
Left atrial enlargement, mild: echo	AF	5
Left atrial enlargement, mild: echo	AR	4
Left atrial enlargement, mild: echo	SFP	3, 4
Left atrial enlargement, mild: echo	VSD	1
Left atrial enlargement, severe: echo	AF	2
Left atrial enlargement, severe: echo	IE	2

Features of interest	Short name	Case No
Left atrial enlargement, severe: echo	VMD	4, 6
Left heart failure: clinical signs	IE	2
Left heart failure: clinical signs	VMD	2
Left ventricle, hyperkinesis	AR	2, 3, 4, 5
Left ventricle, hyperkinesis	IE	2
Left ventricular dyskinesis: echo	VT	1, 2
Left ventricular ejection time, low output states: echo	AF	2
Left ventricular ejection time, low output states: echo	CN	1
Left ventricular ejection time, low output states: echo	PC	1
Left ventricular ejection time, low output states: echo	VMD	2, 4
Left ventricular ejection time, low output states: echo	VT	2
Left ventricular failure: echo	IE	2
Left ventricular failure: echo	VMD	2, 6
Left ventricular hyperkinesis: echo	AR	2, 3, 4, 5
Left ventricular hyperkinesis: echo	VMD	4, 6
Left ventricular volume overload: echo	AF	2
Left ventricular volume overload: echo	AR	2,3,4, 5
Left ventricular volume overload: echo	CCC	1, 2
Left ventricular volume overload: echo	IE	1
Left ventricular volume overload: echo	RCT	1, 3, 4
Left ventricular volume overload: echo	VMD	3
Lignocaine/lidocaine: therapeutic use	ACF	1
Lignocaine/lidocaine: therapeutic use	VT	1, 2, 3
Lymphocoma: echo	CN	1
Lymphoma: cytology	CN	1
Lymphoma: pathology	CN	1
Magnesium sulphate, therapeutic use	ACF	2
Magnesium sulphate, therapeutic use	AF	4
Magnesium sulphate, therapeutic use	VT	2
Mare reproductive loss syndrome	PC	case series
Membranous VSD, determining prognosis: echo	VSD	1,2
Membranous VSD: echo	VSD	1,2,3
Mesenteric vessel congestion: ultrasonography	VMD	6
Mitral infective endocarditis: echo	IE	1, 2, 3
Mitral infective endocarditis: echo	RCT	3
Mitral infective endocarditis: pathology	IE	1, 2
Mitral regurgitation, lesion-orientated images: echo	VMD	3
Mitral regurgitation, mild/moderate: echo	AF	4, 5
Mitral regurgitation, mild/moderate: echo	AR	4
Mitral regurgitation, mild/moderate: echo	RSD	1
Mitral regurgitation, mild/moderate: echo	SFP	3, 4, 5
Mitral regurgitation, mild/moderate: echo	VMD	1, 5
Mitral regurgitation, mild/moderate: echo	VSD	1
Mitral regurgitation, murmur: auscultation	AF	2, 4
Mitral regurgitation, murmur: auscultation	AR	1, 4
Mitral regurgitation, murmur: auscultation	IE	1
Mitral regurgitation, murmur: auscultation	RCT	1
Mitral regurgitation, murmur: auscultation	RSD	1
Mitral regurgitation, murmur: auscultation	SFP	3, 4, 5
Mitral regurgitation, murmur: auscultation	VMD	4, 5, 6
Mitral regurgitation, physiological: echo	AF	3, 7
Mitral regurgitation, physiological: echo	AR	1
Mitral regurgitation, physiological: echo	ET	2
Mitral regurgitation, physiological: echo	SFP	1

Features of interest	Short name	Case No
Pericarditis: clinical signs	PC	1
Pleural effusion: ultrasonography	CN	1
Pleural effusion: ultrasonography	PC	1, case series
Pleural effusion: ultrasonography	VMD	6
Prednisolone, therapeutic use	VMD	5
Pressure gradients: estimation from CW echo	AF	2
Pressure gradients: estimation from CW echo	CCC	1, 4
Pressure gradients: estimation from CW echo	RCT	1
Pressure gradients: estimation from CW echo	VSD	2,3,4
Propafenone: therapeutic use	VT	1, 2
Propanolol, therapeutic use	AF	4
Proximal flow convergence: echo	AR	2
Proximal flow convergence: echo	RCT	1
Proximal flow convergence: echo	VMD	4
Pulmonary hypertension: echo	AF	2
Pulmonary hypertension: echo	CCC	3
Pulmonary hypertension: echo	IE	2, 3
Pulmonary hypertension: echo	PH	1,2
Pulmonary hypertension: echo	RCT	4
Pulmonary hypertension: echo	VMD	2
Pulmonary oedema: radiography	AF	2
Pulmonary oedema: radiography	IE	2
Pulmonary oedema: radiography	VMD	2, 4
Pulmonic regurgitation, physiological: echo	AF	5
Pulmonic regurgitation, physiological: echo	ET	2
Pulmonic stenosis: echo	CCC	6
Quinidine gluconate: therapeutic use	ACF	2
Quinidine gluconate: therapeutic use	VT	1
Quinidine sulphate: therapeutic use	AF	1
Recumbent sleep deprivation: clinical signs	RSD	1
Recurrent airway obstruction: clinical signs	PH	1
Recurrent airway obstruction: cytology	PH	1
Recurrent airway obstruction: endoscopic findings	PH	1
Recurrent airway obstruction: radiography	PH	1
Recurrent largyngeal neuropathy: endoscopy	AF	6
Renal failure: laboratory findings	PC	1
Renal failure: laboratory findings	VMD	2
Rib fractures: computed tomography	HP	2,3
Rib fractures: radiography	HP	1
Rib fractures: ultrasonography	HP	1
Right atrial appendage: echo	VSD	6
Right heart failure: clinical signs	ACF	1
Right heart failure: clinical signs	VMD	2
Right heat failure: clinical signs	PH	1
Right ventricular dilation: echo	AF	5
Right ventricular dilation: echo	CCC	1, 3
Right ventricular dilation: echo	PH	1
Right ventricular dilation: echo	VMD	2, 6
Right ventricular dilation: echo	VSD	3,4
Right ventricular wall thickening: echo	CCC	6
Right ventricular wall thickening: echo	CN	2, 3
Right ventricular wall thickening: echo	VMD	4
R-on-T phenomenon: ECG	AR	3
R-on-T phenomenon: ECG	VT	1

Index